Veterinary Treatment for Working Equines

This book is dedicated to my two children, Henry and Amelia

Veterinary Treatment for Working Equines

2nd edition

Graham R. Duncanson
BVSc, MSc (VetGP), DProf, FRCVS

CABI

CABI is a trading name of CAB International

CABI
Nosworthy Way
Wallingford
Oxfordshire OX10 8DE
UK

Tel: +44 (0)1491 832111
E-mail: info@cabi.org
Website: www.cabi.org

CABI
200 Portland Street
Boston
MA 02114
USA

Tel: +1 (617)682-9015
E-mail: cabi-nao@cabi.org

A catalogue record for this book is available from the British Library, London, UK.

ISBN-13: 9781800624269 (hardback)
9781800624276 (ePDF)
9781800624283 (ePub)

DOI: 10.1079/9781800624283.0000

Commissioning Editor: Alexandra Lainsbury
Editorial Assistant: Lauren Davies
Production Editor: Rosie Hayden

Typeset by Straive, Pondicherry, India

Contents

Author's Note

The author would like to apologize to the vast army of very competent equine veterinary surgeons for the deficiencies in this book. It is not intended as a definitive textbook of equine medicine or surgery, but is rather a quick guide to help equine practitioners in the field worldwide, particularly those who have no access to sophisticated equipment. The author would be very grateful for feedback to vetdunc@ukonline.co.uk so that he can improve his own practice and enhance any subsequent editions of this book.

The practice of veterinary medicine has evolved continually over the past 45 years, and will continue to evolve at an accelerating rate in the years to come. The author has carefully checked the dosages of the medicines advised in this book. However, readers are strongly advised to check the data sheets of all medicines for current dosage advice. Many medicines are not licensed for use in the horse: these are human preparations and, although they have been used by the author, dosages are empirical. The publisher and the author cannot be held responsible for misuse or misapplication of the material in this work.

Foreword

Veterinary challenges vary around the world, but at the heart of the work, veterinarians and paraprofessionals play a pivotal role in supporting the welfare of working equids (horses, donkeys and mules). Worldwide, there are estimated to be over 100 million working equids who contribute to the daily lives and livelihoods of so many families, including performing tasks such as collecting water and firewood, the transport of people in remote places, ploughing fields and providing direct and indirect income to people who rely on them. The working conditions for both equids and their owners are arduous, such as living with reduced economic resources and navigating challenging climatic conditions. The role equids play usually goes unnoticed, and local services often do not have the capacity to deal with equine welfare, including limited accessibility of veterinary drugs, facilities, training and compensation from governments.

Veterinarians are just one part of the jigsaw for improving working equid welfare, and veterinary work needs to be considered within the wider systems and looking at what is being done to bring about long-lasting improvements for equine welfare. This can be done through a variety of methods, including community and equine owner engagement, capacity building of pre-existing systems and lobbying government and other organizations to bring about change. Ultimately, reducing reliance in equine-owning communities on outside expertise is an important aspect to consider, and ensuring that any veterinary work carried out overseas leaves a lasting legacy. At World Horse Welfare, we work with 16 local partner organizations across the world, in Latin America, Africa and Asia, taking this holistic approach with the aim of creating long-lasting sustainable change for equids and the communities that rely on them. As with any veterinary work, one of the fundamental aspects of working in this environment is working with people, understanding the local context and challenges and changing people's perceptions to make an impact on equine welfare.

Working within the context outlined above, this book is a valuable companion for any vet working in low- or middle-income countries and can act as a useful reference to give confidence and the ability to adapt to resource-limited settings across the world. It covers all aspects of veterinary medicine and surgery relevant to clinicians in the field, as well as providing plenty of practical tips on how to cope with some of the day-to-day problems any clinician will face. It is not intended to be a definitive textbook, but offers plenty of thoughts on further reading at the end of each chapter.

Graham Duncanson is very well placed to write this book, having had a lifelong association with working equines. After qualifying at Bristol Veterinary School, Graham spent 8 years working in Kenya. In 1975 he moved to Norfolk to work in a large animal practice. However, over the past four decades he has travelled extensively to support working equines all over the world, mainly in Africa but also in the Middle East, India, Myanmar and Central America. Latterly, he has devoted an increasing amount of time to teaching younger veterinary colleagues.

I hope that you draw great inspiration from this book, now updated in a second edition, and that it will provide invaluable assistance to you as you go about treating these extraordinary beasts of burden. It is intended as a quick and practical reference to help you face the many challenges that lie ahead.

Roly Owers MRCVS
Chief Executive, World Horse Welfare
www.worldhorsewelfare.org

Introduction

The first known contact between early humans and equines was in approximately 15,000 BC (see Fig. I.1). Equines are depicted in wall paintings in the Lascaux caves in France; at that stage equines represented only a source of food. A skull, dated to c. 4000 BC and showing evidence of wear from the use of a bit on the first cheek teeth, has been found near the Black Sea. Was this a riding horse or was it used to pull a chariot? We have no way of knowing. However, it is likely the animal was used for a warlike purpose. Mercifully, we do not involve equines in war situations today, but, on the other hand, millions of horses, donkeys and mules are used as working animals throughout the world.

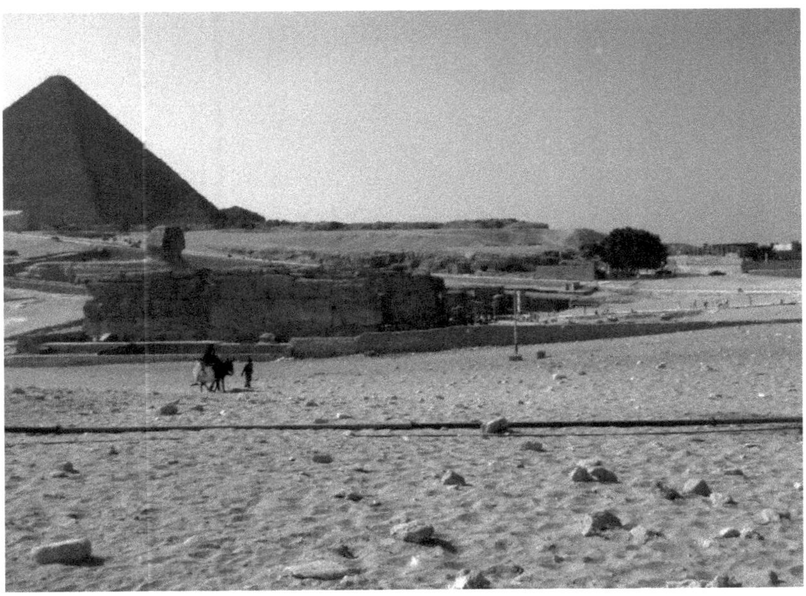

Fig. I.1. Equines have been used by humans for thousands of years.

I define a working animal as one used by humans to carry out a working task – this normally means pulling or carrying. I have excluded all riding horses used to carry a rider for pleasure only, and so therefore no references to pleasure horses or racehorses will be found. Nonetheless, I am sure that the various treatments described in this book will be, in many cases, applicable to such horses. However, the main purpose is to provide a handy guide for veterinarians and others who are called on to treat working animals worldwide, my main aim being to improve the welfare of these animals. It might be argued that in many instances there are severe problems with human rights for the owners of those animals, but these I cannot alter and so I have concentrated on the working equine.

It is well recognized that, although horses and donkeys have very many similarities, they also exhibit certain differences. As the sterile progeny of the two species, the mule and the hinny inherit properties from both, but these in turn have differences. To help clarity, the text will be based on the horse, with any subtle differences seen in ponies mentioned. More fundamental differences in donkeys and mules will be fully explained.

Acknowledgements

The author would like to thank all the very many equine veterinary surgeons, both academics and practitioners, who have taught and guided him over the past 57 years. They are too numerous to mention individually, except for Laura Quiney BVSc MRCVS, who is employed by IMV imaging, Bellshill, ML4 3NJ, UK. Laura has written the subsection on imaging in Chapter 4 and supplied all the images.

The author would like to thank Avice O'Connor MVB, MRCVS and World Horse Welfare for the use of some of their images; also Alex Lainsbury and the rest of the staff at CABI, who have made the publication of this book possible.

Abbreviations

ADH	Antidiuretic hormone
Ad lib	As much as desired
AGID	Agar gel immunodiffusion
AI	Artificial insemination
ASF	African swine fever
ASIT	Allergen-specific immunotherapy
AST	Aspartate aminotransferase
BAL	Bronchoalveolar lavage
BCS	Body condition score
BDV	Border disease virus
BHV	Bovine herpes virus
bid	Twice daily
BTV	Blue tongue virus
BUN	Blood urea nitrogen
BVD	Bovine virus diarrhoea
BWT	Body weight
C	Celsius
CAE	Caprine arthritis and encephalitis
cal	Calorie
CCN	Cerebro-cortico-necrosis
CEM	Contagious equine metritis
CFT	Complement fixation test
CK	Creatinekinase
CLA	Caseous lymphadenitis
cm	Centimetre
CNS	Central nervous system
C-NS	Coagulase-negative staphylococci
CN V	Central nerve number 5
CPD	Contagious pustular dermatitis
CSF	Cerebrospinal fluid
CT	Computed tomography/Controlled test
cu	Cubic
Cu	Copper

DM	Dry matter
DNA	Deoxyribonucleic acid
EAE	Enzootic abortion of ewes
EBM	Evidence-based medicine
ECG	Electrocardiogram
EDTA	Ethylene diamine tetra-acetic acid
e.g.	For example
EGGD	Equine glandular gastric disease
EGUS	Equine gastric ulcer syndrome
EHA	Egg hatch assay
EHV	Equine herpes virus
EIA	Equine infectious anaemia
ELISA	Enzyme-linked immunosorbent assay
EP	Equine piroplasmosis
EPG	Eggs per gram
ERU	Equine recurrent uveitis
ETR	Excessive transverse ridges
EU	European Union
EVA	Equine viral arteritis
F	Fahrenheit
FAT	Fluorescent antibody test
FCE	Feed conversion efficiency
FCR	Feed conversion ratio
FECRT	Faecal egg count reduction test
FMD	Foot and mouth disease
FPT	Failure of passive transfer
ft	Feet (measurement)
g	Gram
GA	General anaesthetic
GG	Glycerol guaiacolate
GGT	Gamma glutamyltransferase
GI	Gastrointestinal
GLDH	Glutamate dehydrogenase
GnRH	Gonadotropin-releasing hormone
Hb	Haemoglobin
IBH	Insect bite hypersensitivity
i.e.	That is
IgE	Immunoglobulin E
IgG	Immunoglobulin G
i/m	Intramuscularly
IO	Intraoribital
ip	Intraperitoneally
IU	International units
i/v	Intravenously
kg	Kilogram
l	Litre
LAT	Latex agglutination test
LDT	Larval development test
LN	Lymph node
MCF	Malignant catarrhal fever
MCH	Mean corpuscular haemoglobin

MCHC	Mean corpuscular haemoglobin concentration
MCV	Mean corpuscular volume
ME	Metabolizable energy
mg	Milligram
min	Minute
MJ	Megajoules
ml	Millilitre
MOET	Multiple ovulation and embryo transfer
MRCT	Malignant round cell tumours
MRI	Magnetic resonance imaging
MV	Maedi-visna
NGT	Nasogastric tube
NMS	Neonatal maladjustment syndrome
NSAID	Non-steroidal anti-inflammatory drug
OIE	Office International des Epizooties
PAS	Perinatal asphyxia syndrome
PBS	Phosphate-buffered saline
PCR	Polymerase chain reaction
PCV	Packed cell volume
PE	Proliferative enteropathy
per os	Orally
PET	Positron emission tomography
pH	Negative logarithm of hydrogen ion activity
PHE	Proliferative haemorrhagic enteropathy
PLR	Papillary light reflex
pme	Post-mortem examination
PMN	Polymorphic nuclear cell
PMSG	Pregnant mare serum gonadotrophin
PPID	Pituitary pars intermedia dysfunction (Cushing's disease)
ppm	Part(s) per million
PRA	Progressive retinal atrophy
PUBH	Polymerized ultrapurified bovine haemoglobin
PUPD	Polyuria-polydipsia
qid	Four times daily
RAO	Recurrent airway obstruction
RBC	Red blood cell
RFI	Residual feed intake
RNA	Ribonucleic acid
RPM	Revolutions per minute
RT-PCR	Reverse transcriptase polymerase chain reaction
s/c	Subcutaneous
SCV	Small cell variant
SG	Specific gravity
sid	Once a day
SNT	Serum neutralization test
TB	Tuberculosis
TDN	Total digestible nutrients
tid	Three times daily
TMH	Trigeminal-mediated headshaking
TMS	Trimethoprim-sulphadoxine

TPR	Temperature, pulse and respiration
UK	United Kingdom
USA	United States of America
VDS	Veterinary Defence Society
VLA	Veterinary Laboratory Agency
VNT	Virus neutralization test
vol	Volume
WBC	White blood cell
wt	Weight
ZN	Ziehl-Neelsen

Glossary

Abortion the premature birth of young, which may be alive or dead.
Annual a plant which grows from seed, flowers and dies within a year.
Anthelmintics drugs that expel parasitic worms from the body, generally by paralysing or starving them.
Antigen a molecule or part of a molecule that is recognized by components of the host immune system.
Autosome chromosome a non-sex chromosome.
Awn a bristle or hair-like appendage to a fruit or to a glume, as in barley and some other grasses.
Bacteraemia bacteria in the blood.
Base pairs in DNA the four bases pair up to form the internal structure of DNA. Adenine with guanine and thymine with cysteine.
Biennial a plant which flowers and dies in the second year after growing from a seed.
Bradycardia decrease in heart rate.
Bruxism grinding of teeth.
Calculi stones formed in the urinary system.
Cerebral relating to the cerebrum, the largest part of the brain.
Cestodes parasitic flatworms, commonly called tapeworms, which usually live in the digestive tract of vertebrates as adults and in the bodies of various intermediate hosts as juvenile stages.
Codon-3 nucleotide sequences that encode a specific single amino acid.
Colitis inflammation of the colon, often used to describe an inflammation of the large intestine.
Coma profound unconsciousness from which the patient cannot be roused.
Congestion the presence of an abnormal amount of blood in an organ or part.
Contusions bruises.
Convulsion a violent involuntary contraction of muscles.
Corm underground bulbous root.
Cryptorchid rig.
Cystitis inflammation of the bladder.
Deciduous plants those which shed all their leaves annually.
Detoxicate to render a poison harmless.
Distension the filling of a hollow organ to more than its usual capacity.
Diuresis excessive urination.

DNA fingerprinting much like the fingerprint used in human identification, but done with unique DNA characters for each individual animal. Utilizes PCR to replicate small samples.
Drenching giving an anthelmintic dose by mouth.
Dysentery an illness characterized by diarrhoea with blood in the faeces.
Dysphagia difficulty in swallowing.
Dysphonia hoarseness heard when vocalizing.
Dyspnoea difficulty in breathing.
Dystocia difficulty at parturition.
Egg reappearance period the time taken (usually expressed in weeks) for eggs to reappear in faeces after anthelmintic treatment. Usually this is described for drug-sensitive worm populations at the time of product licensing.
ELISA (enzyme-linked immunosorbent assay) a technique used primarily in immunology to detect the presence of an antibody or an antigen in a sample. Basically, an unknown amount of antigen is bound to the surface of a plastic well, then a specific antibody is added and if specific will bind the antigen. This antibody is linked to an enzyme or is detected by incubation with a second antibody that is linked to an enzyme. In the final step a substance is added that the enzyme can convert to some detectable signal (usually a colour change which is detectable by a spectrophotometer).
Emaciation excessive body wasting.
Emesis vomiting.
Emetic a substance which causes vomiting.
Emphysema air or gas in the interstices of a tissue.
Enema rectal injection.
Epidemiology the study of factors affecting the health of populations and often how diseases are transmitted.
Exon the coding part of a gene.
FECRT (faecal egg count reduction test) a test that measures the effect on faecal egg output of anthelmintic treatment. Generally, efficacy is assessed by comparing FECs obtained on the day of treatment with those obtained 14 days after treatment. This is an important tool in detecting anthelmintic resistance in the field.
Fistulous withers suppurating fistula on the withers of a horse.
Foetid malodorous.
Gelding castrated equine.
Gene mapping the gene on a given chromosome.
Genetic engineering the direct manipulation of genes to alter the physical appearance of an animal. Also used in recombinant vaccine technology.
Genome an organism's entire hereditary information, encoded either in DNA or, for some types of virus, in RNA. The genome includes the genes that code the proteins and non-coding sequences of the DNA.
Genotype the inherited instructions organisms carry in their genetic code.
Glabrous without hair of any kind.
Granules small grains.
Gravid the pregnant horn of a uterus.
Haematuria blood in the urine.
Haemoglobinuria haemoglobin in the urine.
Haemolytic a substance which causes breakdown of red blood corpuscles.
Helminths a group of eukaryotic parasites that live inside their host. They are worm-like and live and feed off animals.
Hepatitis inflammation of the liver.
Herbaceous perennials plants in which the greater part dies after flowering, leaving only the rootstock to produce next year's growth.
Heterozygous a genotype consisting of two different alleles at a given locus.

Homozygous a genotype consisting of two identical alleles at a given locus.
Iatrogenic resulting from treatment.
Ileus failure of peristalsis.
In foal a pregnant mare or filly.
In vitro in the test tube.
In vivo in the living body.
Indigenous native of the country in which it was produced.
Intron the non-coding part of a gene.
Jaundice a disease in which bile pigments stain the mucous membranes.
Larvae juvenile forms that many animals undergo before the mature adult stage. Larvae are frequently adapted to environments different to those adult stages live in.
Leucocytosis increase in WBC in the blood.
Leucopenia decrease in WBC in the blood.
Linear leaves those that are long and narrow.
Lumen the inner space of a tubular structure, such as the intestine.
Markers a short tandem repeat (STR) that may be used to aid in the identification of a trait.
Mediastinum space in the chest between the lungs.
Melaena dark tarry faeces indicating bleeding high in the intestinal tract.
Metritis inflammation of the uterus.
Microsatellite a stretch of DNA that is repeated several times in a row. These are located at random throughout a chromosome. The variation in these markers allows for the parentage verification and other forensic activities.
Micturition the passing of urine.
Mitochondrial DNA DNA found only in the mitochondria. Only provided by the female. Controls cellular metabolism.
Monoecious when male and female flowers are separate, but on the same plant.
Mutations alterations in DNA sequence in a genome that spontaneously occur during meiosis or DNA replication are caused by factors such as by radiation, viruses or chemicals.
Myiasis fly strike.
Narcosis sleep induced by a drug or poison.
Nematodes roundworms, one of the most diverse phyla of all animals.
Nodule a small round lump.
Non-gravid the non-pregnant horn of a uterus.
Nuclear DNA DNA found in the nucleus of all cells of the body. A copy is provided by each parent. This DNA carries the code for phenotype (physical characteristics).
Nucleotide the building blocks of DNA. Composed of deoxyribose sugars, a phosphate and one of four nitrogenous bases.
Orchitis inflammation of the testicle.
Ovoid egg-shaped.
Panacea a cure-all.
Paracentesis the technique of puncturing a body cavity.
Pathogenicity the ability of a pathogen to produce signs of disease in an organism.
Pathognomonic a single specific sign of a disease.
Pediculosis lice infestation.
Phenotype any observable characteristic or trait of an organism, such as its morphology, development, biochemical or physiological properties or behaviour. Phenotypes result from the expression of an organism's genes, as well as the influence of environmental factors and possible interactions between the two.
Poll evil an infection in the atlantal bursa creating a fistula at the poll. It is normally caused by an injury. It is not caused by *Brucella abortus* as was historically postulated.
Polydactyly having an extra limb.
Polydipsia excessive drinking.

Polymerase chain reaction (PCR) a technique to amplify a single or a few copies of a piece of DNA by several orders of magnitude, generating thousands to millions of copies of a particular sequence. Polymerase chain reaction relies on cycles of repeated heating and cooling of DNA which cause melting and enzymatic replication of DNA. Primers (short DNA fragments) containing sequences complementary to the target region along with a DNA polymerase (after which the method is named) are key components to enable selective and repeated amplification. As PCR progresses, DNA generated is used as a template for replication, setting in motion a chain reaction in which the template is exponentially amplified.
Polyphagia excessive eating.
Premix medicine available in a concentrated form to be added to food.
Primer several thousand copies of short sequences of DNA that are complementary to part of the DNA to be sequenced.
Proctitis inflammation of the rectum.
Proctocloclysis administration of fluid per rectum.
Ptyalism excess saliva production.
Purgative a strong laxative.
Pyelectasia urine pooling in the kidney.
Pyrexia raised rectal temperature.
Recumbency unable to get up.
Rhinitis inflammation of the nose.
Rig a male in which one or both testicles have not descended into the scrotum.
Ringwomb failure of the cervix to dilate.
Rostral towards the nose.
Ryegrass a commonly grown grass, *Lolium perenne*.
Schistosomus reflexus a deformity of a fetus in which the spine is bent backwards.
Sclerosis hardening of a tissue.
Septicaemia pathogenic bacteria in the blood.
Short Tandem Reprints (STR) sections of DNA arranged in back-to-back repetition.
Slough dead tissue which drops away from living tissue.
Spasm involuntary contraction of a muscle.
Staggers an erratic gait.
Stomatitis inflammation of the mouth and gums.
Stricture a narrowing of a tubular organ.
Subclinical when the symptoms are not evident.
Syncope fainting.
Syndrome a group of symptoms.
Tachycardia increased heart rate.
Tachypnoea increased respiratory rate.
Tenesmus straining to pass urine or faeces.
Teratoma a developmental embryological deformity.
Torpid sluggish.
Tourniquet an appliance for temporary stoppage of the circulation in a limb.
Trismus locking of the jaw.
Tympanic distended with gas.
Typhilitis inflammation of the caecum.
Ubiquitous everywhere.
Udder mammary gland.
Ureter the tube connecting the kidney to the bladder.
Urethra the tube leading from the bladder to outside.
Urethritis inflammation of the urethra.
Urine scald inflammation of the skin caused by persistent wetting with urine.

Urolithiasis the formation of stones in the urinary system.
Urticaria an acute inflammatory reaction of the skin.
Vaginitis inflammation of the vagina.
Vagus 10th cranial nerve.
Venereal disease a disease spread by coitus.
Vesicle a collection of fluid in the surface layers of the skin or of a mucous membrane.
Viraemia virus particles in the blood.
Volatile a substance which evaporates rapidly.
Zoonoses diseases communicable between animals and humans.

1

Vital Signs and Normal Values

Abstract

This chapter gives the reader a framework on which to interpret abnormal signs and values from what is considered to be normal. However, most textbooks give ranges taken from sports horses and racehorses. The practitioner is strongly advised to establish the normals from the population of working horses being treated in the area.

1.1 Introduction

Many textbooks assume that vital signs and normal values are the same the world over. This is, broadly, not very helpful. This chapter will give a very broad range in tabular form so that the reader can adapt this book by adding narrower ranges for the environment of the individual's practice and from the laboratory available. The term 'reference range' is now widely used, rather than 'normal range'. Classically, a normal animal is said to be within the 95% normal range. By definition, 5% of normal animals will not appear to be normal. Thus, if 20 tests are carried out, every animal is likely to have one value outside the normal range. Therefore, there is a strong argument for carrying out only specific tests for the parameters in which the clinician is particularly interested. Laboratories on the whole do not like this arrangement, as they favour a blanket approach, which they find easier and cheaper. Clinicians are urged therefore to work closely with their particular laboratory so that a compromise regarding cost and relevance is reached.

The author is well aware that getting samples to laboratories will not be easy or quick in many parts of the world. High temperatures are likely to be a problem. The logistics should be considered with the laboratory. Fresh samples are likely to be the most difficult, so swabs for bacteriology in transport medium should be taken. Bacteria can be plated out and grown in the field. Only then can they be submitted for identification. Equally, smears can be made and microscopic evaluation can be carried out in the field after appropriate staining. These slides can then easily be referred to a more experienced pathologist. Antibiotic sensitivity testing can easily be carried out in the field. Relevant antibiotic testing discs can be used. There is little point in knowing the sensitivity of an isolated organism to an antibiotic that is not available.

Serum samples after centrifugation can be submitted rather than whole blood. Packed cell volume (PCV) can be measured easily with a bench hand-driven centrifuge. Thick and thin blood smears can be used to search for protozoal infections. Dung samples can be examined for bowel worms, lungworms and even liver fluke

2nd Edition (G.R. Duncanson)
DOI: 10.1079/9781800624283.0001

eggs. Coccidial oocysts can be included in this screening, although their pathogenicity may be in doubt. Fungi can also be grown. To help, practitioners can submit photographs of post-mortems to referral pathologists. If e-mail is available, this can be carried out throughout the world. Obviously, histological samples will be extremely helpful in tropical climates, as they will withstand higher temperatures. Care should be taken when packing these, as any contamination from the formalin onto bacteriological samples will be disastrous.

Vital signs will vary from climate to climate, similarly to normal values, and will show a similar bell-shaped distribution curve. Clinicians will routinely carry out full clinical examinations and build up their own range of normal values. Experience will show how climate variations in temperature, air movement and humidity will affect these values. Naturally, the physical attribute of the equine will have a marked effect: type, age, gender, pregnancy, etc. The state of the individual, e.g. stressed, recently transported, etc., will also cause variation.

1.2 Normal Temperature, Pulse and Respiration (TPR)

Normal TPR values for a range of equines are shown in Table 1.1.

Capillary refill time is a good vital sign to record. In all types and ages, the normal value should be less than 2 s. Auscultation of the chest is helpful. In a normal equine, no sounds should be heard from the lungs. Often it is more convenient to take a heart rate rather than a pulse. The abdomen should be mentally divided into four quadrants for auscultation: these are upper and lower, right and left.

1.3 Collecting Blood Samples

When collecting blood samples, it is important to collect into the right anticoagulant for the type of analysis required. The correct volume of blood for the amount of anticoagulant in the bottle is also important. Blood should be collected from the jugular vein with as little excitement for the animal as possible, although this may be difficult with certain individuals. Needles and syringes must be clean and not contaminated with medicines. It is important to remember that the carotid artery lies just deep to the jugular in the caudal aspect of the neck, so this area should be avoided, i.e. the jugular should be entered in the neck nearer to the head than the shoulder.

For haematological samples, the anticoagulant required is EDTA (these bottles often come with a lilac-coloured stopper). Haematological samples will provide measures of haemoglobin and the number of red blood cells. These figures will be higher in very fit horses and heavy horses. It is important to note that if a haematocrit tube is not filled from the top of the sample immediately before it is allowed to stand, the haematocrit will have a lower reading, i.e. there will seem to be fewer red blood cells in the sample than are actually present. Anaemia may then be misdiagnosed. Even in profound cases of anaemia, normoblasts are very rarely seen in peripheral blood. The number of platelets will be reported. The total number of white blood cells will be given, which is then broken down into the total number of neutrophils, eosinophils, basophils, lymphocytes and monocytes. These can be shown as percentages, but this may be misleading. Total numbers are a better figure for study. Unsegmented neutrophils do not normally appear in peripheral blood; if they are reported it is an indication of a shift to the right,

Table 1.1. A guide to normal TPR values in various equines.

Equine type	Temperature (°C)	Pulse (beats/min)	Respiration (breaths/min)
Newborn foal	38.5–39.5	100–125	14–15
Newborn donkey foal	38.0–39.5	80–120	16–60
Older foal	37.5–38.0	60–100	14–15
Older donkey foal	36.6–38.9	44–80	16–48
Pony	37.5–38.0	45–55	12–15
Horse	37.5–38.0	20–40	10–15
Donkey	36.2–37.8	36–68	12–44

i.e. their presence indicates that the neutrophils are immature and therefore there has been extra usage of neutrophils by the horse. This is likely to indicate a bacterial infection. Total numbers of white blood cells are often higher in young horses. Foals particularly will show an increase in the number of neutrophils.

1.4 Normal Haematological Values

Erythrocyte parameters for the horse are as follows:

- PCV (%): 33–46;
- RBC (10^{12}/l): 6.0–9.6;
- Hb (g/dl): 11.0–16.5;
- MCHC (g/dl): 33–36;
- MCV (fl): 44–58; and
- MCH (pg): 14.1–19.3.

Erythrocyte parameters for the donkey are as follows:

- PCV (%): 25–38;
- RBC (10^{12}/l): 4.0–7.3;
- Hb (g/dl): 9.0–15.3;
- MCHC (g/dl): 31.4–39.1;
- MCV (fl): 57–79; and
- MCH (pg): 18.9–28.6.

The PCV is the most useful measure of dehydration and haemoconcentration. If the total number of RBCs is high, this is consistent with haemoconcentration; if it is low, it is consistent with anaemia. The amount of haemoglobin will mirror these trends. The mean corpuscular haemoglobin concentration (MCHC), the mean corpuscular volume (MCV) or the mean corpuscular haemoglobin (MCH) values are not very useful parameters in the horse.

Leucocyte parameters

The normal range of total leucocyte numbers is 6–12 × 10^9/l, and the ratio of neutrophils to lymphocytes is 60:40. If the total number is low, that is called leucopenia and indicates endotoxaemia or septicaemia. It may in fact indicate the start of any bacterial infection. As such an infection progresses, the animal will produce more leucocytes and so develop leucocytosis. As these will be immature neutrophils, such a rise is called a shift to the left. It can occur with acute inflammation without bacterial involvement. A drop in the numbers of lymphocytes is termed lymphopenia and occurs at the start of a viral attack. A drop in the number of neutrophils is termed neutrophilia, which can be seen if corticosteroids have been administered. A rise in the number of eosinophils may be seen in severe cases of parasitism or allergic conditions. Eosinophils are slightly more common in the peripheral blood of the donkey than the horse. Basophils are rarely seen in peripheral blood in the donkey. Monocyte numbers are normally low, but these may increase in a horse with either a chronic suppurative condition or a granulomatous inflammation; this is called monocytosis. Monocytosis may also be seen on recovery from an upper respiratory viral attack.

We should include under this heading the platelets, also termed thrombocytes. These may show an increase in bacterial infection, termed thrombocytosis. However, the reverse is much more commonly seen, i.e. thrombocytopenia, which is often an artefact created as the platelets have clumped together in the EDTA. However, it also occurs in disseminated intravascular coagulopathy (DIC), immune-mediated thrombocytopenia (IMTP), equine infectious anaemia (EIA), endotoxaemia, equine ehrlichiosis and neoplasia, or as a result of severe haemorrhage.

The ranges of percentages of leucocytes are given below:

- neutrophils: 45–55 (range much wider in the donkey, i.e. 28–78);
- eosinophils: 0–5 (range 1–10 in the donkey);
- basophils: 0–1;
- lymphocytes: 35–50 (range wider in the donkey, i.e. 17–65);
- monocytes: 0–3 (up to 5 is normal in the donkey); and
- thrombocytes (platelets x 10^{10}/l): 24–55.

1.5 Biochemical Parameters

For measurement of biochemical parameters, e.g. enzymes, triglycerides, bile acids, no anticoagulant is required, i.e. just serum (these bottles, without anticoagulant, often come with a red-coloured stopper). Table 1.2 lists the main

Table 1.2. Biological parameters in the equine.

Parameter	Range	Interpretation of results
ALP (IU/l)	<560	Raised in chronic biliary obstructive liver damage, bone marrow and intestinal disease
AST (IU/l)	<400	Raised in acute muscle and liver damage
Amylase (IU/l)	<24	Raised in pancreatitis
Bile acids (IU/l)	<20	Raised in cholelithiasis (bile stones), acute liver disease and chronic cirrhosis
CK (IU/l)	<50	Raised in myopathies
GGT (IU/l)	<79	Raised in acute hepatitis, chronic cirrhosis and pancreatitis
GLDH (IU/l)	<14	Raised in cellular damage and liver, intestinal and sometimes skin damage
Tbil (pmol/l)	<27	Raised in anorexia and intestinal damage
TP (g/l)	<80	Best to split into albumin and globulin fractions; raised in dehydration
Albumin (g/l)	60–70	Low in diarrhoea, liver failure, renal disease and severe inflammation
Globulin (g/l)	20–35	Raised in parasitism, infection, inflammation and liver failure
Urea (mmol/l)	3–5	Raised (uraemia) in dehydration, tissue breakdown, high-protein diet and kidney failure
Creatine (pmol/l)	<200	Raised in kidney disease
Sodium (mmol/l)	140	Low in diarrhoea
Potassium (mmol/l)	4	Low in diarrhoea and anorexia or starvation
Chloride (mmol/l)	100	Low in diarrhoea or high obstruction and in increased sweating; high in dehydration
Calcium (mmol/l)	3	Low in decreased food intake

parameters measured, their normal range in the equine and interpretation of results.

Triglyceride measurement is very important in donkeys and small ponies. Any value over 1 mmol/l is significant and indicates hyperlipaemia.

The anticoagulant required for trace element sampling is lithium heparin (these bottles often come with a green stopper). The exception is for zinc estimation; no stopper containing rubber should be used, as rubber contains low levels of zinc and this will contaminate the sample. Normally, plastic stoppers are used for zinc estimation. Selenium is incorporated into the glutathione peroxidase (GSH-Px) of red blood cells. Testing will measure its availability.

Glucose estimation requires fluoride oxalate as an anticoagulant (these bottles often come with a grey stopper). To be meaningful, immediate separation of red blood cells is required as red cells will use up the glucose. The normal glucose value is 3.5–6.0 mmol/l.

1.6 Other Blood Tests

For estimation of clotting times, blood needs to be collected into sodium citrate. No other anticoagulant is acceptable. Normal clotting time (the better term is prothrombin time) will be given by the laboratory. The value for the individual patient should be compared with this.

All serological samples need to be taken in a plain tube. Ideally, these should be spun down so that the serum can be harvested. However, equine blood settles very well so the serum can be drawn off without centrifugation, but naturally the yield is less. Whole blood cannot be frozen without causing a breakdown of red blood cells. However, serum and indeed plasma may be frozen with no deleterious effect. This is often the preferred mode of transport in hot climates. The diagnoses that can be expected from serum samples will vary enormously between laboratories. In many conditions two samples taken 10 days apart give a more meaningful reading than a single sample, since rising or falling titres can be recorded. This would be important in rare conditions such as brucellosis or Lyme disease (borreliosis).

Field estimation of PCV can be obtained by allowing an EDTA sample to stand. The normal PCV will be 40%. Very fit horses will have a higher figure, while ponies will have a lower figure.

In cases of severe hyperlipaemia, the fat in the blood can be seen in an EDTA sample. A more subtle measurement can be gained from serum triglyceride values.

To summarize the choice of sampling vessels, plain tubes (normally with a red stopper) should be used for:

- urea;
- total protein;
- bilirubin;
- bile acids;
- triglycerides;
- creatinine;
- copper;
- electrolytes;
- enzymes;
- hormones; and
- serology.

Tubes containing EDTA (normally with a purple stopper) should be used for:

- haematology; and
- platelets.

Tubes containing heparin (normally with a green stopper) should be used for:

- fibrinogen; and
- bicarbonate.

Tubes containing oxalate (normally with a grey stopper) should be used for:

- glucose; and
- phosphate.

Tubes containing sodium citrate should be used for:

- clotting time.

Tubes with stoppers not containing rubber should be used for:

- zinc.

Serum Amyloid A (SAA), a protein produced in response to inflammation, is released into the blood stream to alert the immune system that there is an infection or injury present. As SAA is the fastest marker to rise in response to inflammation, it provides useful insight for detecting inflammation, monitoring health status and observing response to treatment. There are now available relatively inexpensive stable-side testing machines, e.g. the VeraSTAT-V device.

There are several other body fluids that may be helpful to the clinician for diagnostic purposes, e.g. cerebrospinal fluid (CSF), peritoneal fluid and synovial fluid. These will be discussed under the relevant body systems.

1.7 Urine Tests

Urine is a sample that is easy to collect and assess. It should be collected in clean, sugar-free bottles (jam jars should not be used). Ideally, new sterile containers should be used. Urine is often cloudy or turbid due to the presence of calcium carbonate crystals; this is normal. Normal urinary pH range is 7.5–9.5. There should be no blood or sugar present and the specific gravity should be between 1.020 and 1.060. The appearance of the urine will vary depending on time of collection; normally it is initially clear, becoming cloudier. Diet will affect the amount of calcium carbonate in the urine and hence the cloudiness. Foods containing high levels of calcium, e.g. lucerne, will give a cloudier urine. Normal urine can also appear mucoid, due to the presence of detectable protein. Such results are not significant. Enzymes found in the urine will be discussed under kidney disease.

1.8 Faeces Tests

Faeces is also an easy sample to collect. Obviously, parasite eggs may appear, and their significance will be discussed later. It is important that the sample is adequate in size (200 g) and is collected from a minimum of five sites from the faeces pile. It is important that the sample is less than four hours old. The sample should be stored in a bag with the minimum amount of air at below 40°C. The sample should be thoroughly macerated before testing. It is vital that sensitivity is high as this will influence treatment planning, particularly when egg counts are high. Due to natural variation in the egg output of individual horses, if faecal egg counts (FECs) are used to evaluate a whole group then it is vital that as many horses are tested as possible. In adult groups which are well managed 20% of animals will contribute to 80% of the total egg output. In temperate climates (this includes high altitude areas in the tropics), adults can be managed with targeted anthelmintic treatments during the periods of high egg outputs (the warmer months in temperate climates and the rainy months in high-altitude tropical climates). With this regime, testing needs to be performed ideally at 8-week intervals with an adulticidal anthelmintic administered only to high shedders, such as animals producing more than 200 eggs/g of faeces. Target regimes are not advocated in groups of horses under 3 years of age.

It is important to realize that egg counts do not give a quantitative indication of numbers of adults in the gut. This is particularly important with cyathostominosis. Worms may accumulate over several years in the gut mucosa in an encysted form. FECs are therefore of limited value. The trigger that reactivates encysted larvae is still not known. The signs are rapid weight loss and diarrhoea. This leads to a protein losing enteropathy. The condition is most common in animals under 6 years of age in late winter (towards the end of the rains in tropical countries). Mortality can be high. The use of Moxidectin is recommended before the condition is likely to occur. A low FEC will not be a reliable indicator as to the level of encysted larvae.

Faecal egg count reduction tests (FECTs) should be performed regularly with each parasite species to alert horse keepers to the efficiency of anthelmintic drugs.

However, there are other tests on faeces that can be performed simply. Naturally, the consistency should be noted. The presence of long fibre particles and whole grains is indicative of dental problems. Sand is easily tested: 250 g of faeces is mixed with water in a polythene bag and allowed to stand; sand particles will readily be seen at the bottom after a few minutes. The presence of a small amount of hidden blood is normal; however, larger amounts of hidden (or so-called occult) blood should be investigated. Blood can be found by dissolving a small amount of faeces in water and testing with a urine dipstick. Isolation of bacteria is not straightforward. Rectal swabs are unreliable and fresh faecal samples are better. At least five should be taken on separate occasions to rule out a salmonella infection. Rotavirus can be isolated from the faeces of foals, and there are several methods available. Practitioners would need to contact an appropriate laboratory for this test. Freshness and intercountry posting would pose considerable problems in most parts of the world where equines are used for work.

Further Reading

Dyson, S.J. (1992) Self-assessment picture tests in veterinary medicine. In: Dyson, S.J. (ed.) *Equine Practice*. Wolfe Publishing Ltd, Prescott, Arizona.

Reinemeyer, C.R. and Neilson, M.K. (2013) *Handbook of Equine Parasite Control*. Wiley, Chichester, UK.

2

Simple Diagnostic Tests

Abstract

This chapter describes simple tests to aid the equine clinician in the field to reach a diagnosis without having to perform more invasive investigations.

2.1 Passing a Nasogastric Tube

A pertinent old quote

'If you have never given a horse a nosebleed from passing a nasogastric tube then you have never passed one!' Advise owners of the inherent danger.

Before starting, hold the tube beside the horse's head with the end level with the pharynx. With a permanent marker, mark the position of the nostril on the tube. When passing the tube, when you reach your mark, the end will be level with the pharynx.

Stand beside the horse, having used a twitch or sedation as appropriate, with the lubricated tube out of the way over your shoulder. Use one hand to control the nose and the other to hold the tube. Push caudally on the nose to flex the neck. Push in the tube, being careful to keep it out of the false nostril.

You will feel some resistance as you come to the mark and then push on the tube as the horse swallows. As you advance the tube you may see it in the oesophagus in thin-skinned horses. To aid the passing, you can blow into the tube. Listen in the tube. You should hear stomach sounds, but not hear or feel air from the lungs. Should you hear or feel air, or the horse is persistently coughing, you have gone into the trachea. You should withdraw the tube to the pharynx and try again. If you fail a second time, I advise you to totally remove the tube and immerse it in cold water so that it becomes more rigid, as this will aid you when you try again, making sure the neck is fully flexed.

Should there be haemorrhage, there is no need to treat as it will be from the nasal mucosa and will be self-limiting.

2.2 Glucose Absorption Test

This is a useful test when trying to clarify a diagnosis with the thin horse or the animal with chronic diarrhoea. It is equally as useful in mules and donkeys. It is easy to perform in the field and is not expensive, but is rather time-consuming. The horse is starved for 12 h, usually overnight. A blood sample is then taken for immediate glucose estimation. A human glucometer, as used for diabetic patients, is ideal. The

DOI: 10.1079/9781800624283.0002

horse is then stomach-tubed with glucose dissolved in water (1 g/kg body weight). The volume should be 1 ml/kg. Thus a 500 kg horse should receive 0.5 kg of glucose dissolved in 0.5 l. The horse should be starved throughout the test. A second sample should be taken after 2 h and then at hourly intervals for a further 2 h. The blood glucose level in a normal horse will be ~8 mmol/l at the start, which should rise to >12 mmol/l within 2 h. This level will slowly decline, but will still be >10 mmol/l after 4 h. On the other hand, in a horse with a malabsorption problem, e.g. a generalized intestinal lymphosarcoma, the level will never reach 10 mmol/l and will return to preglucose levels within 4 h. Sadly, the outcome for a horse with low glucose absorption is bad. However, it does mean that the clinician can advise euthanasia earlier in the course of a disease and thus prevent further suffering.

2.3 Serum Amyloid A

Serum Amyloid A is a major acute-phase protein (APP) produced in the liver in response to inflammation. It is the fastest biomarker to rise in response to inflammatory stimuli. It can be measured in the stable by a small machine, e.g. a Vera STAT-V (available from Randox Laboratories Ltd, 55 Diamond Road, Crumlin, County Antrim BT29 4QY, UK, +44 (0) 2894422413, marketing@randox.com).

2.4 Zinc Sulfate Turbidity Test

Foals are born with no effective immunity. Their survival depends on obtaining the effective passive transfer of immunoglobulins via the colostrum of the mare, as soon after birth as possible. This has to be ingested quickly as the tiny portals of entry, in the foal's intestine, for such large protein particles close within 24 h. The ideal scenario is for adequate colostrum to be ingested within 3 h; however, 6 h is the accepted cut-off point. Obviously, colostrum obtained after this time is still beneficial, but it may not be life-saving. The quality of the colostrum is important: sick or debilitated mares will have poor-quality colostrum. A test for colostrum quality is described later. Also, some mares, particularly multiparous mares, will produce milk several days before birth; ideally, this should be stored in a refrigerator pending the birth of the foal. There is a fine balance with heavily pregnant mares; the udder should be left completely alone to avoid this milk flow. An occasional small degree of milk flow should be ignored. Trying to catch this small, worthless sample will only stimulate the mare to produce more and therefore defeat the whole exercise. If mares are foaling in groups, it is very sensible to collect some colostrum from an older mare with plenty of colostrum. Obviously, the older mare must be allowed to give her own foal sufficient colostrum, but after 6 h some 250 ml can be collected and then stored in a deep-freeze unit. Should this colostrum be required, it should be defrosted, either at ambient temperature in hot countries or in a bowl of hot water in colder climates. Colostrum may be defrosted in a microwave, but only at the defrosting setting. If it is defrosted at a higher cooking setting, vital proteins will be denatured.

Ideally, therefore, we need an estimation of the foal's immunological status as early as possible. The zinc sulfate turbidity test can be performed at 12 h. The value of performing the test at this stage is great. Most foals will not develop septicaemia and show signs of illness until 24–48 h. Antibiotics given early systemically are beneficial, but not nearly as beneficial as good quality colostrum or serum from an immune donor. There are other tests available, but these are expensive and difficult to perform. If the serum is sent away to a laboratory the result will be received too late. Obviously, if it is known that the foal has not received colostrum in the first 6 h because the mare has died, the foal has not become ambulatory or the mare has totally rejected the foal, there is no need to perform the test as the immune status of the foal is known, i.e. it is naive. Alternative measures have then to be implemented. It is only when the immune status is unknown that there is a need to perform the zinc sulfate turbidity test.

Dissolve 250 ml zinc sulfate in 1 l of freshly boiled water. Place 6 ml of the solution into several plain vacuum tubes (usually these have a red stopper). These tubes will last for months, so may easily be prepared and stored at room temperature. Carbon dioxide, which causes cloudiness, is the main problem. However, this will have been removed by boiling, and the vacuum in the tubes will prevent any contamination.

Add 0.1 ml serum or plasma (an insulin syringe is ideal for this purpose) to the tube. Mix by inverting the tube. If the foal has received adequate colostrum, the tube will become markedly turbid within 10 min. For a more accurate measurement, if the tube is not turbid after 10 min, the tube can be left for 60 min. If the writing in this book cannot be seen through the tube, then the immune status is adequate. If the clinician thinks that there is going to be a problem in interpretation of the result, a sample of plasma from the mare should be taken. If the foal has received adequate colostrum, the two zinc sulfate tubes should have equal turbidity. The test is, however, unreliable if the foal is already sick or if the sample is haemolysed. Once again, I stress the need for the needle to be clean when taking the sample. If the practitioner thinks that it will be difficult to access the vein twice in a foal, i.e. there is a need to inject intravenously as well as taking a blood sample, the following procedure should be adopted. The fluid to be injected is drawn up into a syringe and the needle is discarded. A new needle is attached to a clean new syringe. The vein is located and the needle attached to the syringe is placed in the vein. The blood sample is drawn up into the syringe. The syringe is disconnected and the needle is left in the vein. The fluid in the previously prepared syringe is injected into the vein and the needle is withdrawn. A new clean needle is placed onto the syringe containing the blood sample, and the blood is slowly injected into the appropriate vacuum tubes. If non-coagulated blood is required, then there is some haste required in getting the blood into the tube with the anticoagulant and commencing inversion of the tube.

2.5 Cryptorchid or Rig Test

When a possible rig (cryptorchid) is presented to the clinician, great care and thought should go into the case. It is not just a matter of carrying out a simple blood test. A careful palpation and visualization of the scrotal area should be performed. We will consider all the scenarios.

1. If the animal has one normal testicle in the scrotum and a second palpable in the inguinal ring, the sides should be noted. Although this animal is a rig, it is likely that with a good general anaesthetic (GA), both testicles will be able to be removed. The surgeon should remove the testicle in the inguinal ring first. If that cannot be removed, on no account should the normal testicle be removed. The animal should be referred to another surgeon. There is no need to carry out a rig test.

2. If the animal has one normal testicle in the scrotum and no testicle can be felt in the inguinal ring on the other side, it should be examined for scars. This may require deep sedation or even a GA in fractious animals. If there is no scar, then the animal is definitely a rig. The side of the normal testicle should be noted. Rig surgery will need to be carried out. In my experience, if the normal testicle is on the left side, the right testicle is likely to be found just inside the inguinal ring. On the other hand, if the normal testicle is on the right side the left testicle might be just inside the inguinal ring or it might be further up in the abdomen. Once again there is no need to carry out a rig test.

3. If the animal has one normal testicle in the scrotum and no testicle can be felt in the inguinal ring on the other side, it should be examined for scars. If there is a scar, this scar must be examined carefully. If the scar is just in the skin, then the animal is definitely a rig. The side of the normal testicle should be noted. Rig surgery will need to be carried out. There is no need to carry out a rig test.

4. If the animal has one normal testicle in the scrotum and no testicle can be felt in the inguinal ring on the other side, it should be examined for scars. If there is a scar, this scar must be examined carefully. If the scar is attached to a deep structure not just in the skin, then the animal is unlikely to be a rig. One testicle is likely to have been removed previously. The side of the normal testicle should be noted. Normal surgery to remove that testicle will need to be carried out. If after a few weeks the animal stops showing stallion-like behaviour, there is no need to carry out a rig test. On other hand, if the stallion-like behaviour persists then a rig test should be carried out. If this test is positive, then the side with the earlier scar will need to be investigated.

5. If the animal has no normal testicles in the scrotum but two testicles can be felt in the inguinal rings, it is a rig. However, with a good

GA it is likely that both testicles can be removed. There is no need for a rig test.

6. If the animal has no normal testicles in the scrotum and one testicle palpable in the inguinal ring (the side of this testicle should be noted), this animal is a rig. At this stage a rig blood test would not be appropriate, as the practitioner already knows there is a testicle, albeit abnormal, present. On the other hand, appropriate surgery should be carried out. The side without the palpable testicle should be investigated for scars. If there is a scar with adhesions deeper than the skin, it is likely that the testicle on that side has been removed. The surgeon can then remove the other testicle with some confidence. If after some time the stallion-like behaviour persists, then a rig test should be carried out. If this is positive, then further surgery will be required to investigate the side where no previous testicle was located.

7. If the animal has no normal testicles in the scrotum and no palpable testicles in the inguinal rings, I think it is reasonable to carry out a rig test without investigating the scars.

It is hoped that any animal presented to the clinician will be over 3 years of age (the exception to this rule is the donkey). A rig blood test is simple. A single sample for oestrone sulfate can be taken, with a normal male showing a level of oestrone sulfate >10 ng/l; a cryptorchid will have a value between 0.1 and 10 ng/l; a gelding will have a value of <0.02 ng/l.

Complications arise with animals under 3 years of age or in the donkey. First, a clotted blood sample needs to be taken (normally in a red-topped tube). 6000 IU of human chorionic gonadotrophin (hCG) is given intravenously; 30–120 min later a second sample should taken. A normal gelding will have a level of 0.15–0.30 nmol/l testosterone, which will decrease following injection of hCG. On the other hand, a rig will start with a level of 0.3–4.3 nmol/l, which will rise to 1.0–12.9 nmol/l following injection.

2.6 Water Deprivation Test

This test must not be performed on dehydrated horses. It is used to differentiate between horses suffering from the common condition of psychogenic polydipsia (often called 'box wetting') and the very rare diabetes insipidus. It is only necessary if the urine specific gravity (SG) is <1.025. Should this occur, water is withheld overnight (12 h). Dry hay or straw may be fed. Urine is then tested in the morning. If the SG is >1.025, then diabetes is not likely; if <1.025, then a second urine sample should be taken after 4 h. It may be necessary to catheterize the animal to obtain this sample. If the SG is then still <1.025, a presumptive diagnosis of diabetes insipidus may be made.

2.7 Vasopressin Challenge Test

This test is required to diagnose the cause of diabetes insipidus. Vasopressin (60 IU) is injected intramuscularly (i/m) if urinary SG is <1.025. If the cause of diabetes insipidus is neurological, the so-called central form of diabetes insipidus, the SG will rise to >1.025 within 6 h. In renal diabetes insipidus the SG will not rise, as the tubules are unable to concentrate the urine.

2.8 Overnight Dexamethasone Suppression Test (ODST)

This test is used for pituitary pars intermedia dysfunction (PPID), more commonly known as equine Cushing's disease. A basal serum cortisol concentration is taken at 5.00 pm. This is followed by an intravenous (i/v) injection of dexamethasone at 2 mg/50 kg body weight. A second serum cortisol test is taken at 11.00 am the following morning. The pars distalis (the main site of adrenocorticotrophic hormone (ACTH) synthesis) of the normal horse is suppressed by dexamethasone, leading to post-dexamethasone cortisol concentrations of <27 nmol/l (often zero). In contrast, a dysfunctional pars intermedia (a significant source of ACTH and other adrenocorticotrophic substances) is not susceptible to dexamethasone suppression, and therefore a post-dexamethasone cortisol concentration >27 nmol/l is expected in PPID cases. The ODST can be combined with the thyroid-releasing hormone (TRH) stimulation test for added accuracy. However, in practice, the diagnosis of equine Cushing's disease should be made on clinical signs, as these two tests are very expensive. In temperate climates the measurement of ACTH is a simpler and less expensive test. It is 100% accurate in the northern hemisphere when taken in the autumn, and can still act as a guide at other times of the year.

2.9 Schirmer Tear Test

Although this test will show the presence of both excessive and reduced production of tears, it is normally reserved for the diagnosis of keratoconjunctivitis sicca. There are standard Schirmer tear test strips available. However, in the field a 6.5 cm length of No. 1 filter paper, 0.5 cm wide, can be used; a fold should be placed 0.5 cm from one end. The paper strip is placed into the conjunctival sac so that the fold rests on the margin of the lower eyelid. The eye is allowed to close and the paper is left for 60 s. The distance the wetness has advanced down the paper from the fold is measured accurately. In a normal horse this will be between 12–28 mm; <10 mm would indicate keratoconjunctivitis sicca. For this test to be valid no local anaesthetic should be used and all medication should be withdrawn 6 h before the test. A horse with blocked tear ducts will produce a normal amount of tears. Tear ducts can be tested for patency by putting fluorescein dye into the eye and waiting for 45 min. The dye will appear in the nostril if the duct is patent.

2.10 Phenylephrine Equine Dysautonomia (Grass Sickness) Test

This test is very useful in field situations where the diagnosis of grass sickness is difficult. The horse should be examined from the front and the degree of drooping of the upper eyelids (ptosis) should be assessed. An experienced clinician may be aware that the drooping is more pronounced in a case of grass sickness. It is important that the horse has not received sedation within the previous 6 h. A 0.5% solution of epinephrine (adrenaline) is prepared and 0.5 ml is instilled into one eye. When examined 30 min later the eye containing the epinephrine will appear normal, i.e. less drooping of the upper eyelid, but the other eye will still show a drooping upper eyelid in a case of grass sickness. In a normal horse the epinephrine will have no effect.

2.11 Alpha-2 Adrenoreceptor Agonist Test for Horner's Syndrome

This condition of autonomic dysfunction in the head and neck region is rare in the horse. On the affected side there are areas of sweating. These areas will become dry 15 min after a sedative dose of an alpha-2 adrenoreceptor agonist. In many cases the sweating will be transferred to the other side.

2.12 Tracheal Wash

Obtaining a sample

Use a 1.2–1.5 m endoscope and a sterile catheter to obtain a sample. Use the specific endoscope providers instructions which may vary depending on the diameter of the endoscope biopsy channel. Clinicians should use a standard technique for obtaining and processing a tracheal wash sample, both for developing an understanding of sample interpretation and for repeated testing of a single horse (Smith, 2019). Important points are:

1. Unless the sample is highly cellular, it is necessary to concentrate the sample using sedimentation or cytocentrifugation.
2. Diff-Quick staining is not appropriate as there is poor staining of mast cells.
3. Specialist clinical pathologists will be helpful.
4. The sample should contain some mucous. Increased turbidity suggests increased white blood cell count and red/brown tinge suggests recent haemorrhage.
5. The presence of epithelial cells is normal.
6. Nasopharyngeal contamination should be avoided by a neat, rapid sampling technique to avoid coughing.
7. Acute haemorrhage is indicated by the presence of free red blood cells.
8. Chronic haemorrhage is indicated by the presence of haemosiderophages containing haemosiderin.
9. More than 20% neutrophyls is considered to be abnormal.
10. More than 2% eosinophyls is abnormal.
11. More than 1% mast cells is abnormal.
12. More than 10% lymphocytes is abnormal.

13. More than 80% macrophages is abnormal.
14. The presence of bacteria without clinical signs is not totally indicative of infection.
15. Presence of fungi hyphae is rare, but any are abnormal.
16. The presence of intracytoplasmic bacteria is consistent with infection.
17. Presence of *Pseudomonas* indicates poor cleaning of the scope.
18. Presence of *Dictyocaulus arnfieldi* larvae is significant.

2.13 Thoracis Ultrasonography

This is well worthwhile, particularly in foals, to reveal *Rhodococcus* infection. It is helpful in adults to reveal a fluid line. Radiography might be appropriate in foals but is not indicated in adults.

2.14 Bronchial Alveolar Lavage (BAL)

This procedure may cause severe coughing and so standing sedation is advised. With the neck extended pass the Fogatty BAL catheter through the ventral nasal meatus into the trachea. Continue passing the inner catheter as far as possible so that it blocks a bronchus. Then inflate the cuff. Introduce 3 × 60 ml of sterile phosphate buffered saline (PBS) prepared in advance. Withdraw the fluid into plain and EDTA tubes; hopefully there will be as much as 90 ml of frothy fluid. This can be sent for cytology and bacteriology. The advantage of a BAL over a tracheal wash is that an endoscope is not required. The disadvantage is that it is more invasive.

2.15 Peritoneal Tap

This is often referred to as a 'belly tap'. The correct term is abdomino centisis (or abdominal paracentesis). It is a useful test to help with diagnosis in abdominal disease, both in acute disease, usually in animals showing colic, and also in more chronic conditions. It will reveal evidence of peritonitis, haemoperitoneum and abdominal neoplasia. It should be preceded by a rectal examination to make sure there are no extremely over-filled organs, usually the caecum, to avoid inadvertent enterocentisis. The site is the most dependent point of the abdomen. The area should be clipped and cleaned. A very small incision should be made with a scalpel, and a bovine teat cannula should be pushed vertically upwards. Peritoneal fluid will start to run out and should be collected in a tube containing EDTA for cytological analysis (normally with a purple top) and a plain tube (normally with a red top) for culture and sensitivity. If no very full organ has been felt on rectal examination, it is simpler not to cut the skin but use a one-and-half-inch 18-gauge needle (normally with a pink hub). Normal peritoneal fluid is straw-coloured and clear. It does not clot. RBCs should not be present in any quantity. Peritoneal fluid with the same PCV as blood from the jugular is likely to be from a blood vessel.

If the PCV is very high, it will have come from the spleen. If it is slightly less, it indicates peritoneal bleeding as contrasted to a very low PCV, which indicates a strangulating or infarctive lesion.

If bacterial culture is required, a sample should be collected straight into a blood culture medium.

2.16 Blondheim Test for Myoglobin in Urine

Equine urine is normally pigmented. This test allows the clinician to differentiate haemoglobin and myoglobin from each other and from other pigments that are non-protein in nature. First the urine must be either fresh or stored in a sealed container in a refrigerator. Urine (1 ml) is added to 3 ml of 3% sulfosalicylic acid. The liquid is then centrifuged. If the urine becomes clear and is of a normal colour, the pigment was either haemoglobin or myoglobin. To differentiate between them, 2.8 g ammonium sulfate is mixed well with a further 5 ml sample of urine. After centrifugation, if the urine becomes clear the pigment was haemoglobin. Myoglobin will remain as a pigment even with the addition of ammonium sulfate.

2.17 Synovial and Tendon Sheath Fluid

It is vital that this is collected aseptically. Contamination with blood is common. It should be collected into both a plain and an EDTA tube, or if culture is required, then direct into a blood culture tube. It should show viscosity with a stringy appearance. The volume will be related to the site.

2.18 Punch Biopsy

1. Restrain horse. Sedate if necessary.
2. Clip, if necessary. If hair is short and fine avoid clipping.
3. Do not scrub or prepare the site unless to reduce surface contaminants for samples being submitted for bacterial culture.
4. Inject 2–3 ml local anaesthetic under the skin at each site for biopsy (three or four sites minimum) and wait a few minutes.
5. Use the largest biopsy punch possible (ideally 8 mm) to cut through the skin. Ensure the punch goes through the dermis as well as the epidermis. The two layers can separate, and it is possible to leave the dermis in situ.
6. If necessary, hold the edge of the biopsy with tissue forceps and lift it to enable it to be cut from deeper tissues with a scalpel blade. It is important the sample is grasped from the edge and not crushed.
7. Place the samples in 10% formalin for histology.
8. If bacterial culture is required, wrap the samples in swabs moistened with sterile saline or macerate them in a sterile manner and place them in a bacterial culture broth for transport to the laboratory.
9. Staple or suture each biopsy site to close the skin defect.

References and Further Reading

Knottenbelt, D.C. (2006) *Equine Formulary*. Elsevier Saunders, St Louis, Missouri.

Mair, T., Divers, T. and Ducharme, N. (2002) *Manual of Equine Gastroenterology*. Harcourt Publishers, Edinburgh, UK.

Roberts, V. (2016) Nasogastric intubation in horses. *Vet Times* 43(14), 11 April.

Smith, S. (2019) Interpretation of tracheal wash samples in horses. *In Practice* 41: 220–226.

3

Behaviour and Restraint

Abstract

Normal and abnormal equine behaviour is discussed, particularly in relation to restraint. The book concentrates on the ambulatory equine practitioner. However, it is reasonable to assume that the veterinarian will have a base that has a stable and a treatment area containing a set of stocks.

3.1 Introduction

Sadly, most tasks we want a working horse to perform are alien to its nature. We work behind it in its blind zone. We do not let it go when it is startled. We confine it and, even worse, tie up its head. Yet we can make a horse do most tasks if we approach the problem in the correct manner. We just have to remember that they are big and strong, but are also sensitive. We must also bear in mind that they are social herbivores.

3.2 Physiology

An equine has very good, almost total, all-round vision. Vision is marginal very close to the rump and absent right behind the tail. They are bifocal in that they can see very well grazing near to the ground, but they also have a wide field of view for movement on the horizon. However, they rely on head movement for accurate focusing and judgement of distances. This is very relevant for head carriage when pulling a cart. They have good night vision, but this takes longer for adaptation than for a human. Therefore, they should not be turned out suddenly from a well-lit area in darkness.

They can hear much lower-frequency sound waves than can humans, e.g. they are aware of imminent earthquakes. Their most sensitive range is the same as in the human, so they are quite capable of hearing and distinguishing words. They can hear much higher-pitched sounds than can humans. Sixteen muscles control the equine ear. However, when their ears are back their hearing is impaired. Horse calls are within the human hearing range. The pitch increases as the horse becomes more frightened or aroused.

A horse's sense of touch varies with the area involved. They are most sensitive around the head, particularly muzzle, lips, ears and around the eyes. Particularly good areas to calm a horse are the withers and neck crest. One should imitate other horses and scratch, rub or stroke that area. Although it is customary to pat a horse on the neck to reward it, this action actually raises the heart rate and so is counterproductive.

DOI: 10.1079/9781800624283.0003

A horse has a much more sensitive sense of smell than does a human. Applying strong, volatile, non-irritating substances around the nostrils can mask this strong sense of smell. It is their strong sense of smell rather than taste that makes them refuse medicines in their food. Normally, the keeping of these medicines in the refrigerator will lessen their smell.

Horses have a more sensitive sense of taste than do humans. However, they are similar in that they reject acids (pH <3) but like sugar (10 g sucrose/100 ml water). Although they like salt, they will reject solutions containing >60 g salt/100 ml water.

Humans who are said to 'have a way with horses' are not magicians, but naturally understand a horse's body language and respond accordingly.

Looking at a horse's ears, we can easily pick up signals. If they are lying flat backwards it indicates either anger or fear; a lesser angle will indicate less fear or even submission. It is obviously possible that the horse has its attention focused backwards. And this is more likely to be true if the ears are only partially back, a position that can indicate submission but, more likely, drowsiness. Extreme drowsiness is shown when the ears are really drooping laterally. If the ears are pricked the horse is paying attention to the front. If highly pricked it is likely that the horse is startled. Constantly changing ear movements will indicate confusion.

The tail can give us more useful information. If it is tucked between the legs, the horse is definitely unhappy. This may indicate submission to fear or a defensive attack. A backward kick is a possibility. If the tail is just hanging down, sleep is possible, or even illness; slightly raised indicates some alertness – the horse may be about to move or urinate. If it is already moving it will accelerate. If the tail is raised up to halfway, then it is excited or about to defecate. It may be greeting another horse or starting to show courtship display, but there may also be an element of fear. If the tail is held high up, then the horse is definitely excited. It may challenge another horse or run away. Violent swishing of the tail can be confusing: it may mean pain or annoyance – the more violent the more annoyed. Obviously, flying insects will annoy all horses. A horse needs a good long tail, which should not be trimmed unless it is rubbing on the ground. It goes without saying that it should *never* be docked, except on extremely strong clinical grounds.

The nostrils, if dilated, can indicate fear or alarm. If they are wrinkled that is normally because the horse does not like what it smells, but it can also indicate mild anger. If the horse is drowsy its lower lip will drop. This can also mean submission. If the mouth is open, then this indicates anger and likelihood of biting. If only the lips are parted, then this is submission. If the upper lip is curled back, this is the flehmen signal. Classically, stallions smelling mares exhibit this, but it may also be made if a horse does not like a particular smell. Yawning can be confusing, as it may mean either mild abdominal pain or drowsiness.

I believe that some authors read too much into a horse's head carriage. Certainly, they nudge for food and stretch out their heads with anger. However, nodding can mean so many things that it is a very confusing signal. Often the carriage of the head is simply the horse trying to focus on the ground at the optimal focal distance. Body shape and carriage can also be very confusing; the indications for an observer are not very helpful.

3.3 Effect of Husbandry on Behaviour

The horse will naturally eat 18 h/day and be constantly moving, except for one or possibly two periods of rest. Normally, only one of these periods involves actually lying down in sternal recumbency or, much more commonly, lateral recumbency. If a horse is physically restricted, particularly if it is isolated, its behaviour will be adversely affected. These effects are increased if the feeding is altered. Ideally, the horse should be eating long-fibre food for 18 h out of the 24 h in a day. If this is replaced by short-fibre feed, then adverse behaviour may be increased. In consequence, the animal will become frustrated and increasingly aroused. This will lead to a decrease in the threshold for stimulation and increased energy. This is a vicious circle, as increased energy will once again lead to increased frustration and so on. The spin-off from this cycle is handling difficulties, aggression and stereotypies.

Research has indicated that horses at pasture and feral horses spend similar times in their daily activities of feeding, standing, lying, walking and socially interacting. To some extent horses in a stall, on an ad-lib long-fibre diet, mimic this. However, for obvious reasons horses in stalls spend less time moving and reacting socially. The occasional horse will exhibit abnormal behaviour patterns in this situation. The majority of our problems arise when concentrates are fed.

Obviously, considerably less time is spent on eating. We have already stated that less time is spent on locomotion and reacting with other horses. This leaves almost half of the time free, so to speak. It is during this time that horses behave abnormally. And thus, we cause an adverse effect if we do not feed long fibre. These detrimental effects are made worse the higher the percentage of protein in the diet. There is a direct correlation between protein levels and abnormal behaviour.

3.4 Age of the Horse and Its Ability to Learn

A foal under 1 month of age tends to be unafraid of novelty, provided it can be near to and follow its mother. Horses are very rarely frightened of thunder (unlike dogs) when they first experience thunder with a mother that is not afraid of thunder. As horses age they become more suspicious of novelty as they distance themselves from their mothers. To some extent their peers are a substitute for their mothers, but their suspicions are not nearly so easily calmed. However, their exploration instinct increases with age but their submission to threat also decreases. From 2 to 4 years of age there is a movement away from the harem of mares, accompanied by more exploration with their peers. This is the time when 'breaking' (a dreadful word) takes place. It is only after 4 years of age that they settle down as adults.

3.5 Stereotypies and Stable Vices

There is some confusion with these terms. There is some crossover but there are also some problems, e.g. head shaking, which are neither. The classical stereotypies are crib-biting, wind-sucking, weaving, box-walking, rug-tearing and head-banging. These are also stable vices. However, some stable vices, such as pawing, kicking, wood-chewing and hay-dipping are not stereotypies. The traditional methods of control are usually physical, using tack and gadgetry. Sometimes surgery is resorted to. Others favour limiting the damage by environmental manipulation, while more recent control methods use counter-conditioning. All these methods have varying success rates. However, they normally fail because there is increased frustration and a decrease in the level of arousal.

Most success has been accomplished by changing the husbandry to decrease frustration and increase the level of arousal. Ideally, the stable environment should be changed to provide a more suitable social environment. Exercise should be increased and, most important of all, more long fibre should be fed to increase eating time; making it more difficult for the horse to obtain its food can increase eating time. Small-mesh hay nets can also be used. High-fibre nuts can be put in plastic balls with small holes so that the ball has to be moved before a nut drops out. Horses can be fitted with electronic devices so that they have to move round an area and can obtain food only at preselected intervals.

3.6 Classical Conditioning

The horse will receive both conditioned and unconditioned stimuli and will then show a response. An example of an unconditioned stimulus is a painful injection. An example of a conditioned stimulus is the sight of the vet approaching. The horse's response to both stimuli is to attempt to escape.

3.7 Generalization

The horse will associate different conditioned stimuli. The man in an overall or the man carrying a black bag will both equal vet. The man in an old coat or carrying a bucket will both equal groom. The unconditioned stimulus will be food. The conditioned stimuli will be the sight of a man in a green jacket or a man carrying a bucket. The response will be relaxation. This awareness of the horse can be put to good use. Conditional stimuli can be strung together. So, to make a horse back up, one can say 'back up' (first stimulus), raise the hand (second stimulus) and wave a hand in front of the horse's eyes (third stimulus). The unconditional stimulus would be to push the horse away.

3.8 Trial and Error Learning

This is a common method by which horses can learn to intimidate their owners. The chance action or trial might be for the horse to move quickly towards the owner or towards the vet. The owner or vet quickly moves back. The horse learns this very quickly! Extinction learning is required to stop this behaviour. The following sequence is common: calling the horse (conditional stimulus), it comes towards you (the reaction) and is given food (the reward). However, such a sequence is not actually desired. What is wanted is to call the horse and it comes. Therefore, what is needed is to remove the reward by extinction. Sadly, horses learn bad behaviour quickly, but extinction takes time. Another example would be door-banging. This starts as a chance action. The owner with a yell inadvertently rewards the action. It is vital that the banging is ignored. Worst of all is to feed the horse that is banging. Rewards for good behaviour should be random.

3.9 Habituation

This is a process whereby the horse learns to ignore stimuli that are normally frightening or painful. The First Nations employed this form of training to good effect when they used to 'sack' a horse. The handler takes the young horse on a halter into a box, then holds the end of the halter lead rope loosely in one hand and a blanket in the other. The blanket is flicked at the horse (the unconditional stimulus), and the horse reacts by moving away. The horse calms down again and the blanket is again flicked. With most horses the learning curve is very steep. They very soon realize that the blanket is not frightening, so that it can be flicked all over and under the horse without it moving. This procedure is very like extinction where, instead of a reward not following the stimulus, the expected punishment does not follow. The 'sacking' is actually termed saturation therapy, and obviously with other stimuli is dangerous and stressful.

Perhaps a better therapy is 'systematic desensitization'. In this therapy there is a careful and very gradual progressive manipulation of the fearful stimuli and/or the time the horse is exposed to it. Ideally, care is taken to stop the training session just before the horse shows signs of apprehension. If the horse does not show extreme apprehension or if the stimulus is not too severe, then a procedure called 'counter-conditioning' can be used. The confident, relaxed horse that needs retraining can be conditioned to associate the instinctive or conditioned noxious stimulus with a positive reward in lieu of 'punishment'. This can be very effective in the short term with the normally relaxed horse that does not like injections. Remember that the conditioned stimulus is the approach or touch of the vet holding the needle. The unconditioned stimulus is the pain, and the response is a sudden flinch (which is actually going to cause more pain). Hold the needle between your thumb and first finger, pointing away from the palm with a clenched fist. Rhythmically press the injection site with the base of the hand many times until flinching stops. Then turn the hand, maintaining the same rhythm to place the needle.

3.10 Shaping

This therapy uses a reward for a preliminary response to a desired action or a reward for an action that is similar to the desired action. Rewards have to be given in a careful sequence. An example would be the horse that does not like loading and in fact positively backs away from the trailer. Initially the reward, which can be a small morsel of food or even a soft voice, is given when the horse stands still. When the horse has understood this response the next phase is the reward, which is given when the horse looks towards the trailer. It must be remembered that the reward is given only when the horse looks towards the trailer and not when it just stands still, i.e. when the horse achieves the second response. When this is fully appreciated by the horse, the third phase is begun, i.e. the horse steps towards the trailer. It must be remembered from then on that the reward is given *only* when the horse carries out this third response. This procedure is carried out with each phase until the horse is loaded.

3.11 Punishment and Reward

Punishment has to be used with great care, for welfare reasons. In addition, punishment may be associated by the horse with the handler, and this is to be avoided. Also, it takes very careful timing to ensure that the horse associates the punishment only with the bad behaviour. However, if the punishment can be removed from the handler and the timing is right, then this method can be very effective. If we use punishment in the previous scenario, i.e. difficulty in loading, we need a long cane with a noisy piece of polythene attached to the far end. The horse is walked towards the trailer, and immediately it stops the polythene is rustled. As soon as the horse continues the rustling is stopped. Timing is everything. It is important when loading not to 'reward' the horse that goes to the side of the trailer, by turning it around and walking away to align it straight again. This sends the wrong message to the horse, i.e. bad behaviour results in the reward of turning away from the trailer. Horses are quite capable of turning in very small circles. You do not need to walk the horse away to turn it.

Another example of remote punishment is the horse that backs away when tied up and breaks the lead rope. In this scenario the horse is rewarding itself, i.e. when it behaves badly by backing away it gains its freedom. The old-fashioned training method would be to put on an unbreakably strong rope halter and tie the young horse to a big tree. The horse would pull back and would punish itself by having the halter tighten on its head. Although this may be effective, there are grave welfare considerations. A better method is to use a small length of bicycle inner tube. With the horse in a small enclosure, this is attached firmly to the head collar, but not so firmly to the lead rope, which is then tied up in the normal manner. The horse is then left alone. When it pulls back, the attachment of the inner tube to the lead rope will break. Instantly, it will be punished by a slap with the inner tube. The horse is caught and tied up again. It will pull away again and receive another slap. Horses learn over varying lengths of time.

Fundamentals of this type of training

It is important to identify the reward that the horse is actually giving to itself for bad behaviour. In the previous example it is gaining its freedom. Another example is the horse that is difficult to catch. It is so easy to endorse this bad behaviour with food: the horse comes to the handler and gets a little food, the reward, and immediately moves away before he can be caught. He is rewarding himself. The handler can inadvertently reward the horse when trying to catch it. It moves away and the handler says 'good boy' in a soft voice, again the reward. Remember that the reward may be to avoid discomfort or pain, e.g. the inner tube. The handler has to manipulate the environment so that reward comes only with the desired behaviour.

Thought has to go into training. It is important to differentiate between an unwelcome response due to fear or anxiety and a learnt response. This is particularly important when studying the horse's response to a piece of tack: is the horse genuinely fearful or even hurt by a piece of tack, or is this a learned response? Has the horse learned through a certain type of behaviour that the tack will be removed?

3.12 Fundamental Rules in Handling

The fundamental rules in handling can be summarized as:

- Speak softly before approaching.
- Approach from the side towards the shoulder.
- Move slowly, steadily and consistently.
- Carefully read the postural signs given by the horse.
- Be aware of the limits of the horse's perception.
- Avoid entanglement with tack.
- Be confident.

3.13 Loading Aids

I previously described two aids for loading horses through reward and non-connected punishment.

However, there are other methods that may help. It must be remembered that continual bullying will make the horse more frightened and harder to load. Horses are naturally frightened of going into a small, dark place, with no chance of escape. Make the trailer as bright and well-lit as possible, and move the partition aside so that it creates as wide an opening as possible. Lessen the slope as much as possible by parking the trailer downhill. Make the ramp as quiet as possible by having the trailer well-secured, with the ramp covered in carpet or straw. All these measures are important for young horses that have not been loaded before. However, these methods are not so useful for the horse that has already learnt bad behaviour. Loading a companion first is always a useful ploy. Loading next to a wall is also recommended, as there is only one side exposed. Obviously, loading down an alleyway is ideal. This works on the same principle as a jumping lane to stop horses jumping out. Remember that the horse needs its head down to visualize the ramp if it is walking forward out of the trailer. Mistakenly, handlers often hold a horse's head down to prevent it hitting the top of its head. This is counterproductive.

3.14 The Barging Horse

We have said that most bad behaviour carried out by a horse results from fear. However, a very few acts of bad behaviour are of an aggressive nature. The horse that tries to barge the handler in the stable is one of these. The trick to train a horse to stop this behaviour is very simple. The handler should obtain a short, stout piece of wood that cannot be broken. The length needs to be about 15 cm (6 in) longer than the width of the handler's pelvis. Wearing a pair of good strong boots and a belt, the handler enters the stable, with the stout stick in the belt pointing upwards. The horse is caught. When it then tries to barge the handler against the wall of the stable the stick is turned in the belt so that one end of the stick is pointing into the horse and the other end of the stick is pointing into the wall of the stable. Then the harder the horse pushes the more severe will be his punishment, i.e. the stick sticking into the horses ribs. The handler is unaffected, as his pelvis cannot be crushed.

3.15 Methods of Restraint

Hobbling

Hobbling of horses with ropes, to prevent either kicking or straying, is not humane and therefore such methods should not be used. Equally, with the advent of modern anaesthetic agents and sedatives, there is no need to use hobbles to cast a horse. Traditionally, horses could be cast using sidelines (another procedure involving rope), but there is no need for this procedure nowadays. However, a single sideline does still have a purpose in drawing forward a hind leg that has a permanently locked patella (upward fixation of the patella, or kneecap). If this is not possible then an emergency sectioning of the median patellar ligament has to be performed (the surgical method is described in Section 12.7).

Controlling the head

This can be carried out with a halter or a head collar. Extra control can be given by passing the lead rope of the head collar over the nose and then threaded back through the head collar, as shown in Fig. 3.1.

A bridle will give even more control, particularly if the reins are removed and a lead rope is attached to one side of the bit and passed through the other side of the bit, as shown in Fig. 3.2.

For more control, particularly in the stallion, a chain can be used instead of a lead rope. A very short chain on the end of a 1.2-m (4-ft) pole can be used. This is often called a stallion pole and is useful in the horse that is liable to bite. Such a pole is, however, not suitable for the horse that is liable to rear, as the holder of the pole is put in danger from the front legs. With such animals it is advisable to use a very long lead rope or a lungeing line. A Chifney bit, as shown in Fig. 3.3, is also useful in such cases; in fact it is often called an anti-rearing bit. The bit has a shallow, inverted port mouthpiece; it has three rings, one in the middle for the lead rope and two on the sides for the two cheekpieces.

The twitch

The twitch is a device for gripping and exerting pressure on the horse's upper lip. It has long

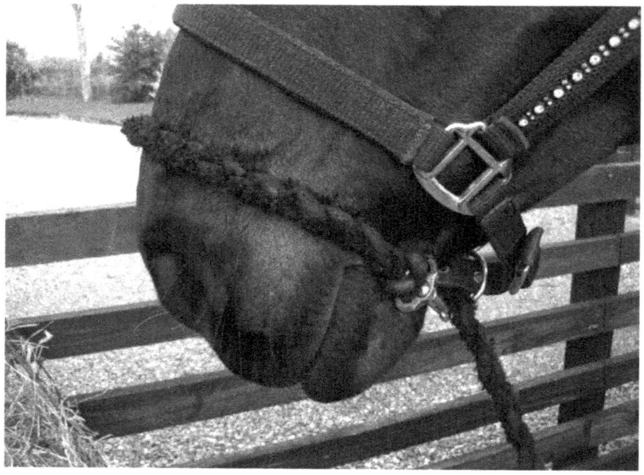

Fig. 3.1. Rope over the nose.

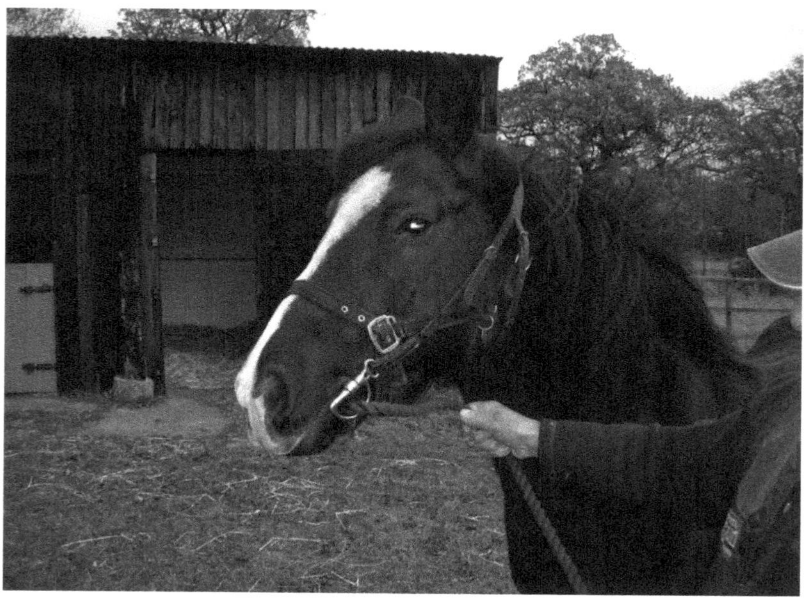

Fig. 3.2. Leading rope through the bit.

been recognized that most equines are effectively restrained from fractious behaviour by a twitch. Its mode of action is not clear. Originally it was thought merely to cause diversionary pain and discourage movement. However, some authorities now think that it causes a natural release of endorphins to relax the horse. Certainly, it is best to apply the twitch and wait for a couple of minutes for it to take effect. The effect of the twitch becomes less after approximately 15 min.

There are various types of twitch. The most common is a wooden pole, either short for one-handed use or long for double-handed grip, with a loop of string through one end. The loop is passed over a hand gripping the upper lip and tightened by twisting the pole. Some twitches

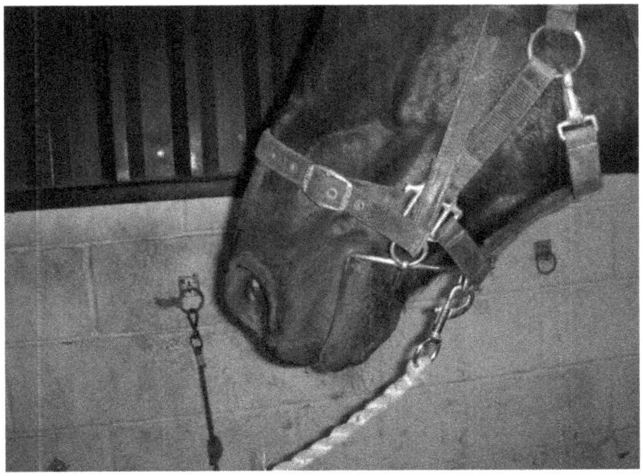

Fig. 3.3. Chifney bit.

are made with a loop of chain. The writer's preference is for a long pole with a rope loop. This can be applied single-handedly by grasping the upper lip as described, passing the loop over the hand and then twisting up using the other hand and gripping the long pole between the thighs. The danger with a long pole is that if it slips from the holder's grasp it is thrown violently round by the horse's head. This can be made less dangerous by having a length of strong yet light alkathene water pipe. Also available is a humane, or hand-held, twitch made of two short aluminium handles hinged at one end. This can be applied to the upper lip, a cord is wrapped round the two handles and the end of the cord tied or clipped to the head collar. The twitch then no longer needs to be held. Twitches of this nature should not be applied to the ear or tongue on welfare grounds. The ear can be held by one hand to help control a horse briefly for a quick, delicate task, e.g. a nerve block to a facial nerve. When examining the mouth, the tongue can be held to aid visualization of the teeth, but it should never be pulled on account of possible damage to the hyoid apparatus. The tongue can be held, but not pulled, in foaling mares to lessen abdominal contractions, so that malpresentations of the foal can be corrected. Last a skin twitch can be applied to the skin on the neck with the hand, to aid in administering of injections.

Further Reading

Kiley-Worthington, M. (1997) *The Behaviour of Horses*. J.A. Allen & Co., London.

4

Veterinary Equipment

Abstract
A full list of veterinary equipment is given in this chapter. In many developing countries second-hand human medicine equipment is available, but in essence the author has concentrated on equipment which is not going to cost a large amount.

4.1 General

Advances in equipment in the medical field have been very rapid in recent years and will continue to be so. Advances in the veterinary field are not very far behind. This chapter will therefore be out of date in some respects before this book has been published. However, the whole ethos of this book is the treatment of working equines worldwide. In most parts of the world sophisticated equipment is not available; in fact, it is not really required. It certainly would not be the best use of resources. Therefore, I will concentrate on equipment required for the ambulatory veterinary surgeon. I will mention certain items that are available and could be included if funds allow.

4.2 Equipment for Handling

The ambulatory veterinary surgeon does not need sophisticated items of tack; these will be described in Chapter 21, which is devoted to harness and tack.

A twitch is vital, and a Chifney bit is sometimes helpful. However, a good handler is the key. Good horsepersons are not born – they are made. They learn to anticipate the horse and respond in the appropriate manner. A lungeing line is sometimes useful. However, a good, long rope will suffice and can be used for many other tasks. Ideally it should be made of soft cotton. To sum up, the ambulatory practitioner needs a long rope and a simple twitch, made from a piece of string and a length of wood.

4.3 Equipment for Diagnosis

1. Thermometer. A clinical thermometer is vital. The traditional glass thermometers will last for years if kept carefully in a plastic case. However, there are now digital thermometers available. The clinician needs to choose whether the thermometer reads in Celsius or Fahrenheit – either is appropriate.
2. Stethoscope. This is the second vital piece of diagnostic equipment. Ideally, it needs to be slim so that auscultation is possible under the muscles caudal to the shoulder. Also, ideally, both a bell and a diaphragm should be present. Obviously, there are sophisticated stethoscopes

2nd Edition (G.R. Duncanson)
DOI: 10.1079/9781800624283.0004

available, e.g. the Littman model. However, the inexpensive models are quite adequate.

3. Biopsy punch. There are sophisticated biopsy gadgets available that are vital for certain biopsies, e.g. liver. However, the small 8-mm disposable punches are useful for both skin biopsies and pinch skin grafts

4. Microscope. A microscope is a delicate piece of equipment. I do not recommend that one be carried in the vehicle as a routine. However, the use of a microscope at one's base is vital. It needs to be equipped for oil emersion. 'Diff-Quick' slides are useful. Gram stain and methylene blue are the standard stains used.

5. McMaster slide. This glass slide used for carrying out faecal worm egg counts is vital. Great care should be taken when handling the coverslip (with the squares), as this is delicate and expensive.

6. Urine dipsticks. These are useful occasionally and are relatively cheap.

7. Haematocrit centrifuge tubes. These can be used without a centrifuge to obtain a quick idea of a PCV. However, a mini-centrifuge is useful and relatively inexpensive. A hand-driven centrifuge for larger tubes is very cheap and can give adequate results.

8. Blood slides and coverslips. These are essential items.

9. Stomach tube (nasogastric tube, NGT). Obviously, a nasogastric tube will be used for treatment. However, I consider it to be a vital piece of equipment for aiding in the diagnosis of certain colics. The clinician will require two sizes, one for horses and one for ponies, donkeys and foals.

10. Arm-length sleeves. These are essential for performing rectal and vaginal explorations.

4.4 Equipment for the Feet

1. Hoof pick. The ideal hoof pick has a small brush on the opposite side to the pick so that the surface of the hoof and the sulci of the frog can be brushed really clean before examination.

2. Hoof testers. These are absolutely essential.

3. Hoof knife. The type of knife used is a very individual choice. There are knives for either left or right hand. Equally, there are double-sided knives that can be used in either hand. Looped knives are useful for dealing with the softer parts of the hoof, i.e. the frog.

4. Hoof trimmers. Like hoof knives, expensive hoof trimmers are required – you only get what you pay for. Cheap hoof trimmers are too stiff for one-handed use and will rust unless used and oiled constantly.

5. Hoof rasp. This can be without handles, which makes its use hard for veterinarians with small hands. It normally has two surfaces, one of which is less abrasive.

6. Hammer. Any type of hammer is suitable for use with the buffer. However, a claw hammer can be useful for removing non-shoeing nails that have become embedded in the hoof.

7. Buffer. This small and inexpensive item is vital for removing shoes.

8. Shoe puller. This item is not essential if you have an individual nail puller. However, once the use of a shoe puller has been mastered, it speeds up shoe removal.

9. Nail puller. I consider this to be essential. Removal of individual nails from the hoof using the shoe as a point of leverage is the safest method of shoe removal.

10. Roofing gutter tape. A roll of this tape is very useful for making bandages waterproof in the hoof area. It is also useful for covering poultices on the feet.

4.5 Equipment for the Limbs

1. Splints. Where funds are tight, there is no need for sophisticated splints. Smooth lengths of wood or plastic guttering are quite adequate. Any sharp ends can be rasped smooth and covered with gutter tape.

2. Oscillating saw. This might be considered non-essential, as a hand-held plaster saw can be used. However, modern plastering materials are very hard, and it is seriously hard work to remove them without an oscillating saw. The horse will eventually stop standing still. An oscillating saw is quick and accurate.

4.6 Equipment for the Eyes

1. Ophthalmoscope. This is an expensive piece of equipment, but is important to the equine clinician. Much can be found out by examining the eyes carefully with a bright small torch and a magnifying glass. Sadly, however, some pathological conditions will be missed. Although a slit lamp is very useful for examining a dog's eyes, it is not required for equine medicine.

2. Fluorescein strips. These are inexpensive and vital, not only for revealing the presence of deep corneal ulcers but also for testing the patency of the tear ducts. It should be remembered that it can take up to 45 min for the fluorescein stain to reach the nasal end of the tear ducts in the horse after instillation in the eye (see Fig. 4.1).

3. Schirmer tear test strips. The condition of dry eye is extremely rare in the horse. However, these test strips are required to diagnose the condition. Home-made strips can be made from filter paper marked off into sections 2 mm wide.

4. Canine urethral catheter. These catheters, designed for catheterization of the urethra of the male dog, are useful for unblocking equine tear ducts. The most useful sizes are 16 and 18 gauge.

4.7 Equipment for Dentistry and Sinoscopy

1. Full-mouth speculum. There are a variety of these on the market. The Hausmann-type gag is quite sufficient for ambulatory dentistry – one size will fit all sizes of horse or donkey. It is important that it is made of steel; those made from cast iron may shatter when dropped or, more seriously, may shear when in the mouth. Some operators use a Butler gag. However, this tends to obstruct the use of dental equipment, and its use should be restricted to aiding the passage of an endotracheal tube in the anaesthetized horse. The old-fashioned Swales gag should never be used, for two reasons. First, there is a danger of damaging an individual cheek tooth, as the whole force of the jaw is focused on a single tooth. Second, the gag can shatter and the resulting sharp metal shards can penetrate the palatine artery. Should the palatine artery be severed for any reason, there is helpful advice here for the practitioner: digital pressure will stop the haemorrhage; however, as soon as it is released the haemorrhage will start again. The artery that runs palatially to the upper cheek teeth rows is too tightly adherent to the hard palate to be grasped with artery forceps. Therefore, after sedation, a small towel should be rolled up and placed between the upper cheek teeth rows and held tightly in position with a headcollar that is too small. This will moderate the haemorrhage, which is not life-threatening. The headcollar can be removed in 30 min.

2. Head light. There are some seriously bright torches available with heavy battery packs.

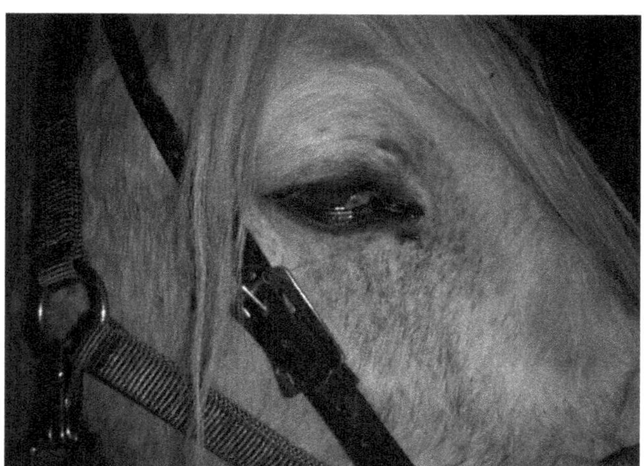

Fig. 4.1. Fluorescein staining of the eye.

These are not really required, and a light that is easily taken on and off is preferable.

3. Dental picks. These should be strong to allow the practitioner to pick out the food matter compacted between the teeth in diastemata (gaps between teeth). There are water picks available, but these are unnecessary for the ambulatory practitioner.

4. Dental probes. These are important in gauging the depth of dental caries and the patency of infundibulae.

5. Dental mirror. This piece of dental equipment needs to be handled and carried with care. It is important to visualize the possible pathology on the caudal and occlusal surfaces of the cheek teeth. Mirrors tend to fog up in the mouth, but this can be avoided by immersing them in warm water. There is good evidence that more pathological lesions are observed if a rigid video endoscope is used for this purpose. However, this is an unnecessary expense.

6. Dental bucket. This is usually made of stainless steel with a brush attached at the side. However, a plastic bucket with a scrubbing brush is quite adequate.

7. 'Wolf' teeth removal equipment. This is very much personal preference. There are many different elevators on the market. The short elevators, which have a concave blade, or the round Burgess/Musgrave type are the safest, as they can be kept in contact with the tooth more easily. A simple pair of elevators is also required. Rongeur forceps are useful for removing very small 'wolf' teeth or fragments, but these are not essential.

8. Mouth washing syringe. There are many types of this; none of them is expensive. Ideally, the type used should be that which can be used one-handedly.

9. Cheek retractor. This is inexpensive but not essential.

10. Dental arcade speculum. This is also inexpensive but not essential.

11. Dental elevators. As stated above, short dental elevators are required for the loosening of 'wolf' teeth. If cheek teeth are to be removed, elevators on a long shaft are required to separate the gingival margin.

12. Molar spreaders. These are required to insert between the cheek teeth to aid extraction. In an ideal world several pairs are required, each thicker than the previous. However, they are expensive, and with skilled use a dental elevator can do a similar job if positioned between the teeth.

13. Molar extraction forceps. All new molar extraction forceps, which are made from high-quality stainless steel, are expensive. This is a pity, as some of the old models made of ordinary steel 70 years ago are as good as or even better than these new models. There are a large number of models, varying in length and size. There is a basic requirement of two models, one for the upper and one for the lower cheek teeth row, and these should be the standard box shape. Models for use in the older horse having three claws to grip the tooth either from left or right are extremely useful. There are specific forceps for removal of caps; however, these are only necessary when dealing with the young horse.

14. Trephine. Hopefully, all cheek tooth extraction will be performed per os. However, a trephine is a useful back-up with a dental punch in case oral extraction fails. A trephine is also useful for sinus surgery.

15. Steinmann pins. These are inexpensive and useful for making smaller holes into the sinuses.

16. Dental halter. This is useful when manpower is limited.

17. Headstand. This is not an expensive luxury, but is conducive for good dentistry.

18. Tracheostomy tube. This can be lifesaving; however, the stainless steel variety is very expensive. An inexpensive option can be made from the handle of a 1-litre plastic container.

19. Dental syringe with 27G needles. This can be obtained from human medical suppliers with local anaesthetic cartridges and is useful for anaesthetising the mucosa when extracting teeth, particularly wolf teeth.

Dental rasps

There is a multitude of different rasps available, but first there are several factors to be considered.

1. The handle must be comfortable for the operator. It should not be too bulky or indeed too slim. Plastic tends to be slippery. Wood is difficult to clean and sterilize. Foam rubber handles are very comfortable to use, but when on shorter rasps they tend to get waterlogged when the handle is immersed in water. The ideal are the

hard rubber-composite handles. However, some people prefer pistol grips.
2. The length of shaft will depend on whether the rostral or caudal cheek teeth are the targets. Obviously, the shaft must be long enough.
3. The type of shaft is variable. Flat shafts are preferable for less experienced operators, as it is easy for them to see at a glance the angle of the head of the rasp when it is in the mouth. This problem can be solved when round shafts are used by having a small, flattened area near to the handle at the same angle as the head.
4. The type of head is also very important. It needs to be slim for the back of the mouth, but should be small for ponies and donkeys. It may be concave in a lateral plane and convex in a caudal rostral plain – the Gledhill rasp. This is a particularly useful tool for rasping a single, over-erupted cheek tooth.
5. The angle of the head varies with the purpose required. The middle of the arcade requires a straight head; the back of the mouth requires a slightly upturned angle, in the region of 15°; for the front an offset or downturned angle is best.
6. They will not shatter or loosen teeth. However, once they are blunt they are disposable. The blades used most commonly are the tungsten carbide blades. These are harder and more abrasive than the grit type, and they therefore do the job more quickly, but they are very slightly harder to use for the inexperienced. They are brittle and so they need handling with care. Plastic tubes are required in the rasping bucket to avoid breakages. Tungsten carbide blades are more expensive but can be resharpened. They rasp in only one direction, and therefore the operator must decide whether to rasp on the 'push' or the 'pull'; normally, they are set on 'pull' for the back of the mouth and on 'push' for the front. There are blades called 'Tru cut', which, like the grit blades, cut both ways. These are made up of small steel teeth, which can be damaged by the action of the horse's teeth biting down on them. Tungsten carbide blades have largely replaced these. The most abrasive of all blades are the 'caps floats', but they are also the most expensive. They are purchased as ten triangular blades, so they can be rotated, giving three times the life of a plain blade. They tend to be rather bulky. The final type of blade, which gives the best finish of all, is the diamond-coated blade. This is expensive but slim, very abrasive and seems very well tolerated by the horse.
7. The rasps so far described are in the standard form of a handle, a shaft and a head. However, there are also S-shaped rasps, which can be covered in either tungsten chips or diamond coating. These are very versatile.

Summary of dental rasping equipment

This long list is confusing for the inexperienced, but below is a list containing the essential items for routine ambulatory dental work, when extractions are not going to be carried out:

- Hausmann gag;
- head light;
- plastic bucket and scrubbing brush;
- six rasps:
  - long, flat;
  - short, offset;
  - long, flat with small head;
  - long, with small, upturned head;
  - Gledhill;
  - small, diamond-coated S-shaped;
- dental syringe;
- dental pick; and
- dental mirror.

4.8 Equipment for Stitching

These items are self-explanatory. This is a complete list. However, the clinician can actually manage with very few.

1. Scalpel handle. It is important that the scalpel handle is the same size as the blades.
2. Scalpel blades. These come in different sizes and shapes for different procedures.
3. Dressing scissors. A pair of curved, blunt-ended scissors need to be readily available for trimming hair. However, a straight pair with pointed ends is required for a stitch-up kit. There are various different sizes.
4. Stitch-cutting scissors. These small scissors need to be available for removing sutures.
5. Dressing forceps. The ends of these forceps are important; they can be either flat or 'rat-toothed'; one pair of each would be required.
6. Tissue forceps. These forceps are for lifting tissue. A minimum of two pairs are required.
7. Artery forceps. These can be straight or curved. Several pairs are required.

8. Bowel clamps. These are not required by the ambulatory clinician. However, they would be vital if colic surgery is undertaken.
9. Towel clips. These are not normally required by the ambulatory clinician unless surgery is going to be performed under a GA.
10. Suture needles. These come in various shapes. They are also either cutting or non-cutting. On the whole, cutting needles will be required for the skin and non-cutting for soft tissue.
11. Suture material. This maybe absorbable or non-absorbable, also either monofilament or braided. On the whole, monofilament non-absorbable will be required for skin wounds.
12. Needle holders. There are various types. The most convenient for stitching up wounds are the combination of cutting and holding type called Gillies.
13. Clippers. These are a luxury. However, they make stitching and wound management so much cleaner and easier, particularly in rough-haired horses and donkeys. The ideal is the rechargeable battery type.
14. Drapes. A single sterile drape is required as a tray cloth by the ambulatory clinician. However, drapes will be required for other types of surgery.
15. Swabs. Sets of sterile swabs are required for a variety of tasks.

4.9 Equipment for the Reproductive System

1. Emasculators. These are required for castrations when ligatures are not being used.
2. Vaginal speculum. This can be disposable and used with a small hand torch. It may be non-disposable, with a special light source. The duck-billed type affords the very best visibility.
3. Uterine biopsy forceps. These forceps are designed for reproductive work and are not required for normal ambulatory veterinary work. They are required to obtain a rectal biopsy. However, this can easily be obtained with a crown bottle cap.

4.10 Equipment for Post-mortem Examination

These articles are not normally carried by an ambulatory clinician. Nevertheless, they should be available in a clean state at the clinic:

- post-mortem knife;
- meat saw;
- sampling equipment;
- enterotomy scissors; and
- sieves.

4.11 Specialist Equipment

I have included these items for completeness. It would be very useful to have access to some of these items of equipment. Nonetheless, within the scope of this book a full description would not be worthwhile. Throughout the text a suitable alternative will be suggested wherever possible to save on financial investment:

- arthroscope;
- flexible endoscope;
- rigid endoscope;
- surgical laser;
- electro-thermocautery;
- motorized dental equipment;
- gaseous anaesthetic machine;
- sophisticated monitoring equipment;
- ECG;
- ultrasound scanner;
- X-ray machine;
- operating table;
- hobbles and winch;
- blood analyser;
- centrifuge;
- refractometer;
- stomach pump;
- cuffed nasogastric tube;
- monkey splint;
- neck cradle;
- slings;
- pole syringe;
- padded blinkers; and
- equine boots.

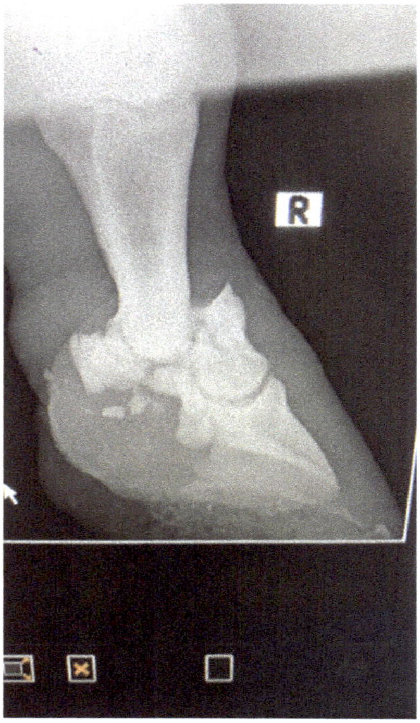

Fig. 4.2. Lateral view of a catastrophic fracture of P2.

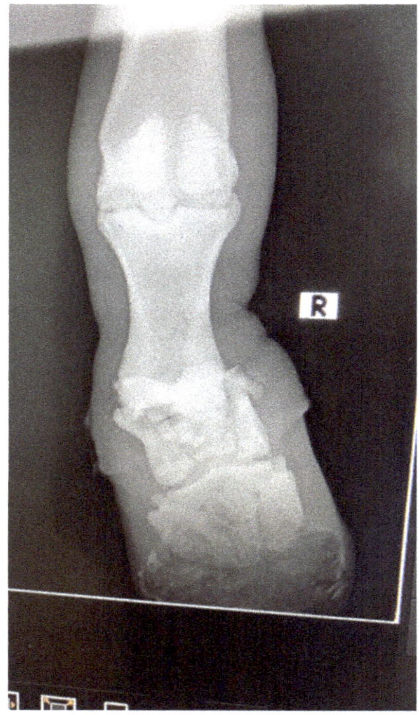

Fig. 4.3. Palmar dorsal view of fracture of P2, often called a 'bag of ice fracture'.

Further Reading

Knottenbelt, D.C. (2006) *Equine Formulary*. Elsevier Saunders, St Louis, Missouri.

5

Diagnostic Imaging

Laura Quiney, IMV imaging

Abstract

This chapter describes imaging, both ultrasonography and radiography, as many equine charities worldwide dealing with working horses have these facilities. However, MRI and CT are outside of the remit of this book.

5.1 Ultrasonography

Ultrasonography is a valuable modality with a plethora of applications for the evaluation of soft tissues, internal organs and bone surfaces. Common indications include, but are not limited to, evaluation of masses (e.g. can distinguish soft tissue masses and abscessation), suspected fractures (discontinuity of bone surfaces may be visible), abdominal pain (can accurately distinguish between 'surgical' and 'medical' colic), evaluation of the musculoskeletal system (diagnosis of the cause of lameness) and wound assessment (presence of foreign material, extent of a penetrative injury).

Basic principles of image formation

Ultrasonography is a dynamic modality, whereby longitudinal (ultrasound) waves are emitted from a transducer, transmit through the patient and may be reflected at tissue interfaces (echoes). Returning echoes are detected by the transducer. The resultant graphical image is formed of dots of varying shades of grey, which represent the reflected portion of the ultrasound wave. The shade of grey mainly indicates the proportion of wave reflected; a high degree of reflection, e.g. at soft tissue–bone or soft tissue–gas interfaces, is represented by light grey or white (hyperechoic), whereas a low degree of reflection, e.g. in fluid, is represented as very dark grey (hypoechoic) or black (anechoic; no echoes detected). The shade of grey will also be influenced by other causes of attenuation. The further away from the transducer the beam has travelled, the more it will be affected by attenuation and therefore the image may appear darker in far field in comparison with the near field.

Transducers

There are several types of transducers. The two main differences to consider are footprint size (influences field of view (FOV)) and frequency range (influences depth of penetration and image resolution). Convex transducers (curved footprint) produce a wide, wedge-shaped FOV;

 Veterinary Treatment for Working Equines, 2nd Edition (G.R. Duncanson)
DOI: 10.1079/9781800624283.0005

linear transducers (flat footprint) produce a smaller rectangular FOV. Low-frequency transducers will have better penetration, and are best for imaging deep structures, but image resolution is compromised. High-frequency transducers offer improved image resolution, but penetration is poor and only more superficial structures can be examined.

Machine functions

1. Depth

The depth function alters the depth of image displayed. It will not alter the depth of penetration of the ultrasound wave.

Rule of thumb: depth should be selected so that the area of interest occupies approximately 75% of the FOV.

2. Frequency

Modern transducers can function at a range of frequencies, whereas older transducers may operate at a fixed frequency. Higher frequencies give good axial resolution, but less depth of penetration. Lower frequencies give poorer axial resolution, but greater depth of penetration.

Rule of thumb: select the highest frequency that gives the depth of penetration required.

3. Focal point

The focal point is usually displayed on the depth scale, as a triangular or egg timer-shaped marker. At the location of the focal point, lateral resolution is the best. The location of the focal point can be adjusted to the area of interest. A standoff pad can be used to position superficial structures of interest deeper within the image and therefore in the focal zone. Although multiple focal zones can be selected to increase the area of maximum resolution, the frame rate will be reduced and the image will become dynamically slow.

Rule of thumb: place the focal zone at the level of, or just below, the area of interest.

4. Gain and time-gain-compensation (TGC)

In order to compensate for attenuation, the returning signal can be amplified by altering the overall gain. Increasing the gain will result in overall brightening (whitening) of the image, whereas if the gain is reduced the image will become darker. If gain is too low, detail is lost as low energy echoes are not correctly represented and, if gain is too high, contrast resolution and detail are lost due to amplification of background noise. The gain setting will depend to some extent upon the light level of the scanning environment (a dark scanning area is best) and personal preference. Altering the TGC (usually multiple sliders) allows amplification of the near, mid and far fields of the image. Ideally, the gain should appear the same throughout the image. If there has been significant attenuation from deep structures (the image appears dark at the bottom), the far field gain should be increased to compensate.

Patient preparation

Preparation is essential to avoid contact artefact, which is most commonly caused by air between the transducer and patient. Contact artefact is caused by poor ultrasound penetration, and the image will appear diffusely hypoechoic. Ideally, the hair coat over the area to be scanned should be clipped, the skin degreased (shampoo or chlorhexidine) and ultrasound gel applied liberally. Ultrasound gel should be topped up throughout the examination to maintain good contact. If the hair coat is fine, or if abdominal examination is to be performed, applying copious amounts of isopropyl alcohol will provide good contact. When isopropyl alcohol is used, the transducer should be wiped down with a damp cloth after use.

Common artefacts

An artefact is something on the image that does not accurately represent what is being imaged (the patient). They can be operator-induced, or as a result of ultrasound physics. It is important to recognize them in order to avoid misinterpretation; however, they can also be used to our advantage and give valuable information.

1. Distal acoustic shadowing

Acoustic shadowing results from complete reflection or absorption of the ultrasound wave, resulting in a hyperechoic (white) interface and a deep shadow of black caused by the lack of wave penetration. This commonly occurs at interfaces between soft tissue and bone (Fig. 5.1), ossification, mineralization or foreign material.

2. Distal acoustic enhancement

This artefact occurs when the ultrasound wave passes through material which causes minimal attenuation, such as fluid (Fig. 5.2). Deep to the body of fluid will be a localized hyperechoic (lighter grey/whiter) area (Fig. 5.3). The collection of fluid needs to be at least 1 cm in diameter in order to visibly produce this effect.

3. Reverberation

Reverberation artefact occurs as a result of wave 'excitation' and delayed, multiple echo return, and is commonly associated with a gas–soft tissue interface (Fig. 5.4). Because depth is derived from the time taken between emission and

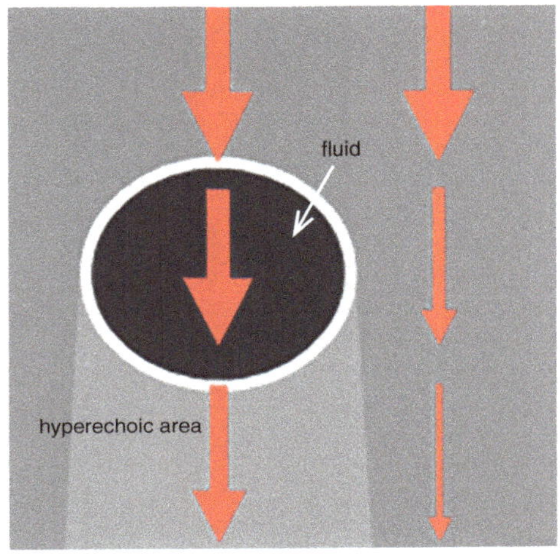

Fig. 5.2. Schematic diagram of distal acoustic enhancement.

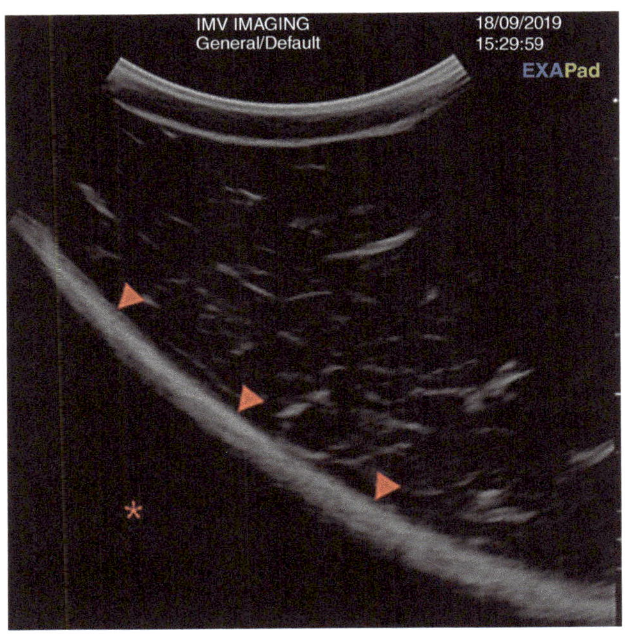

Fig. 5.1. Image of the ilial wing. There is distal acoustic shadowing (*) deep to the soft tissue–bone interface of the ilial wing, which appears as a hyperechoic line (arrowheads).

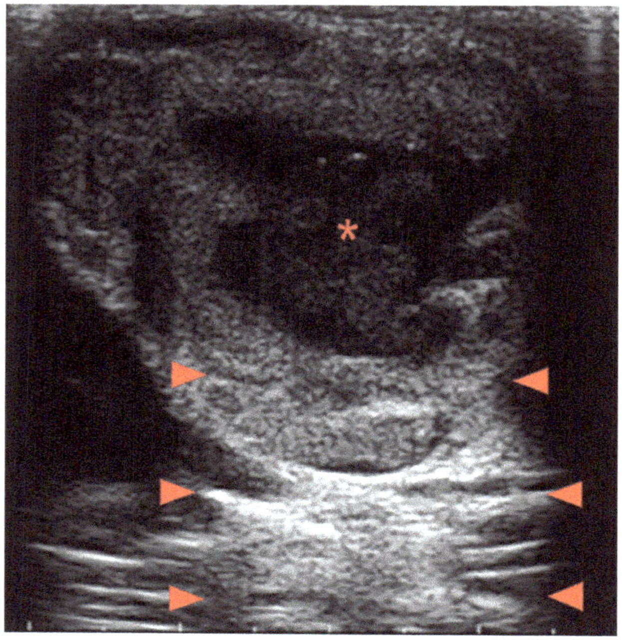

Fig. 5.3. Acoustic enhancement (arrowheads) deep to a collection of fluid (*; purulent material in a pulmonary abscess).

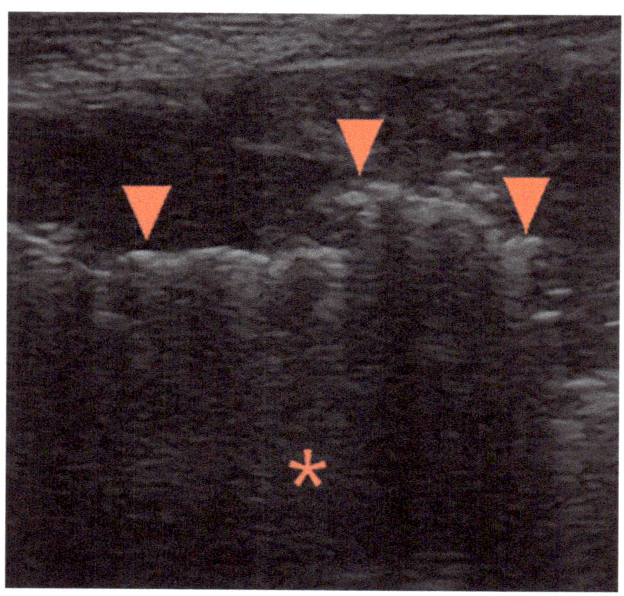

Fig. 5.4. Air within a wound. The fluid (oedema/haemorrhage)–gas interface appears as an irregular hyperechoic line (arrowheads). Deep to the interface are ring-down reverberation artefacts (*).

detection of a wave, multiple deep reflections will be displayed, giving a so-called 'ring-down' artefact.

4. Edge shadowing (refraction)

Refraction of the ultrasound beam at the margin of a curved echogenic structure causes shadowing deep to the edges of the structure (Fig. 5.5). It is commonly seen at the edges of blood vessels (Fig. 5.6), small intestinal loops and tendons/ligaments when viewed in transverse section.

5. Off-incidence artefact

Ligaments and tendons with longitudinal (normal) fibre alignment are subject to the off-incidence artefact in the transverse imaging plane; a diffuse hypoechoic (dark) appearance caused by a non-perpendicular transducer (Fig. 5.7). This should not be mistaken for diffuse pathology. Irregular fibre alignment and fibrous tissue are not subject to this artefact, and remain echoic relative to normal tendon/ligament when the transducer is tilted off-incidence.

Basic machine maintenance

It is essential to care for the ultrasound machine and transducer(s) in order to maximize its longevity. Hair, dust and grit can easily contaminate the internal workings through the fan inlet or outlet, and will compromise the machine's ability to cool, and eventually to function. Keeping the machine covered when not in use, using it on a clean table rather than the ground, regularly wiping the machine (with a dry or minimally damp cloth) and hoovering the fan inlet/outlet is important.

Transducers are easily damaged and cannot be repaired. Irreparable damage can occur if the transducer sustains a sharp impact (e.g. being dropped or kicked), is submerged in water, if surgical spirit is left in contact with the rubber footprint or if the rubber footprint is physically damaged.

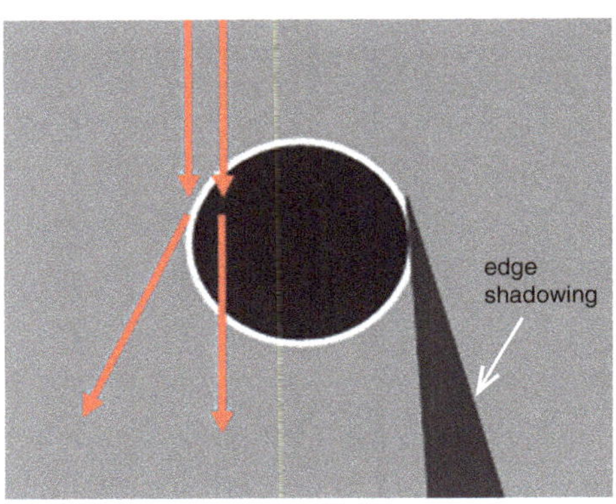

Fig. 5.5. Schematic diagram of edge refraction.

5.2 Radiography

Radiography for the diagnosis and prescribing of prognoses and treatment for working equines is of huge value. Since the first application of conventional film-screen radiography in equine veterinary medicine over 100 years ago, there have been significant technological advances. Digital imaging systems (computed radiography (CR) and more recently direct digital radiograph (DR)) have superseded conventional radiography (film-screen) in some parts of the world

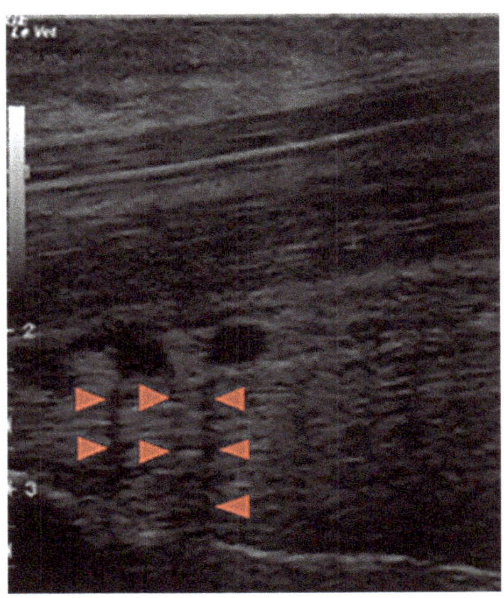

Fig. 5.6. Edge refraction artefacts (arrowheads) within the suspensory ligament, emanating from the margins of two blood vessels in transverse section.

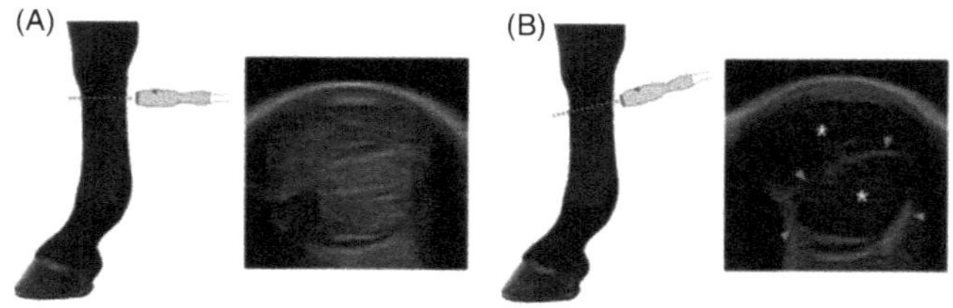

Fig. 5.7. (A) On-incidence ultrasonography, with the transducer perpendicular to the flexor tendons of the metacarpus. (B) Off-incidence ultrasonography. The bodies of the flexor tendons are hypoechoic (*), whilst the border and surrounding fascia remain echoic (arrowheads).

and offer superior image quality and reduced radiation requirements. Though the equipment and methods for processing, viewing and storing images differ, the principles of radiation safety, preparation, positioning, exposure values, centring and collimation are the same for conventional and digital radiography alike. Common indications for radiography include evaluation of the musculoskeletal system (lameness which has been localized to a joint or region), the spine and the head (including teeth and sinuses). Abdominal radiography can be a useful tool for diagnosing large intestinal impaction with sand (sand colic).

Basic principles of image formation

All radiography systems consist of a source (the 'generator') of electromagnetic radiation ('X-ray photons') and a detector ('cassette'). Generators produce a primary beam of radiation over a defined, usually short, period of time, which is directed at the area of interest. The cassette is placed behind the area of interest in the path of the primary beam and detects the X-ray photons. The differential attenuation of X-rays by tissues and materials of different densities and thickness influences the number of X-rays reaching the cassette. Dense tissues or materials have a greater attenuating effect than less dense tissues or materials, and no (or few) X-rays reaching the cassette results in a radiopaque (white or whiter) area of the image, e.g. osseous tissue (bone), metal. Less dense tissues or materials appear radiolucent (black), e.g. fat, air. Tissues of intermediate density, e.g. muscle, appear grey.

Radiation safety

Protection from radiation is extremely important. Codes and rules of practice will vary among countries, and personnel acquiring radiographs must be aware of and observe them. The risk of receiving a radiation dose is through exposure to the primary beam and exposure to scatter. The key principles to follow are:

1. ***No person (or any body part of a person) should ever be in the path of the primary beam.***

- When holding the patient, e.g. a limb, hands must never be within (or near) the area of collimation (primary beam).
- Use a cassette holder. If the cassette must be held by hand, ensure that hands and arms are not within the area of collimation (primary beam), nor behind the cassette, for the primary beam will continue to pass through the cassette. Personal protective equipment (PPE), e.g. lead gloves, will not protect the wearer from radiation in the primary beam.
- Ideally, direct the beam towards a solid wall behind the patient. If that is not possible, assume that the primary beam will continue for ~25 m and ensure no person is near the path, or in the vicinity, of the primary beam.

2. ***Only essential personnel should be involved.***

- People under 18 or who are pregnant should never be involved.

3. ***Personnel should be protected from scatter.***

- All involved personnel should be provided with PPE (lead gown, lead thyroid protector).
- If holding a limb in position, lead gloves should be worn.

- Scatter emanates from the generator and the patient; distance from these areas should be maximized as much as possible and a generator stand should be used.
- Involved personnel would ideally be monitored with a dosimeter system, if available, and a record of involvement kept.

4. *Minimize the amount of radiation produced.*

- Ensure the exposure factors are correct for the region and patient size.
- Take care with technique to avoid unnecessary retakes.
- Ensure the patient is adequately restrained.
- Collimate well – avoid large areas of collimation beyond the region of interest and ensure the area of collimation is never larger than the cassette.

Exposure factors

Selecting appropriate exposure factors is fundamental for diagnostic quality images (Fig. 5.8; Table 5.1). The opacity (whiteness versus blackness, resulting from the amount of X-ray photons reaching the cassette) is governed by the milliampere (mA; number of X-ray photons produced) and exposure duration in seconds (s). Some generators have separate mA and s controls, however many have a combined mAs control. Image contrast is governed by the kilovoltage (kV), which determines the energy of, and therefore the penetrative properties of, the X-ray photons.

Developing an exposure chart is recommended. To do this, record the exposures (kV and mAs) used to acquire diagnostic quality images, according to region, view and size of horse. This provides a guide for exposure setting selection and will improve efficiency. It is vital to use a consistent film-focal distance (FFD), which is the distance between the generator and the cassette. Because of photon attenuation with increasing distance, inconsistent FFD will have a substantial impact on exposure. An FFD of 90 cm is recommended, but different systems can be optimized for ranges of 60–100 cm.

Patient preparation

The horse should be restrained as necessary to ensure the patient is still. This is important for personnel safety, equipment safety and for acquisition of diagnostic quality images. Light chemical sedation is beneficial for many patients, but this will be dictated by patient temperament and the radiographs being acquired.

The region being radiographed should be free of tack or other equipment, and gross contamination, e.g. dirt, should be removed.

Technique

The specific projections required will depend upon the region being radiographed and the suspected pathology. A minimum of two orthogonal views must be acquired, e.g. a lateromedial and a dorsopalmar view of a front fetlock. The basic principles are as follows:

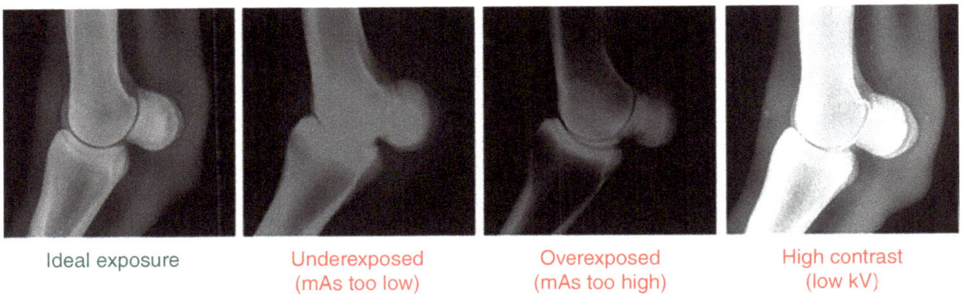

Fig. 5.8. Four lateromedial radiographs of the metacarpophalangeal joint (fetlock) of a horse, acquired using different exposure factors.

Table 5.1. The effect of too high and too low milliamperes/seconds (mAs) and kilovoltage (kV) exposure factors upon x-ray images.

	mAs (opacity)	kV (contrast)
Too high	Overexposure Black 'burnt out' image Soft tissue opacity reduced or lost	Low contrast Lower critical effect on image quality due to high exposure latitude
Too low	Underexposure White image Poor osseous detail (quantum mottle artefact in DR systems)	High contrast Poor bone penetration (bone appears excessively white and of poor detail)

1. ***Patient position.***
Where comfort allows, ensure that the horse is standing squarely and weight-bearing evenly. In most instances the region being radiographed should be in a neutral position, e.g. a vertical limb.

2. ***Generator position.***
Switch on the collimation light, which will indicate the extent of the primary beam (denoted by the area of light) and the centre point (denoted by the intersection of a horizontal and vertical line, or a central laser point). Centre over the mid-point of the area of interest. Collimate by adjusting the area of light, so that the area of interest is included, but no more. The light must never exceed the area of the cassette. Check the FFD.

3. ***Cassette position.***
Place the cassette directly behind the area being radiographed. The plate should be perpendicular to the primary beam, and directly in its path.

4. ***Acquisition.***
When the generator and cassette are correctly positioned, the patient is still, and the operator has ensured that radiation safety protocols are being adhered to by all involved personnel, the acquisition can be made.

5. ***Processing.***
This will depend upon the system being used. With DR systems, processing is automated and almost instantaneous. The image will appear on the viewing screen. With CR systems, the cassette is inserted into an automated processor, and again the image will appear on the viewing screen.

With conventional radiography, X-ray film must be processed manually in a darkened room. The chemical solutions should be prepared at the appropriate dilution. First, the film is placed in the developer solution for approximately five minutes (this is temperature dependent, reduce time in high temperatures). Then the film is agitated several times to ensure there are no air bubbles. The film is washed well in water, then placed in a fixing solution. Washing in water is performed again, followed by air drying.

Basic equipment maintenance

The longevity and performance of the radiography system can be maximized with appropriate care. The major risks are physical damage and internal contamination with hair, dust and grit.

- Appropriate patient restraint, and careful use of the equipment, including cassettes, generator, wires and viewer (for CR and DR systems), will reduce the risk of equipment sustaining impacts from accidental drops, kicks or being stood upon.
- Keep the equipment covered when not in use, and wherever possible use in a clean, dust-free environment. Place equipment on clean tables rather than on the ground.
- Wipe equipment regularly using a dry or minimally damp cloth and hoover the fan inlets/outlets to remove hair and dust.
- Grit and dust accumulation on the cassette can cause artefacts on the image. Regularly opening and cleaning them with an appropriate cleaning solution and a lint-free wipe is recommended – refer to the equipment manual wherever possible.

6

Veterinary Medicines

Abstract

This chapter lists veterinary medicines available to an equine practitioner.

6.1 Introduction

The various veterinary medicines will be discussed in the relevant chapters. However, I will generalize in this chapter on anti-infective drugs and anti-inflammatory drugs, both steroidal and non-steroidal. I will end the chapter with a list of medicines I consider should be carried by the ambulatory equine veterinarian.

6.2 Antibiotics

It is vital that equine veterinarians minimize antimicrobial resistance (AMR) in equine practice, as it is already becoming a problem (Isgren *et al.*, 2022). We must be aware of the direct spread of pathogens, e.g. the zoonotic spread of MRSA and the spread of resistance genes. These genes can be passed into different species of bacteria, meaning bacteria once sensitive to a specific antimicrobial become resistant. This adds to the pool of antimicrobial-resistant bacteria in animals, people and the environment.

Antimicrobial-resistant infections in horses are important.

- They will delay effective treatment.
- They will make the treatment ineffective.
- They will make adverse drug effects more common due to multiple treatments.
- They will worsen the prognosis.
- They will increase the cost of treatment.
- They will adversely affect welfare.

Human health can be jeopardized by:

- transmission of contagious primary pathogens;
- transmission of opportunistic pathogens;
- the contamination of environment bacterial carrying AMR-encoded genes.

A small study carried out at an equine congress in Birmingham (UK) showed that equine vets had a higher prevalence of carrying AMR genes in the nasal secretions than non-vets.

Equine vets can help to slow the course of disease which would benefit the use of antimicrobials by:

- Minimizing the transmission of the disease.
    - Quarantining horses on arrival for a minimum of 2 weeks.
    - Good hygiene practices to avoid as much contact as possible.
    - Monitoring temperatures to help early detection of disease.

DOI: 10.1079/9781800624283.0006

  - Isolation planning, so that if signs are detected a plan can be implemented immediately.
  - Vaccination against relevant diseases.
- Addressing predisposing factors for bacterial infection.
  - Making sure foals receive an adequate intake of colostrum.
  - Arranging early vaccination of foals.
  - Making an early diagnosis of chronic conditions in older horses.
  - Arranging earlier treatment of skin disease to prevent secondary infection.
- Decreasing iatrogenic complications by good clinical hygiene.
  - Maintaining good surgical asepsis.
  - Maintaining good catheter management.
  - Hand washing.
  - Good cleansing of equipment.

If antimicrobial usage can be reduced, then the danger of AMR will be minimized. This will be aided by appropriate drug selection, together with using optimal doses and durations of treatment. Naturally a high standard of care should be exercised with the handling of medicines. It is not all bad news. Workers in the UK (Wilson *et al.*, 2023) report, in a recent survey compared to a previous similar study in 2009, that overall antimicrobial usage appeared to be declining in clinical scenarios and that a greater proportion of practices now have stewardship policies. However, the use of high-priority antimicrobials is still relatively common in equine practice in the UK.

There are two types of antibiotics: those that actually kill bacteria are termed bactericidal antibiotics and those that limit the replication of bacteria are termed bacteriostatic antibiotics.

Table 6.1. Classification of antibiotics used in the equine, with respect to their bacterial regulating ability.

Bactericidal	Bacteriostatic
Penicillins	Tetracyclines
Aminoglycosides	Macrolides
Trimethoprim-sulfadoxine (TMS)	Chloramphenicol
Cephalosporins	Rifampicin[a]
Fluoroquinolones	
Metronidazole Rifampicin[a]	

[a]Rifampicin may be either bacteriostatic or bactericidal, depending on the bacterial species involved.

The various families of antibiotics are classified in Table 6.1.

It is important to choose a bactericidal antibiotic in both the foal and the horse with a depressed immune system. Therefore, tetracyclines should not be used in foals or immunodepressed animals. However, we have a dilemma with the macrolides; these drugs are our main treatment for two serious diseases of foals – *Rhodococcus equi* and *Lawsonia intracellularis.* The best treatment for the former is a combination of erythromycin (a macrolide) and rifampicin. Erythromycin should be given per os at the rate of 25 mg/kg four times daily, and rifampicin at the rate of 10 mg/kg twice daily. If resistance to rifampicin is encountered, then neomycin (an aminoglycoside) may be given per os using a formulation normally licensed for pigs. Neomycin can also be given by i/m injection; however, it is irritant and clinicians are advised to avoid this route. One might consider gentamicin would be useful, but it causes severe nephrotoxicity in the foal.

There are several important differences between foals and adult horses which must be considered when selecting antimicrobial drugs for use in foals (Table 6.2). Neonatal foals have a proportionally greater body water content than adult horses, 71–83% compared to 60–70% in adult horses (Andrews *et al.*, 1997; Feilding *et al.*, 2011). Fluid dynamics differ further between mature horses and foals as a result of foals having a relatively smaller intracellular fluid compartment and larger extracellular fluid compartment, as well as higher blood and plasma volumes. This greater body of water means higher dosages of hydrophilic drugs such as aminoglycosides are necessary in foals, whereas the dosages of lipophilic drugs are less affected (Corley and Hollis, 2009).

Sepsis is the most common cause of foal death during the first 7 days of life. Antimicrobial therapy is central to the treatment of sepsis, along with intravenous fluid therapy and other supportive care. When initially selecting antimicrobials for the treatment of sepsis, it is important to select broad spectrum, intravenously administered bactericidal drugs.

Antimicrobial stewardship involves the judicious use of antimicrobials balanced against the requirement to treat the presenting clinical condition (Raidal, 2019). The same principles apply to human medicine, as well as veterinary medicine, including equine medicine. This

Table 6.2. A list of antimicrobials commonly used in neonatal foals.

Antimicrobial	Dosage (mg/kg unless otherwise stated)	Route of administration	Frequency of administration (h)
Procaine penicillin G	20	IM	12
Sodium penicillin	20,000–44,000	IV	6
Sodium ampicillin	20	IV	6
Piperacillin tazobactam	30*	IV	6
Amoxicillin clavulanate	30	PO	8
Ceftiofur sodium	5–10	IV, IM, SC	12
Cefotaxime	40	IV	6
Ceftriaxone	25	IV	12
Amikacin	25	IV	24
Gentamicin	12	IV	36
Oxytetracycline	5–10	IV	12
Doxycycline	10	PO	12
Marbofloxacin	2	IV	24
Marbofloxacin	4	PO	24
Clarithromycin	7.5	PO	12
Rifampin	5	PO	12
Rifampin	10	PO	24
Trimethoprim sulfadiaz ne	5/25	PO	12
Metronidazole	10	IV, PO	12

*Dosage extrapolated from other species

requires a multifactorial approach combining reduction of resistant reservoirs, improved diagnostic techniques for bacterial infection, improved infection control measures, improved preventative health measures and greater insight into the aetiology of infections to reduce dependence on antimicrobials and limit the emergence of antimicrobial resistance.

It is important to remember that results of bacteriological culture and susceptibility testing may differ between geographic regions. Temporal trends in susceptibility and resistance also occur. Continuous local monitoring of culture and susceptibility results is therefore of utmost importance to ensure that empirical selection of drugs for treatment is based on contemporaneous and locally applicable susceptibility results. Bacteriological culture and susceptibility testing in individual cases therefore might not only benefit the individual patient, but also provides the basis for empirical drug selection in future cases.

Lawsonia intracellularis does not seem to respond to any antibiotics other than the macrolides. It is possible that macrolides are bactericidal at higher doses. What is important to remember is that macrolides should never be given intramuscularly in the horse as this causes a very severe local reaction. Erythromycin should be given per os at the rate of 25 mg/kg three times daily, in combination with rifampicin per os at the rate of 10 mg/kg twice daily. This should be carried on for 4 weeks.

Table 6.3. Classification of antibiotics used in the equine, with respect to time and concentration.

Time-dependent	Concentration-dependent
Penicillins	Aminoglycosides
Cephalosporins	Tetracyclines
Fluoroquinolones	Metronidazole
	Trimethoprim-sulfadoxine (TMS)
	Macrolides (not relevant in the adult horse)
	Chloramphenicol[a]
	Rifampicin

[a]Chloramphenicol is not licensed in the horse and is rapidly metabolized. It should therefore be used only for localized ophthalmic treatment.

Antibiotics can also be classified by their mode of action on bacteria: either time-dependent or concentration-dependent (see Table 6.3).

It is important that time-dependent antibiotics are given at the correct frequency interval. Obviously, in a field situation every 24 h is the most convenient for the injectables. Penicillin-Na G Crystapen causes problems, as ideally it should be given every 6 h.

The peak concentration is very important for the concentration-dependent antibiotics. There is also a post-antibiotic effect, so that these antibiotics need only be given once daily. A good example is gentamicin, an aminoglycoside, which is safer from a nephrotoxic point of view if it is given at 6.6 mg/kg once daily rather than as a smaller dose more often. Trimethoprim-sulfadoxine (TMS) is usually given orally, and it is important that owners are instructed to administer it twice daily.

Before deciding on an antibiotic, it is relevant to consider the factors affecting the route of administration. These are:

- hospitalization;
- temperament of the horse;
- ability of the owner; and
- cost.

Even quiet horses will not tolerate long-term courses of i/m injections; i/v injections are the preferred route in this situation. In a hospital situation i/v catheterization is ideal, but in the field this is hazardous. Jugular abscessation is a nightmare; equally, sarcoid formation has been reported.

Below are presented the antibiotics available for injection in the horse.

Benzathine penicillin G

Products containing this type of penicillin are the so-called 'long-acting penicillins'. These products achieve such low plasma concentrations in the horse that they cannot be recommended. They must not be injected i/v and they cause severe reactions following i/m injection. They are best avoided.

Ceftiofur sodium

This cephalosporin antibiotic can be given either i/v or i/m. It has excellent tissue penetration and so has many uses.

Gentamicin

Gentamicin can be given either i/v or i/m. As stated above, it can be nephrotoxic (particularly in foals), so it is best given only once daily.

Oxytetracycline

Oxytetracycline can only be given i/v, and officially lasts for only 12 h. Nonetheless, by common usage it is usually given every 24 h. This drug was wrongly blamed for many post-operative colic deaths; it appeared to be excreted in high doses in the bile, and this was interpreted as meaning that by killing normal, beneficial bacteria it allowed *Salmonella* organisms resident in the bile ducts to multiply and lead to the death of the horse. Its use was then very much reduced. Nevertheless, it is now not thought to be nearly as dangerous. It is useful in young horses for respiratory infections.

As a mycoplasma may well be involved in these cases it is obviously the antibiotic of choice.

Penicillin-Na G Crystapen

This can be given either i/v or i/m. As stated above, it needs to be repeated ideally at 6 h intervals. Certainly, it cannot be expected to last 24 h.

Procaine penicillin G

This can *only* be given i/m. It is often given in combination with streptomycin (an aminoglycoside). However, streptomycin has actually been shown not to be active in the horse. So, although these products are licensed in the horse, their use is questionable. There are very few experienced equine practitioners who have not seen a severe reaction to procaine penicillin G. Therefore, although it may be used in the horse, the fewer times you use it the less likely you are to provoke a reaction.

Trimethoprim-sulfadoxine (TMS)

The i/v and oral routes are both suitable for TMS. Officially it lasts for only 12 h, but common usage for the injectable formulation is once daily. It is very irritant, so should not be given by the intramuscular route. There is a well-documented danger with alpha-2 drugs, so it should not be administered with any of that type of sedative. It is also reportedly ineffective in the presence of pus.

Cost may be an issue: it would not be sensible to quote exact prices, but to guide practitioners I will show the rough relative costs for daily injections for a horse (see Table 6.4).

There are three penicillin-type antibiotics that are used extensively in species other than equines. The first, ampicillin, has been the cause of many anaphylactic episodes in horses and so its use should be restricted to irrigation of chest infections. The other two, amoxicillin and clavulinic acid, administered either separately or in combination, have no place in equine medicine as they must be injected i/m, which causes severe local reactions. The powder form of amoxicillin, for reconstitution with water for i/v use, is no longer available.

Metronidazole is a useful antibiotic in the horse given per os for non-aerophilic bacteria. Sadly, the paste formulation is no longer available so small tablets have to be crushed up in the feed. The dose is 20 mg/kg three times daily. This works out at 50 × 200 mg tablets three times daily for a 500 kg horse.

Eye infections need special consideration in the horse. Chloramphenicol is widely used, but its use in the horse, which is classed as a food-producing animal, is controversial. Gentamicin is the drug of choice. Amikacin, which is difficult to obtain, is useful for subconjunctival injections. It is also used in joints concurrently with steroids, although this use is controversial as it may be irritant It is thought by some authors to be unnecessary if full aseptic procedures in joint surgery are adhered to. Treatment for the very serious condition of melting corneal ulceration is difficult, but current thinking is to use tobramycin (an aminoglycoside) and EDTA (ethylenediaminetetraacetic acid) plasma.

Skin infections in the horse, as in other species, require prolonged treatment, e.g. 21 days.

Table 6.4. Relative costs of injectable antibiotics used commonly in equines.

Antibiotic	Cost, using X as baseline
Procaine penicillin G	X
Oxytetracycline	X
Trimethoprim-sulfadoxine (TMS)	2X
Penicillin/gentamicin	5X
Ceftiofur	8X

Oral treatment is restricted to TMS twice daily. If there is doubt as to the bactericidal effect the normal dose rate may be doubled. If another antibiotic is required enrofloxacin (a fluoroquinolone) can be used, although there is no licensed preparation yet available for the horse. Nevertheless, there is available a 10% oral solution of enrofloxacin licensed for chickens; the daily dose for the horse is 1 ml/kg. There have been recent pharmokinetic studies performed indicating that uptake may not be sufficient. However, it is still widely used and is relatively expensive.

Sadly, antibiotic therapy is not always successful, for many reasons. The owner should be helped to avoid poor compliance. The clinician can prevent problems by making the correct diagnosis and choosing the correct antibiotic. The dosage, route and frequency should be optimal. Obviously, known drug interactions should be avoided. Unfortunately, antibiotics do not dissolve foreign bodies! Naturally, the clinician cannot be blamed for the depressed immune system of the patient or the antibiotic resistance of the bacteria.

6.3 Antifungal Agents

These can be divided into systemic agents given either by i/v injection or orally. There are also topical agents.

Amphotericin

Amphotericin is the only injectable antifungal agent for equines. It is active against yeasts, histoplasmosis and blastomycosis. The drug is supplied in powder form to be reconstituted with water or 5% dextrose saline – in a very dilute solution in order to avoid cardiac toxicity. It must always be kept in the dark as it is extremely light sensitive. It is prudent initially to give a test dose of 0.2 mg/kg; this can then be increased slowly over several days to 1.0 mg/kg. Renal function should be monitored. Adverse reactions should be treated with corticosteroids. If kidney damage is suspected, then the drug may be given every other day.

Griseofulvin

The commonly used griseofulvin is a very effective treatment for *Trichophyton* spp. These infections are normally caught from cattle. Equine animals should be given 5 g/50 kg of 7.5% powder in their feed daily for 7 days. However, griseofulvin is not effective against *Microsporum equi* (equine ringworm). Care should be taken by pregnant women when handling griseofulvin, as it is teratogenic. It should be remembered that ringworm, particularly *Trichophyton* spp., is a zoonosis. Vigorous scrubbing and strong disinfectants that damage the skin should be avoided. Normal washing with soap is preferable. Women and children are particularly susceptible.

Miconazole

Miconazole is a good topical treatment for *M. equi*. It should be used as a shampoo twice weekly, but it is expensive.

Natamycin

Natamycin is also a good topical treatment for *M. equi*, and it too is expensive. It is supplied in powder form for re-suspension. The suspension is then sponged or sprayed on to the affected area every 4–5 days.

Virkon S

The last on this list is a broad-spectrum virucidal disinfectant. It is a very effective disinfectant and also can be used to treat *M. equi*. It should be made up as a 1% solution, i.e. one 50 g sachet/5 1 water. This solution can be used either as a spray or sponged on to affected areas every 48 h. This use is not licensed in the UK but is widely used off-licence. It is relatively inexpensive.

6.4 Antiprotozoal Agents

I will divide these into two groups. The first group is used to treat blood-borne parasites, mainly in the tropics. The second group is used to treat other protozoal conditions.

The drugs used to treat blood-borne parasites have been developed to treat cattle. They are extremely irritant when used in horses. Clinicians are advised to use deep i/m injections. Some clinicians, nevertheless, use the i/v route. My personal experience with this route is favourable. However, others have reported anaphylactic reactions and death. Local conditions should be investigated so that an informed opinion can be given on the risk to the animal and the likelihood of resistance of the protozoan to be treated.

Group 1

Diminazene aceturate

The most hazardous of this group of drugs, it is extremely effective against *Babesia equi* and *Babesia caballi*. However, as less dangerous drugs are available to treat these protozoans, they should be considered. On the other hand, it is the most effective drug to treat trypanosomiasis used by the author. This includes *Trypanosoma brucei* (surra), *Trypanosoma vivax* (acute 'fly'), *Trypanosoma congolense* (chronic 'fly'), *Trypanosoma evansi* (camel 'fly') and *Trypanosoma equiperdum* (dourine). The first three of these trypanosomes are spread only by tsetse fly. Therefore, you will only see them in a tsetse area. In areas with a high density of tsetse fly only game animals can survive. Workers in The Gambia have reported that they found diminazene aceturate was as good as isometamidine for treating *T. vivax* but not as useful for treating *T. congolense* or *T. brucei* (personal communication). Cattle can be kept for short periods under prophylactic treatment with trypanocidal drugs used prophylactically. Donkeys and mules can be kept in the same manner for short periods. Nonetheless, it is too dangerous to treat horses prophylactically and therefore such areas should be avoided by horses. If trypanosomiasis is suspected in the equine a diagnosis should be made rapidly from a blood smear. Treatment should only be carried out if the diagnosis is certain. *Trypanosoma evansi* is spread by biting flies outside of tsetse areas. Donkeys, and to some extent mules, appear to develop a pre-munity and do not readily succumb to the infection. However, the organism is very serious in horses.

Once again, a rapid diagnosis should be made on blood smears, and treatment should then be carried out. *Trypanosoma equiperdum* is a venereal disease of horses, mules and donkeys. The trypanosomes can be found with care in the pus coming from the vulva and the urethral opening in males.

Diminazene aceturate can be used to cure all these infections. It is supplied in 1.05 g sachets for reconstitution in 12.5 ml water to make a 12.5% solution. This is the normal dose for an adult cow. Often this is made up in a non-sterile manner, which can cause abscesses in cattle. It will cause massive problems if given in such a manner to horses. A protocol for treatment of a 500 kg horse is to dissolve the 1.05 g sachet in 50 ml warm, sterile water in the most aseptic manner possible. This is then injected i/v at blood temperature, as slowly as possible, preferably though a catheter unless the horse is so ill that it is unlikely to move.

Imidocarb

This would be the drug of choice for treating *B. equi* and *B. caballi*. These protozoans are spread by ticks. Imidocarb is supplied in a 12% solution in a 100 ml multidose vial. The risk of abscessation is much less than with diminazene. A dose of 1.2 mg/kg should be given by deep i/m injection on 2 separate days (5 ml for a 500 kg horse). Certain authors suggest a higher dose – 2 mg/kg on 2 separate days. This drug should be used only for treatment.

Isometamidium

Formerly a useful drug in cattle to treat *T. brucei, T. congolense* and *T. vivax*, widespread resistance has since been encountered in cattle and so I would not advise its use in the horse.

Melarsomine

Normally, this medicine is used intravenously in dogs to treat heartworm. However, it has been used in The Gambia to treat trypanosomiasis, but it is not as useful as diminazene or isometamidine (personal communication).

Quinapyramine

Also formerly used in cattle as either the sulfate or chloride preparation, there is now widespread resistance in infections of *T. brucei, T. congolense* and *T. vivax*. I do not advise its use for these infections in the horse, but it has been used to treat *T. equiperdum*. I would not advise its use because it favours the formation of a carrier state. It also causes severe abscessation when given i/m. It is a suspension and on no account should it be given i/v.

Suramin

Suramin can be used to treat *T. evansi* and *T. equiperdum*. However, resistance is widespread and therefore I cannot advise its use.

Group 2

Metronidazole

Metronidazole can be used to treat protozoal diseases, but its principal use in horses is to treat anaerobic bacteria. These may be in the alimentary system, wounds or pedal infections. The best method of administration is by mouth, at the rate of 15 mg/kg every 8 h. The drug is supplied in 500 mg tablets. It may cause inappetence, which is a difficult side effect to deal with as often the owners are unable to get sufficient medicine into the horse. Metronidazole is also supplied as a 20 mg/kg solution in 50 ml sachets. This solution is best used topically on wounds or hoof infections. Nevertheless, some workers have used it i/v at 20 mg/kg every 24 h for 3–5 days to treat clostridial enteritis and peritonitis. The drug per se can cause diarrhoea, so this side effect is very worrying in horses with existing enteric problems. I would advise against i/v use.

Nitazoxanide

Nitazoxanide can also be used to treat EPM and is almost as effective as ponazuril. However, it may cause side effects and so should be given at half the normal dose rate, i.e. 25 mg/kg daily by mouth for 5 days. If all is well, a dose of 50 mg/kg should be given for a further 23 days.

Ponazuril

Ponazuril is the drug of choice for EPM, having a cure rate of 70%. It should be given by mouth at

5 mg/kg every day for 28 days. It is now available in paste form.

Pyrimethamine

Pyrimethamine can be used to treat toxoplasmosis and equine protozoal myeloencephalitis (EPM). There is a synergism between pyrimethamine and potentiated sulfonamides, and so the two drugs are often given together. Pyrimethamine should be given by mouth at 0.1–0.2 mg/kg daily. Sulfonamides should be given at the normal dose rate of 15 mg/kg. This regime may be given for several months until a cure is effected.

6.5 Anthelmintics

Rather than give a long list of the anthelmintics available, I will describe the helminths that cause problems and then suggest methods of control. This will include the strategic use of anthelmintics, bearing in mind the widespread resistance in other herbivores.

Lungworm (*Dictyocaulus arnfieldi*)

Dictyocaulus lives in donkeys without causing symptoms. Nevertheless, the donkey can act as a carrier and infect mules and horses. The presence of this worm will cause coughing in these species. It is readily controlled by ivermectin paste given by mouth at 0.2 mg/kg. It is not controlled by moxidectin paste or any other family of anthelmintics. Some practitioners give ivermectin by i/v injection or in the cattle pour-on formulation. Both these methods of administration are not advised. No resistance to ivermectin has been recorded in lungworm.

Large bowel worms (*Strongylus vulgaris, Strongylus edentatus* and *Strongylus equinus*)

These species are still a problem in many parts of the world, but very rare nowadays in the UK. Forty years ago, damage from the migration of third-stage larvae of these worms through the mesenteric arteries accounted for 95% of colics. Infestation by these large strongyles is very serious, with considerable bowel damage and blood loss often resulting in severe anaemia. However, modern anthelmintics of all classes seem to be very effective in their elimination, and there appears to be little problem with resistant strains. We should, nevertheless, not be complacent: they should be treated and eliminated if they are found to be present. On the other hand, we must not overuse anthelmintics and bring about resistance. These large bowel worms will excrete their eggs into the gut and will be readily seen on a faecal egg count (FEC). However, definitive testing requires coprocultures and examination of third-stage larvae, although polymerase chain reaction and a serum enzyme-linked immunosorbent assay have been developed for research purposes.

Foal worm (*Strongyloides westeri*)

Strongyloides is now, in the author's experience, rarely seen in the UK, but it can cause diarrhoea in foals that will be persistent unless the worm burden is eliminated. A report from Ireland indicates its presence on a stud farm (Kirtland *et al.*, 2023). This indicates an increased incidence between 2014 and 2019, which was then controlled by a peripartum ivermectin treatment of the dams. This parasite is sensitive to all classes of modern anthelmintics and no resistance has been recorded.

Horse ascarid (*Parascaris equorum*)

The horse ascarid worm can occur in both foals and adults. However, horses generally acquire immunity in the first 12 to 18 months, so this is only an issue in foals and yearlings. There are reports of it becoming resistant to certain wormers, but there are no reports of resistance to pyrantel wormer at normal doses so this must be the drug of choice. Piperazine is also effective and no resistance has been reported. A dose rate of 250 mg/kg should be given by nasogastric tube. It is very unlikely that a group of these worms will obstruct the small intestine (SI) of the young foal, although it is possible. Diagnosis may be made with ultrasonography. The adults live in the SI. The larvae migrate through the lungs and are coughed up and so return to the SI, taking approximately 17 days. A 5-day regimen of fenbendazole given at a dose of 10 mg/kg BWT can be used for treating not only adult worms in the SI, but also migrating larvae in the lungs.

Horse pin worm (*Oxyuris equi*)

Oxyuris is seen in the foal but very rarely in the adult. However, the adult female is voided from the rectum and lays its eggs around the anus, causing acute irritation to the horse – the signs of sweet itch, where only the tail is affected. Spread is mainly from foal to foal. Foals will show a loss in condition. There is thought to be an immunity developed, as the adult horse may have the parasite, but large numbers are not seen (see Fig. 6.1). It is important to remove the eggs from the environment by good hygiene. This will help to combat the widespread resistance of this worm to anthelmintics.

Small bowel worms (cyathostomes)

These worms, thanks to their ability to encyst in the mucosa of the large bowel, can not only cause the normal signs of intestinal parasitism but also more importantly cause very severe disease. This occurs when vast numbers of encysted larvae suddenly emerge into the lumen of the large bowel, causing severe damage to the mucosa. Death is a likely result. When the worms have become encysted their presence will not be detected on FEC. Their elimination is difficult. Moxidectin or a double-dose, 5-day course of fenbendazole are the anthelmintics of choice. Nevertheless, prevention of large numbers becoming encysted in the first instance is the ideal control method. Veterinarians should be aware that there is widespread resistance reported to the benzimidazole group of anthelmintics given at standard dosage; this group includes thiabendazole, mebendazole, fenbendazole and oxibendazole.

Equine tapeworm (*Anoplocephala perfoliata*)

There now is a very effective blood test for the diagnosis of this tapeworm, based on antibody detection. This is greatly superior to the rather hit-and-miss faecal examination. The blood test not only shows the presence of tapeworms but also the approximate numbers, and therefore treatment can be much better controlled. If large numbers are present then it is advisable to use a low dose of pyrantel, i.e. 19 mg/kg (this the normal dose of pyrantel that will control large and small strongyles but not fully control tapeworms,

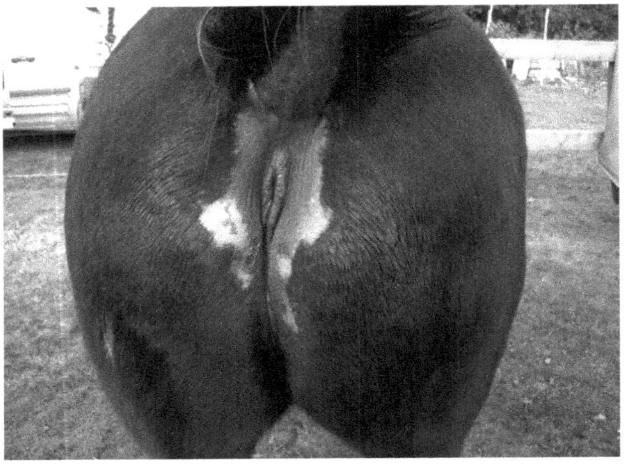

Fig. 6.1. Horse with *Oxyuris* infection (not sweet itch).

where the so-called double dose of 38 mg/kg is required). The low dose of pyrantel will decimate the numbers of tapeworms, hopefully without causing colic. Three weeks later a standard dose of praziquantel, i.e. 1 mg/kg can be given to totally eliminate the remainder of the tapeworms.

The dogma 40 years ago was that tapeworms did not cause problems in the horse: *this is not the case*. It has been shown that the presence of tapeworms is a definite risk factor when considering the colic case. They can cause ileocaecal disease, impaction, intussusception and spasmodic colic. So, the take-home message is that either you treat your horse once a year for tapeworms, or 'best practice' would be to blood test the horse and tailor the treatment of tapeworms according to the result.

Bot fly (*Gastrophilus equinus*)

Bot flies are mainly active in the autumn in the northern hemisphere. The eggs on the coat may be readily seen, and are very sensitive to ivermectins and moxidectins. However, they cannot all be eliminated. Standard practice seems to be to use a moxidectin in the late autumn to eliminate the latent infection of third-stage cyathostome larvae. This is very laudable, but it is often given before there has been a hard frost; it must be remembered that frost kills only the adult flies. The eggs are still viable and will certainly turn into larvae if they are in the warmth of the inside of a horse. The pathogenicity of the bot has always been a cause for debate, but now that we frequently inspect the equine stomach on a regular basis to check for ulcers, we are certainly seeing large numbers of bots. I really cannot believe that in those numbers they are entirely benign.

Liver fluke (*Fasciola hepatica*)

Normally a parasite of ruminants, this species is only rarely seen in the horse. It requires the presence of a water snail as the secondary host. Diagnosis is not easy and relies on raised liver enzymes in a serum sample and then very careful flotation of faeces to visualize the eggs. The presence of one egg is significant. Treatment is by mouth with triclabendazole at 12 mg/kg.

Use of anthelmintics

The answer in the effective use of anthelmintics must be strategic target dosing with faecal collection. This is beneficial for all parties concerned. It is good for the owner of the horse because it is cheaper to do an FEC than to worm the horse regardless of which product is used. Obviously, death of the horse from cyathostomiasis is a financial disaster. Severe weight loss and poor performance is almost as bad. It is good for the manufacturers of anthelmintics as they, in fact, will record higher sales as the horse-owning public are being made much more aware of the dangers of bowel worms. I am sure also that the ethical medicine companies realize the probable long-term disaster of total resistance. These companies do not want short-term high sales of blanket worming only to be faced with a total lack of sales when their products no longer work.

It should be stressed that all holdings are different, and each horse owner/yard owner needs to be counselled carefully and individually. It is ideal to carry out regular FECs on smallholdings where there is no movement of horses coming into the yard; all the horses can be tested at the same time. Those animals with an FEC of <200 eggs/g can be treated. The danger in busy yards with lots of comings and goings of horses is that if not all the horses are tested at the same time, then a high-shedding individual will be missed.

It should be stressed that horses, mules and donkeys should not be treated with anthelmintics prepared for other species without considerable thought. The dosage must be correct. The application of a pour-on is inappropriate. The use of injectable preparations should be extremely carefully considered. Certain anthelmintics intended for other species, e.g. levamisole, are not suitable for equines.

Another totally different class of anthelmintics should be mentioned – the organophosphorus group, examples being haloxon and metriphonate. I consider their use should be avoided. They are an environmental hazard to fish, birds and wildlife, and they have a limited action on parasites. Their therapeutic index is small. They should not be used in pregnant mares or foals. Horses should not be exercised for 48 h following treatment.

In conclusion, it is very important that equine practitioners get the message of strategic targeted dosing across to their clients, otherwise multiple resistances will become widespread.

6.6 Ectoparasiticides

Ivermectins and moxidectin, which are covered under anthelmintics, do have an ectoparasitic action when given by injection. However, this is off-licence and not recommended. Generally, they do not appear to have any ectoparasitic action when given by mouth. The exception to this is injectable doramectin, which is well tolerated by horses when injected i/m at 1 mg/3.3 kg. It is supplied in a 1% solution, so a 500 kg horse requires 15 ml. This will also kill helminths, mange mites and bots. Equines are affected by a large number of ectoparasites, many of which are opportunists from other species. Nevertheless, the main parasitic groups involved can be grouped into mites and ticks, lice, midges, *Culicoides* spp. and flies.

Benzyl benzoate

An acaricide and also a lotion, this compound is very effective against mange mites if applied liberally daily to all the affected areas. If *Chorioptes equi* is involved, the areas must include all four legs, up to and including the knees and hocks. Benzyl benzoate does to some extent control the irritation of midges causing sweet itch; it performs this function by preventing the midge from getting near to the skin. It therefore needs to be applied daily to all areas likely to be infested.

Coumaphos

A so-called louse powder, this preparation is not very effective. It needs to be applied every 5 days to increase its effectiveness but, to avoid toxicity, it should not be applied more frequently than every 14 days. It has no effect on mange mites.

Cypermethrin

Marketed to control nuisance flies, this should be applied every 14 days. It will control midge irritation if applied to affected areas daily, and will also control *Chorioptes equi* if applied daily to all four legs to above the knees and the hocks. It also controls lice.

Diethyltoluidine

An extremely effective midge repellent, but sadly this is washed off by rain, and even in dry conditions is rarely effective for more than 6 h.

Fipronil

This ectoparasiticide is not licensed in the horse, but it is extremely effective against mange mites when the spray is applied to all the affected areas every 14 days. However, it is very expensive.

Piperonyl butoxide

This can be used to control lice if applied every 14 days; however, if it is required to control midge irritation it needs to be applied to the affected areas daily.

6.7 Steroidal Anti-inflammatory Drugs

The use of steroidal anti-inflammatory drugs in equines is highly controversial, though there is no doubt that they have their uses. Equally, they can cause laminitis, a disease which should be avoided at all costs. They should never be used in pregnant animals. Also, it is very important that no preparation containing steroids is used in the eye with a corneal ulcer. Steroids are contraindicated in viral infections and they delay wound healing. Antibiotic cover should always be given when they are used if there is any risk of a bacterial infection.

Beclomethasone

This corticosteroid is available in a formulation suitable for administration via an inhaler to maintain therapy in non-infectious airway inflammatory disease.

Betamethasone

Although this potent corticosteroid is supplied in an aqueous suspension, it should only be injected i/m in the horse. The dose is 4–8 mg/100 kg to treat shock and hypersensitivity reactions. It should not be considered for long-term use as it may precipitate Cushing's disease (see Section 20.16).

Dexamethasone

This is the injectable corticosteroid of choice in the horse, and may be injected either i/v or i/m. The dose can be adjusted between 10 mg/100 kg and 50 mg/100 kg for treatment of a wide variety of inflammatory, hypersensitivity and allergic conditions.

Fluticasone propionate

This corticosteroid is more potent than beclomethasone for inhalation use. It is also much more expensive.

Hydrocortisone

There is no preparation specifically prepared for the horse. Nonetheless, it is available for topical use as both a 1% cream and hydrocortisone aceponate in a cutaneous spray. Both of these preparations are useful for allergic and inflammatory skin conditions.

Methylprednisolone

A corticosteroid suitable for long-term use as a single injection. It is recorded as lasting for up to 4 weeks, but its main use in equine practice is for intrasynovial injection.

Prednisolone

This is the oral long-term corticosteroid of choice in the horse for treating allergies and lymphosarcoma. The dose recommended is 1–2 mg/kg daily by mouth. The difficulty is in formulation: 50 mg tablets are available, but 5 mg tablets work out cheaper. It also is available as a topical gel combined with lidocaine.

Triamcinolone

The intra-articular corticosteroid of choice. Care should be used when injecting several joints, owing to the danger of laminitis. It can also be used to treat eosinophilic granuloma by intradermal injection.

6.8 Non-steroidal Anti-inflammatory Drugs (NSAIDs)

These are the most commonly used drugs for control of pain and inflammation in the horse. Dosage rates vary for the mule and the donkey, and these will be mentioned where they differ from those used in the horse. The most common indications are musculoskeletal and gastrointestinal pain as a result of inflammation. Their primary action is via cyclooxygenase (COX) inhibition of the inflammatory pathway. COX inhibition may have some detrimental adverse effects, which are very complex. However, in practical terms they may have detrimental effects, primarily on the gastric mucosa and secondarily on the kidney.

Aspirin

Aspirin is the oldest known NSAID. It is available as a powder for administration by mouth, although this has a bitter taste and is not palatable. It has a very short half-life in the horse, which is said to be only 7 min, and hence there is a large dosage required (100 mg/kg); this large dosage is also required for donkeys and mules. It has been used by some practitioners for the control of pain in donkeys with laminitis. It can be given on alternate days with phenylbutazone (4.4 mg/kg). It is also available in tablet form.

Carprofen

A useful NSAID for musculoskeletal pain. It is available as a solution for i/v use at the rate of 0.7 mg/kg; as it is supplied as a 50 mg/ml solution, this equates to 1 ml/70 kg. This can be followed up by granules in the food at the same dose rate. It is supplied in sachets that are a daily dose for 300 kg body weight. It clears more slowly from the system in the donkey and so is ideal for once-daily dosing. It has a high safety margin. It is a moderately effective analgesic and anti-inflammatory agent.

Eltenac

Eltenac is available only for i/v use. It is particularly useful for tissue swelling, particularly in tendons. It is supplied in a solution of 50 mg/ml with a dosage rate of 0.5 mg/kg, i.e. 1 ml/100 kg. It is no longer available in the UK.

Firocoxib

This drug has a proven clinical efficacy on pain associated with osteoarthritis which is equal to that of phenylbutazone. It is a unique equine COX-2 selective NSAID which retains its physiological action of COX-1. It is supplied in a tablet form which can be administered either with a small amount of tasty food or just with a horse treat.

Flunixin meglumine

This is the drug of choice for gastrointestinal pain and is the most potent NSAID for abdominal pain. It is also very effective for ocular pain. It is supplied in a solution of 50 mg/ml with a dosage rate in the horse of 1.1 mg/kg daily, i.e. 2 ml/100 kg. It should be given i/v; it may be given i/m but it is irritant. It is cleared twice as fast in the donkey and so the same dosage should be given twice daily. It is useful in cases of endotoxaemia and can be given at a dose rate of 0.25 mg/kg every 8 h. It can also be used at this dose rate in donkeys with hyperlipaemia. It is supplied as granules in 10 g sachets containing 250 mg for oral dosing. In inappetent animals it can be given in paste form; every 10 g contains 500 mg of active ingredient.

Flurbiprofen

A very expensive NSAID solely for ocular use in cases of uveitis and keratitis. It inhibits miosis and provides topical anti-inflammatory effects. It is supplied in 10 × 4 single-unit vials.

Ketoprofen

Ketoprofen is available only for i/v use in equines. It is supplied in a 10% solution with a dosage rate of 2.2 mg/kg, i.e. 10 ml for a 450 kg horse daily. It is cleared much more rapidly in donkeys and so twice-daily administration is required. It is only really useful in abdominal pain. Because it is not as potent as flunixin meglumine it is recommended, as it will not mask surgical colic.

Meclofenamic acid

Supplied for oral use in 10 g sachets of granules, with a daily dosage rate of 2.2 mg/kg. It has antipyretic properties as well as anti-inflammatory and analgesic properties.

Meloxicam

A potent NSAID useful in the alleviation of inflammation and pain relief in acute and chronic soft tissue and orthopaedic disorders. It is available for i/v use in a solution containing 20 mg/ml, with a dosage rate of 0.6 mg/kg, i.e. 3 ml/100 kg body weight daily. This can be continued by oral administration of the fluid at the same dose. The oral suspension is supplied with a dosing syringe showing weight calibration.

Phenylbutazone (PBZ)

This is still the most commonly used NSAID for musculoskeletal pain and inflammation in the equine. The initial loading dose of 4.4 mg/kg should be halved in the horse for continuation, but continued at that dosage in donkeys. It is supplied as a solution containing 200 mg/ml, i.e. 1 ml/50 kg. It must be given intravenously as it is extremely irritant. It is also supplied in both powder and paste forms for oral administration. Tablets of 100 mg and 200 mg are also available for dogs. This NSAID can be used for low-dose treatment in small ponies, and in donkeys for long-term pain control. Occasionally, horses will refuse the medicine in their food; in such cases it is useful to put the medicine in the fridge to reduce the smell.

Suxibuzone

This formulation is available in granular form for oral administration. Its actions are very similar to those of PBZ. It is claimed to cause less stomach wall ulceration than PBZ and therefore is particularly useful for long-term medication. The dose is 12.5 mg/kg daily for 2 days in the horse, and then a reduction to 6.25 mg/kg daily. This reduction should not be used in the donkey, as the drug is cleared faster in this species. Dosage works out at two sachets twice daily for a horse for 2 days, and then it should be reduced to one sachet twice daily. It would appear to be as potent as PBZ.

The clinician has a dilemma with the use of most NSAIDs in pregnant and lactating mares, in foals under 6 weeks of age and equines destined for human consumption. Clinical judgement needs to be used for the good of the patient and its welfare.

6.9 Miscellaneous Medicines Affecting the Respiratory and Cardiovascular Systems

Acetylcysteine

This is a mucolytic that may be used orally for treating recurrent airway obstruction (RAO) at 0.2 mg/kg daily. It can be a useful substance to use as an enema for retained meconium in the foal – 4 g acetylcysteine added to 10 g baking soda ($NaHCO_3$) and dissolved in 100 ml water to make a 4% solution. A suitable dose for a foal is 200 ml instilled per rectum.

Adrenaline

This drug increases systolic blood pressure and can be used for cardiac resuscitation, at 0.2 mg/50 kg. It can also be used on wounds to lessen haemorrhage.

Atropine sulfate

Classified as a parasympatholytic drug, it can be used as a bronchodilator. It should be injected i/v at 1 mg/30 kg as a single, one-off injection in severe cases of 'heaves'. Ileus may be a side effect if further injections are given. Atropine can be given at 20% of this dosage to treat organophosphorus poisoning. It can be used as a mydriatic for a full examination of the inner eye or for treatment of recurrent uveitis.

Bromhexine

This is a mucolytic and can be used to remove excess mucus in respiratory conditions. It should be given orally twice daily at 0.2 mg/kg.

Carbamazepine

Classified as an anticonvulsant, this drug can be used to treat headshaking. Start at 10 mg/kg by mouth and repeat every 6 h. If there is improvement, the dose can be doubled but need only then be given twice per day.

Clenbuterol

Classified as a beta-2 agonist, it can be used for bronchodilation and to supplement mucociliary clearance. It can be used in the treatment of acute 'heaves' by a single i/v injection of 80 μg/100 kg. It is also available as an oral powder, which can be used to follow on from the initial treatment of the acute phase for long-term treatment, at a dosage of 80 μg/100 kg per os.

Cropropamide

This is a respiratory stimulant for the newborn foal. Normally mixed with crotethamide, it should be given on the side of the tongue. It may be repeated within 30 s if not effective.

Dembrexine

Dembrexine is a useful mucolytic for oral use in horses with RAO. It should be given at a dose of 0.3 mg/kg twice daily by mouth, being ideal for in-feed medication.

Doxapram hydrochloride

This is a respiratory stimulant in the foal. Give 1 mg/kg i/v or under the tongue.

Etamphyline camsylate

Another respiratory stimulant in the foal, which should be injected i/v. A normal dose is 700 mg.

Frusemide

Frusemide can be used as a diuretic in the horse to treat oedematous conditions. The dose is 1 mg/kg i/v twice daily.

Hydroxyzine

This is the only antihistamine useful in the horse, and can be used to treat urticaria or sweet itch. It may be helpful in some cases of headshaking. The dose for oral use is 1 mg/kg three times daily. It must be remembered that on no account should this drug be used in the pregnant mare, on account of the risk of abortion.

Salbutamol

A short-acting beta-2 agonist, it can be used via inhalation for acute 'heaves'. It is not suitable for long-term therapy but can be used for strategic dosing just prior to work.

Salmeterol

A long-acting beta-2 agonist, it can be used via inhalation for long-term therapy of RAO.

Sodium cromoglycate

This is a mast cell inhibitor. It can be used via inhalation for prevention of RAO, but not for treatment.

6.10 Therapeutic Iodine

This is said to be useful for treating entrenched chronic infections, particularly in cases of post-castration sepsis. It can be given as sodium iodide slowly i/v. The solution is extremely irritant and so the use of an intravenous catheter is recommended. The daily dose is 44 mg/kg and should be given for 3 days. This can be easily prepared by dissolving 10 g of sodium iodide in 125 ml of boiling water. This is the dose for a horse weighing 440 kg and can be given after cooling to blood heat. Iodine can also be given per os as potassium iodide as a powder in feed. The dose is 16.5 mg/kg daily for ten days.

6.11 Bisphosphonates

These medicines are used to treat navicular disease and spavin. There are two licensed preparations in the UK called Tiludrine and Clodronate. The author has no experience with these medicines, which are notorious for causing colic as a side effect. He is hesitant at recommending them in working horses.

6.12 Injectable Equine Medicines to be Carried by the Equine Ambulatory Practitioner

- Local anaesthetic;
- 2% xylazine;
- detomidine 10 mg/ml;
- acepromazine 10 mg/ml;
- butorphanol tartrate 10 mg/ml;
- ketamine 10 mg/ml;
- NSAIDs;
- 2% dexamethasone;
- antibiotics;
- oxytocin;
- 20% calcium 400 ml; and
- either 4 × 100ml barbiturate euthanasia solution or 2 × 50ml somulose solution (contains 400 mg/ml quinalbarbitone and 25 mg/ml cinchocaine hydrochloride).

6.13 Fluid Therapy

When treating horses with haemodynamic shock, the intravenous route is generally preferred for rapid and direct correction of hydration and electrolyte disturbances. However, i/v fluid therapy is expensive and relatively invasive, requiring the placement of an intravenous catheter, which can itself be associated with complications such as thrombophlebitis. In other situations where rapid fluid resuscitation is not required, such as mild to moderate dehydration or ongoing maintenance support, enteral fluid therapy offers an alternative and there is published evidence demonstrating the advantages of nasogastric tube (NGT) fluid administration in certain clinical situations, such as in the treatment of colonic impactions. When prolonged therapy is required, complications associated with NGT may include pharyngitis and laryngitis and additionally an indwelling nasogastric tube may interfere with eating. Passage of a NGT also requires special expertise, and incorrect placement (or administration of fluid in the face of impaired gastric emptying) is associated with potentially fatal consequences. This makes longer-term fluid therapy via temporary NGT placement (or an indwelling NGT) precarious in the field.

There is a paucity of publications on the administration of fluid per rectum (proctoclysis) in horses, despite this being an accepted method of fluid administration in other species. Except where rapid volume resuscitation is a requirement, the rectal route of fluid administration in horses may offer an inexpensive, safe alternative to i/v fluids, particularly when administration via NGT is contraindicated, such as with anterior enteritis, proximal gastrointestinal obstructions or with pharyngeal or oesophageal disease. If effective, it could also be used as an economical augmentation to fluid administration via other routes.

References and Further Reading

Andrews, F.M., Nadeau, J.A., Saabye, L. and Saxton, A.M. (1997) Measurement of total body water in horses, using deuterium oxide dilution. *American Journal of Veterinary Research* 58: 1060–1064.

Corley, K.T.T. and Hollis, A.R. (2009) Antimicrobial therapy in neonatal foals. *Equine Veterinary Education* 21: 436–448.

Fielding, C.L., Magdesian, K.G. and Edman, J.E. (2011) Determination of body water compartments in neonatal foals by use of indicator dilution techniques and multifrequency bioelectrical impedance analysis. *American Journal of Veterinary Research* 72: 1390–1396.

Fleury, C. (2005) *Guide to Clinical Parasitology in Horses*, vol. 2. Kalianxis, Paris.

Floyd, E.F., Easton-Jones, C.A. and Theelen, M.J.P. (2002) *Equine Veterinary Education* 34(1): 49–56.

Isgren, C.M., Williams, N.J., Fletcher, O.D., Timofte, D., Newton, R.J. *et al.* (2022) Antimicrobial resistance in clinical bacterial isolates from horses in the UK. *Equine Veterinary Journal* 54(2): 390–414.

Khan, A., Hallowell, G.D., Underwood, C. and Van Eps, A.W. (2019) *Equine Veterinary Journal* 51: 767–773.

Kirtland, A., McAloon, C., Walshe, N. and Duggan, V. (2023) *Strongyloides westeri* on a thoroughbred breeding farm in Ireland (2014–2019): Prevalence, risk factors and peripartum ivermectin. *Equine Veterinary Education* 35: 253.

Knottenbelt, D.C. (2006) *Equine Formulary*. Elsevier Saunders, St Louis, Missouri.

Raidal, S.L. (2019) Antimicrobial stewardship in equine practice. *Australian Veterinary Journal* 97: 238–242.

Wilson, A., Mair, T., Williams, N., McGowan, C. and Pinchbeck, G. (2023) Antimicrobial prescribing and antimicrobial resistance surveillance in equine practice. *Equine Veterinary Journal* 55: 494–505.

7

Vaccines

Abstract

This chapter discusses surveillance and notifiable diseases in the UK, after which diseases which are controlled at least by vaccinations are discussed and the reader is provided with details of the vaccines available, as well as notes on the zoonotic concerns.

7.1 Surveillance

This is defined as: 'the systematic collection, analysis and interpretation of health data, dissemination of the information gained and initiation of control action should disease levels rise above a pre-determined threshold' (Colgate, personal communication, 2023).

There are six mechanisms through which surveillance is carried out:

- voluntary notification;
- mandatory notification;
- outbreak investigation;
- sentinel surveillance; and
- census.

7.2 Notifiable Diseases in the UK

- African horse sickness;
- contagious equine metritis (CEM);
- eourine;
- epizootic lymphagitis;
- equine viral arteritis (EVA);
- equine viral encephalomyetis;
- equine infectious anaemia (EIA);
- glanders and farcy;
- rabies;
- vesicular stomatitis; and
- West Nile virus.

7.3 Introduction

The number of diseases that can be controlled by vaccination in horses is relatively small compared with other species. Although the goal may be to prevent infectious disease in the individual horse, if a large enough percentage of horses in a given population can be immunized, then the disease will never reach epidemic proportions. Vaccination programmes are laid down taking into account the horse's age, its use and the likely exposure level. Vaccination is important in pregnant horses to provide passive immunity in the colostrum. Most vaccines have a primary course of two or three doses followed by a half-yearly or annual booster. Young foals may be vaccinated quite early in life if they are born

2nd Edition (G.R. Duncanson)
DOI: 10.1079/9781800624283.0007

to unvaccinated dams. However, if they are born to vaccinated dams and have received a good passive immunity, then vaccination should be delayed. Passive immunity will interfere with the effectiveness of vaccination.

It is very important that practitioners follow the manufacturer's advice, not only regarding storage but also frequency of administration, for any vaccine.

Certain manufacturers combine vaccines for ease of administration. These combinations have not been listed as they are so diverse and numerous. Practitioners are advised to thoroughly investigate the actual risk to their equine patients and vaccinate accordingly, rather than follow a blanket approach which may be more expensive and less effective. All countries, all areas and, indeed, all holdings are different. The clinician needs to be well informed of the availability of vaccines, likely diseases posing a risk and the legislation laid down by that country.

It is sensible to carry out a risk analysis for individual premises.

The practitioner should consider:

- The age and the use of the equines on the premises. (This book is focused on working horses. However, the author is well aware that working horses need to be bred and reared.)
- The likelihood of exposure to an infectious disease from:
  - The arrival of new horses.
  - The arrival of personnel.
  - The arrival of possible infection on transport.
  - The local transmission from high stocking rates of equines in the vicinity.
- A biosecurity plan that reflects the readiness of the premises to an outbreak if one should occur. This would include the availability of an isolation facility and barrier nursing.

General principles of vaccination remain important.

- Primary courses should be given well in advance of likely exposure.
- Boosters should be strategically timed to optimize protection during periods of high risk.

Realistic expectations must be accepted for vaccination.

- Vaccines will work to reduce the risk of infection but will not totally eliminate disease.
- Vaccines will not necessarily impart immunity immediately.
- Specific administration protocols recommended by the manufacturers should be strictly adhered to.
- Not all animals will respond to vaccination as well as others.
- Vaccination should be considered as just one of a list of measures to prevent disease.

7.4 Rabies

Although horses are an end host for this disease, vaccination is useful in endemic areas. Horses can be protected by a single dose of vaccine given at or after 3 months of age. Annual boosters are required. Mares can receive a booster dose before breeding or 4–6 weeks before foaling.

7.5 Encephalomyelitis

There are three types of encephalomyelitis – eastern, western and Venezuelan. It is a viral disease spread by mosquitoes, the reservoir hosts being rodents and reptiles. Vaccination should be timed to coincide with the time of maximum challenge in endemic areas. Vaccination can be started as young as 3 months. An initial three doses separated by 4–6 weeks should be followed by booster doses every 6 months. Pregnant mares should be boosted 4–6 weeks before parturition.

7.6 Tetanus

The tetanus bacterium is found worldwide. Vaccination should be encouraged in all animals, and can start as early as 4 months. The first injection should be followed by a second after 4–6 weeks. With some modern vaccines boosters are required only every 3 years; however, others may require more frequent boosters. Ideally, pregnant mares should receive a booster 4–6 weeks before foaling.

There is a tetanus antitoxin available, which should be given to unvaccinated animals if they are in immediate danger, e.g. from surgery – particularly castration – or if they have received a wound. The first dose of the vaccine should be started at the same time. The dose of antitoxin recommended is very varied, being between 1500 IU and 7500 IU. Clinicians have a dilemma: it is relatively expensive. A successful court case was mounted against a practitioner in the UK who was seen to fail to give the recommended dose of antitoxin and the horse subsequently died of tetanus. The advice must be to give the dose as recommended by the manufacturer for the preparation licensed for use in that country. Very much higher doses, e.g. 50,000 IU, have been recommended for i/v injection in the early stages of the actual disease. However, as the bacillus is very sensitive to penicillin a more cost-effective treatment would be penicillin in high doses.

7.7 Influenza

Practitioners should study not only the vaccine manufacturer's recommendations but also the legislation of that country. Influenza virus demonstrates a good transfer of passive immunity, so that some authorities do not advise vaccination in foals bred from vaccinated mares before 9 months. However, the majority of recommendations are to start vaccination at 5 months of age.

This initial dose should be followed by a second in 4–6 weeks (certain recommendations are for as early as 2 weeks), with a third in a further 6 months. Normal horses should then have a booster annually. However, when there is a high risk of an outbreak then all animals should receive boosters at 6-monthly intervals. Pregnant mares should receive a booster vaccination 4–6 weeks before foaling. There is an intranasal vaccination available in some countries, which may not require the same number of boosters.

7.8 Equine Herpes Virus (EHV)

The main symptoms of herpes virus in the horse are respiratory, musculoskeletal and abortion. Vaccine regimes need to reflect the symptoms likely to occur. On the whole equine herpes virus type 1 causes abortion in susceptible mares. Mares at risk should be vaccinated i/m on three occasions during pregnancy, ideally in the 5th, 7th and 9th months. EHV type 1 can cause neurological and respiratory signs. If there is an outbreak in an area it is safest to advise owners to take a cautious but pragmatic approach. At-risk animals should be placed in isolation for 14 days (to avoid direct and indirect contact with other horses) and undergo daily clinical monitoring (ideally twice daily rectal temperature recording), with a blood sample for serum antibody testing collected at the beginning (this can be stored in the fridge, ideally with the serum separated from the clot, which can be discarded). A second serum sample, together with a nasopharyngeal swab, should be taken at the end, prior to release from isolation. Animals that develop clinical signs whilst in isolation (which may include just fever, inappetence and lethargy but also nasal discharge, coughing and limb oedema through to neurological signs), should undergo veterinary examination with samples taken at the time for EHV-1 testing, especially nasopharyngeal swabs for PCR. Vaccination is *not* advised to animals that may have been exposed EHV-1 and are undergoing this isolation and screening process. EHV type 4 causes respiratory signs and is termed rhinopneumonitis, mainly a disease of young horses. Vaccination can begin at 5 months of age. Two further doses of vaccine should be given at monthly intervals. From then on, young horses at high risk should be boosted at 3-monthly intervals; in lower-risk areas this can be stretched to 6-monthly boosters. Such a course of vaccination will cover older horses against the musculoskeletal form. There is a need for a more effective vaccine to be developed.

7.9 Botulism

Botulism may occur worldwide, but it appears only to be a threat in certain areas or under particular management situations. Therefore, unlike tetanus, ubiquitous vaccination is not recommended. Foals from vaccinated mares should not start their course of vaccination before 5 months, but foals from naive mares may start at any age. The initial course is three doses at monthly intervals. Boosters should be given annually. Pregnant mares should be vaccinated 4–6 weeks before foaling.

7.10 Ehrlichiosis

Vaccination is recommended in endemic areas, with the timing to coincide with periods of greatest risk. Vaccination can start in foals at 5 months of age. This should be followed by a second dose after 3–4 weeks and then annual boosters. Pregnant mares should be vaccinated 4–6 weeks before foaling.

7.11 Viral Arteritis

It should be remembered that this is not a marker vaccine. Therefore, subsequent blood tests of stallions cannot differentiate between vaccination and possible carrier status. Before vaccination of any stallion, it is prudent to obtain a negative blood test in case the stallion needs to be moved. Vaccination can be performed any time after 1 month of age. It is a single i/m injection, which needs to be boosted annually. Ideally, mares and stallions should be vaccinated at least 3 weeks before breeding. Mares should not be vaccinated in the last 2 months of pregnancy.

7.12 Rotavirus

Since this is a disease of the foal, mares should be vaccinated to provide passive transfer of antibodies in the colostrum for the foal. Mares should receive three doses in the last trimester of pregnancy separated by 3–4 weeks.

7.13 West Nile Virus

Its correct name is equine encephalomyelitis. Worldwide this zoonotic disease has a limited distribution. It is spread by various species of mosquito. There is no direct spread between horses, which are considered dead-end hosts. The incubation period is 3–15 days. The non-specific signs are inappetence and pyrexia. It is commonly subclinical. The neurological signs range in severity from mild depression to head-pressing and a state of drowsiness. Additional neurological signs can include behavioural changes, facial twitching, impaired vision, inability to swallow, heightened sensitivity, muscle fasciculations, paresis/paralysis of front/hind limbs, ataxia, aimless wandering, recumbency, coma and death. Diagnosis can be confirmed with a serum sample or infected tissue for RT-PCR (reverse transcription polymerase chain reaction) on post-mortem. However, where it occurs vaccination is recommended, with the first dose being given to foals at 5 months of age and a second dose given 4 weeks later. Foals born early in temperate climates should receive a further dose in the autumn, and this should be followed by an annual booster. Pregnant mares should be vaccinated 4–6 weeks before foaling. The disease is notifiable in the UK. A 2022 case was associated with an import.

7.14 Protozoal Myeloencephalitis

There is no licensed vaccine against this disease at the time of going to press. There are some unlicensed products and hope of a vaccine in the near future. More details of the disease can be found in Section 16.16.

7.15 African Horse Sickness

The vaccine is a live freeze-dried pellet containing eight modified strains covering 43 recognized antigenic types. The dose is 5 ml of vaccine 1 given i/m, followed in 4 weeks by 5 ml of vaccine 2, also given i/m. Boosters need to be given prior to likely challenge. Diagnosis maybe confirmed by a sample of serum for ELISA, complement fixation and virus neutralization or whole unclotted blood and infected tissue for RT-PCR and viral isolation.

7.16 Strangles

There have been many problems over the years with vaccination against strangles, a disease caused by *Streptococcus equi*. The vaccine, which requires 3 i/m injections each separated by 1 month after the age of 5 months, is thought not to be very effective. A vaccine developed to be injected intradermally into the upper lip was found to be too virulent and was discontinued. An intranasal vaccine, which requires an initial course of two doses separated by 1 month followed by an annual booster, can only be started at 11 months of age. Pregnant mares should receive a booster 4–6 weeks before foaling. Strangles vaccination should be restricted to horses at high risk in equine populations where the disease is endemic, and not considered for the general equine population. New strangles vaccines are constantly being developed. Further information on this old but important disease can be found in Section 14.3.

Further Reading

Kahn, C.M. (ed.) (2008) *The Merck Veterinary Manual*, 9th edn. Merck & Co., Inc., Whitehouse Station, New Jersey.

Russell, P.H. and Edington, N. (1986) *Veterinary Viruses*. CAB International, Wallingford, UK.

Whitlock, F, Colgate, V. and Newton, R. (2023) Guide to equine exotic vectorborne diseases and their risks to UK horses. *In Practice* 45(4): 232–238.

8

Sedation, Analgesia, Field Anaesthesia and Euthanasia

Abstract

Individual drugs are discussed in detail, with descriptions of their properties and limitations, together with possible side effects and contraindications. The author draws on his considerable experience in field anaesthesia, having performed over 4000 castrations under general anaesthesia and over 30,000 sedations for dentistry and other procedures. The problems of euthanasia are discussed.

8.1 General

Steroidal and non-steroidal drugs are discussed in Chapter 6. The divergence of dosages for donkeys and mules from horses and ponies is pinpointed. Surprisingly, the sedatives, anaesthetics and medicines for euthanasia are very similar for horses, ponies, mules and donkeys, and they have similar doses. The only exception is etorphine hydrochloride, which is a very potent analgesic with the ability to provide short-term anaesthesia. The use of this drug in mules or donkeys is hazardous. There are the alarming problems with recycling of the drug, and therefore its use in both donkeys and mules needs considerable planning.

Excitable animals are sometimes poor subjects for not only sedation but also for general anaesthesia. To achieve the best results, it is important the animals are not stressed before the giving of the initial sedation. Dosages can be adjusted downwards by up to 50% if the animal is extremely quiet, e.g. heavy horses, or adjusted upwards by 50% if the animal is in a hyperexcited state.

Often sedatives, tranquillizers, analgesics and anticonvulsants are given in combination. I will describe these combinations and cross-reference them under each named drug. I will not include gaseous anaesthetic agents. Medicines for euthanasia will appear at the end of the chapter.

A sedative is a drug producing mental calming through sleepiness, while a tranquillizer achieves mental calming through reduced anxiety and awareness and decreased locomotory activity. Both are often referred to as sedatives. They are usually administered by i/v injection and, less commonly, by i/m injection. Some sedatives provide analgesia, which may be sufficient for the procedure, while at other times additional local or even general anaesthesia will be required. When veterinary attention is absent, oral or sublingual medication may be used.

Post-operation analgesic protocols are important in all equine patients. They are particularly important in donkeys, not only because their often-quiet demeanour may deceive the clinician, but also because of the very real danger of hyperlipaemia in even moderately obese animals.

DOI: 10.1079/9781800624283.0008

Pain may be divided into three categories.

- Nociceptive (physiologic) pain: The result of the physiological process of nociceptive signalling, usually sharp, localized and affecting a well-defined area. This is evoked by high-intensity stimuli and is adaptive and brief. Examples include needle pricks and responses to hoof testers.
- Inflammatory pain: This is evoked by high- and low-intensity stimuli that indicate recovery which is secondary to tissue injury. Sensitization often occurs. This pain is adaptive and reversible and continues until inflammation decreases. Examples include lacerations, synovitis, surgery, tendinitis and desmitis.
- Neuropathic pain: This is maladaptive and persistent. It is evoked by high- and low-intensity stimuli. Central sensitization is sustained and pain can occur in the absence of continued noxious stimuli. Examples are nerve trauma and neuroma formation.

8.2 Recognition of Pain

Identifying pain in equine patients, particularly in donkeys and mules, can be difficult. Without verbal communication, we are relying on the accurate identification of obvious behavioural or locomotory abnormalities and interpretation of physiological indices. Clearly when an animal is demonstrating non-weight-bearing lameness or violent signs of abdominal discomfort, whether the animal is in pain is not in dispute. But what about the more subtle signs related to head carriage, facial expression and asymmetrical ears? Equines are a prey species; they may not overtly demonstrate pain in a situation they perceive to be dangerous. Pain control should be planned by providing multi-modal analgesia.

8.3 Outcomes from General Anaesthetics

These are improving with mortality rates for non-colic cases dropping from 0.9% to 0.6%. The improvement may be attributed to several factors:

- The use of a combination of anaesthesia with inhalation and i/v constant-rate infusion.
- Sedation of the animal with an alpha-2 agonist while the animal is still anaesthetized to help with recovery.
- Improvement of monitoring.
- Assisted induction.
- Assisted recovery.

The main risk factors must be remembered:

- Size: larger equines with a high body mass present with greater risks of myopathy.
- Breed: draught horses are more prone to spinal cord malacia and myopathy.
- Temperament: both excitability and overly relaxed behaviour are risk factors.
- Sex: this is a risk factor in stallions on account of the dangers of the use of acetylpromazine maleate (ACP) causing paraphimosis.
- Age: this is a risk factor at both ends of the spectrum, foals and geriatrics.
- Naturally, the longer the surgery the higher the risk.
- Interestingly, the time of day is a risk as out of hours are riskier.
- Naturally, elective procedures are safer.

Certain actions to be taken should be remembered:

- Food should be restricted.
- Water should be provided.
- The mouth should be washed out if there is going to be intubation.
- Placement of a venous cannular.
- Careful thought should be given to the use of antibiotics prior to and during anaesthesia. A risk analysis is useful.

8.4 Acetylpromazine Maleate (ACP)

A long-established tranquillizer, this can be given either orally or by injection, the preferred route by injection being i/v. The results from subcutaneous (s/c) or i/m injection are less reliable. The drug is available in varying strengths, so the bottle should be checked carefully for the strength before calculating the dosage. It is not a good drug for restraint in the horse as the animal is soon alarmed. Noise should be moderated, as loud noise definitely stimulates the animal. If given by mouth 45 min before sedation is required; it can help to allow i/v administration of a more potent sedative. It is favoured for premedication by anaesthetists – a large survey indicated that anaesthetic mortality was reduced by its use. However, that has not been a universal experience. It is used by some clinicians to lower the blood pressure in cases of laminitis. However, there is little evidence-based medicine (EBM) to back up its use; indeed, some authorities claim it is contraindicated.

The main use is in exteriorizing the penis. It can be given with detomidine and butorphanol to good effect, at a dose rate of 0.1 mg/kg. Its use should be avoided in stallions, as there is a danger of penile prolapse. In fact, there is also a slight danger in geldings. The important procedure to follow is *not* to allow a male horse out of a confined space until the penis is not only withdrawn but also the animal has regained the ability to withdraw the penis at will.

8.5 Butorphanol Tartrate

An extremely potent analgesic that should be given by injection, the preferred route being i/v. However, it can also be given s/c or i/m. When given on its own it should be given at the highest dosage rate, i.e. 0.2 mg/kg. This will give immediate relief from visceral pain, but that only lasts for 45 min. There are two unwanted side effects at this dosage. First, there may be severe ataxia; second, there is a sharp rise in central nervous system (CNS) pressure, so it should not be given in cases of head trauma. On recovery 'box-walking' has been noted, but this is rare. Its principal use is in combination with an alpha-2 agonist to give reliable sedation. The principal alpha-2 agonists are detomidine, romifidine and xylazine. The dosages for these combinations are given under the respective drugs (see below).

In certain countries – but not the UK – this drug has classified status and so special storage and usage rules apply.

8.6 Chloral Hydrate

A long-established drug, chloral hydrate is a hypnotic rather than a sedative. It is supplied as either a crystalline powder or a very concentrated solution; the latter should be diluted to form a 10% solution Reportedly, it can be given orally by stomach tube. This must be painful as it is irritant to mucous membranes, but this effect will be masked by the hypnotic effect; there is no good reason for using the drug in this manner. It has two other uses. The first is in combination with thiopentone sodium (see Section 8.16) to provide anaesthesia, and the second is when it is added to the drinking water to apprehend a very fractious horse. Since oral chloral hydrate is so irritant and bitter, all water needs to be withdrawn for at least 24 h before administration. This, I feel, creates a welfare issue and hopefully an alternative method can be found.

After premedication with acetylpromazine, good anaesthesia can be obtained by giving a 10% solution i/v at the rate of 1 g/100 kg (i.e. a 500 kg horse will be given 5 g). The horse will then be very sleepy and ataxic. A bolus of thiopentone sodium at the rate of 0.3 g/100 kg (i.e. a 500 kg horse will be given 1.5 g) will cause recumbency and anaesthesia. This can be maintained by further boluses of 0.2 g/100 kg of thiopentone sodium. The danger with this regime is that both chloral hydrate and thiopentone sodium are extremely irritant if given perivascularly.

8.7 Detomidine Hydrochloride

The excellent sedative and analgesic properties make this drug ideal for premedication. It is obtained in multi-dose vials containing 10 mg/ml. An i/v dose of 4 mg/100 kg can be given as premedication, to be followed in 5 min by 220 mg/100 kg ketamine given i/v (see Section 8.12). This will give approximately 15 min of anaesthesia, which can then be topped up with incremental half-doses of both drugs given together i/v for more prolonged anaesthesia. Combining it with butorphanol tartrate can enhance its sedative properties; for general standing sedation, 2 mg/100 kg can be given i/v in the same syringe as 2 mg/100 kg butorphanol tartrate. If i/v injection is impossible, this dose can be given fivefold i/m for a similar effect; however, a much longer time is required. Detomidine hydrochloride can be given sublingually at ten times the dose rate for really fractious horses, particularly stallions, which bare their teeth; once again, a long time is required before sedation takes effect.

There is now a gel formulation available in an oral syringe form. It should *not* be given orally but sublingually. The mouth should be empty. Absorption takes up to thirty minutes and is too slow to be topped up. Rubber gloves should be worn. Care should be taken with this drug – like all alpha-2 agonists – in the last trimester of pregnancy. Although not recommended, the clinician is left in a dilemma as this category of drug provides the best and safest sedation. There have never been any problems reported; nevertheless, owners should be well briefed. It is always prudent to delay their use for routine procedures like dentistry until foaling has been completed.

8.8 Diazepam

The use of this drug is mainly as an anticonvulsant, although it does have sedative and muscle relaxant effects. It should be given i/v; it comes in 2 ml vials containing 5 mg/ml. It has two uses. First, it can be given to convulsing foals; a starting bolus of 20 mg should be given i/v. If the foal is still twitching, further diazepam can be given very slowly to effect. Historically, practitioners have used pentobarbitone sodium for this purpose; however, this drug is difficult to obtain except as the triple-strength version for euthanasia (see Section 8.18). Also, it is irritant if given perivascularly, and sadly this is easy to do in a convulsing foal; placing a catheter to prevent this is not easy. However, once the foal is more relaxed, then a catheter should be stitched into place. The second indication for the use of diazepam is to obtain total relaxation of the tongue for complicated dental procedures at the back of the mouth. Diazepam can be given following sedation with an alpha-2 agonist mixed with butorphanol tartrate. An ideal dose is 10 mg for a 500 kg horse (i.e. one 2-ml vial); half this dose is suitable for a pony.

8.9 Etorphine Hydrochloride

Originally called M99, it was said to be 99 times more potent than morphine sulfate. As will be explained later, horses are relatively resistant to morphine sulfate; on the other hand, man is very sensitive to morphine sulfate. This explains why this drug is so dangerous if injected into a human – even a small quantity can be lethal. The human antidote is naloxone. This should be drawn up in a syringe ready for injection *before* etorphine hydrochloride is handled. Just to give the reader an example of the potency of this drug, I will describe its action in the African elephant. Eight milligrams of etorphine hydrochloride will provide anaesthesia to a 350 kg pony if given i/v; 8 mg of etorphine hydrochloride will provide anaesthesia to the biggest African elephant in the world, even if only given i/m; such an elephant is likely to weigh 3500 kg, i.e. ten times as much. Veterinary surgeons *must take care*.

Normally, the drug is supplied with acetylpromazine maleate in 10 ml multi-dose vials. The trade name is Large Animal Immobilon. Each millilitre contains 2.45 mg of etorphine hydrochloride and 10 mg of acetypromazine maleate, and it is coloured yellow. In the same foam container is the horse antidote, Large Animal Revivon. Each millilitre of Large Animal Revivon contains 3.26 mg of diprenorphine hydrochloride and it is coloured blue.

Intravenous injection of the correct dose of Large Animal Immobilon, i.e. 1 ml/100 kg, will result in up to 45 min of anaesthesia. There is some uncoordinated movement and juddering, but no violent movement. An equal volume of Large Animal Revivon given i/v reverses the action. It is also wise to give half the Large Animal Revivon dose i/m concurrently. This prevents recycling of the drug and allows for a more consistent reversal.

It is dangerous in old or debilitated animals, and it can cause severe respiratory depression in the newborn if given at parturition. This can be counteracted to some extent by giving 1 ml of Large Animal Revivon i/v to the newborn foal. It is dangerous in animals with recurrent airway obstruction (RAO). Paraphimosis and priapism can follow its use. For all these reasons and because it is so dangerous in man, I do not feel it should be used in equine practice.

8.10 Fentanyl

This can be a useful post-operative analgesic. The route of administration is transdermal by the use of skin patches.

8.11 Glyceryl Guaiacolate (GG)

A spinally acting muscle relaxant, GG must never be given on its own. However, in combination with thiopentone sodium (see Section 8.16) given as an anaesthetic following acetylpromazine and detomidine premedication, it is a good, safe and inexpensive anaesthetic. A suitable regime for a 500 kg horse would be 50 mg acetylpromazine given i/v, followed in 40 min by 5 mg detomidine; after a further 4 min, the horse should be catheterized. A home-made infusion of GG and thiopentone sodium can then be given via the catheter, to effect. The horse will fall down and the infusion should be continued until a suitable plane of anaesthesia is reached. This can then be topped up to lengthen the anaesthesia. The home-made infusion is made by adding 50 g GG and 1.5 g thiopentone sodium to a warm solution of 5% dextrose. Precipitation will occur if this solution is allowed to fall below 8°C.

Glyceryl guaiacolate can also be used in combination with ketamine (see Section 8.12) and detomidine as a 'triple-drip' infusion; relatively long-term anaesthesia can be obtained by this method.

8.12 Ketamine

This is an excellent short-acting anaesthetic when given in combination with detomidine, romifidine or xylazine (see Section 8.15 and 8.17). Diazepam can be given to increase the duration of anaesthesia, but ketamine must never be given on its own. A suitable induction regime for a 500 kg horse would be 50 mg romifidine given i/v, followed by 1100 mg ketamine given i/v after the sedative effect of the romifidine is seen; the dose of diazepam for a 500 kg horse would be 10 mg. The anaesthesia can be prolonged in anticipation of stimuli by a top-up dose of half the initial dose of both drugs given in the same syringe; this can be repeated up to five times. The normal dose rate of ketamine after sedation with romifidine, detomidine or xylazine is 2.2 mg/kg. However, this may be increased to as much as 5 mg/kg without any untoward side effects.

8.13 Morphine Sulfate

In many countries this is classed as a dangerous drug, and so special storage and usage rules apply. It causes excitement in the horse and should never be given on its own; however, it gives very reliable sedation when administered in combination with alpha-2 agonists. There have been reports of problems with this combination in the donkey, but these have not been substantiated. Care should be taken, as various strengths of solution are supplied. A suitable sedation dose given to a 500 kg horse by i/v injection would be 5 mg of detomidine hydrochloride followed in 5 min by 100 mg morphine sulfate. These should not be given in the same syringe as there is a slight danger of excitement. Some practitioners, however, do feel that although there is a risk it is worthwhile when given for a well-supervised colic surgery recovery case. The fear that it causes post-operative ileus is unfounded. The other main indication is for the relief of severe musculoskeletal pain; once again, it should be given following an alpha-2 agonist.

8.14 Pethidine Hydrochloride

Like morphine sulfate, this opiate should not be given on its own to horses but in combination with acetylpromazine and/or xylazine. A suitable dose for a 500 kg horse would be 1 g given i/m following 500 mg acetylpromazine and 500 mg xylazine given i/v, producing sedation. It gives good relief from both musculoskeletal and gastroenteric pain. *Pethidine should never be given i/v*, as it may cause a violent reaction.

8.15 Romifidine

This is a useful alpha-2 agonist for sedation, both on its own (it will not remove the kick reflex) and in combination with butorphanol tartrate. A suitable dose for a 500 kg horse would be 25 mg romifidine and 10 mg butorphanol tartrate, given i/v. This combination is not licensed, but is perfectly safe given in the same syringe, producing very safe sedation. In fractious horses five times this dose may be given i/m. It can also be used as a premedicant for ketamine anaesthesia, at the dose of 10 mg/100 kg.

8.16 Thiopentone Sodium

This is a very inexpensive, short-acting anaesthetic, although it should never be given without premedication with acetylpromazine. A suitable induction protocol for a 500 kg horse would be 50 mg acetylpromazine i/v, followed by 5 g thiopentone sodium, also given i/v. Great care should be exercised, as thiopentone sodium is extremely irritant perivascularly. There is an alarming period of apnoea, but this passes and then the breathing settles into a normal rhythm. For most practitioners ketamine has superseded thiopentone sodium. However, it is a very safe induction agent and, provided that the horse is maintained on gaseous anaesthesia for a sufficient time, then recovery is not violent. It is no longer available as a veterinary product, although it is still licensed for human use.

8.17 Xylazine

This is also an alpha-2 agonist, but with a stronger analgesic effect than either detomidine or romifidine. It also has a shorter action. A dose of 300 mg xylazine given i/v to a 500 kg horse would be very suitable for short sedation and analgesia, e.g. for rectal examination of a violent colic or placing a hind leg nerve block in a difficult horse. It can be used with pethidine or ACP, as stated earlier, for deeper, more profound sedation. Equally, it can be used with butorphanol tartrate. A suitable dose given i/v for a 500 kg horse would be 150 mg xylazine and 10 mg butorphanol tartrate. Xylazine is particularly useful for sedation in the donkey, when there is a risk of hyperlipaemia from inappetence. The i/v dose of 180 mg for a 150 kg donkey will give short, but useful, sedation.

General anaesthesia in equines carries an inherent risk which is higher than in small animals and humans. Therefore, many surgical procedures are performed in the standing sedated animal, combined with local anaesthesia. Selection of cases that require general anaesthesia in preference to sedation involves individual assessment of the procedure, the temperament of the animal, available facilities and number of trained personnel.

It is beyond the scope of this book to describe gaseous anaesthesia or full indoor surgical facilities or to suggest outside places suitable for general anaesthesia. However, if oxygen could be provided that would be worthwhile. An

Table 8.1. Equine dosing chart for sedation.

	Detomidine 10 mg/ml	+	Butorphanol 10 mg/ml	OR	Xylazine 100 mg/ml	+	Butorphanol 10 mg/ml
Dose	0.012 mg/kg		0.025 mg/kg	OR	0.5 mg/kg		0.1 mg/kg
Route	IM or IV		IV *	OR	IV		IV
Weight	ml		ml	OR	ml		ml
50 kg	0.06	+	0.13	OR	0.25	+	0.5
100 kg	0.12	+	0.25	OR	0.5	+	1
150 kg	0.18	+	0.38	OR	0.75	+	1.5
200 kg	0.24	+	0.5	OR	1	+	2
250 kg	0.3	+	0.63	OR	1.25	+	2.5
300 kg	0.36	+	0.75	OR	1.5	+	3
350 kg	0.42	+	0.88	OR	1.75	+	3.5
400 kg	0.48	+	1	OR	2	+	4
450 kg	0.54	+	1.13	OR	2.25	+	4.5
500 kg	0.6	+	1.25	OR	2.5	+	5
550 kg	0.66	+	1.38	OR	2.75	+	5.5
600 kg	0.72	+	1.5	OR	3	+	6
650 kg	0.78	+	1.63	OR	3.25	+	6.5
700 kg	0.84	+	1.75	OR	3.5	+	7

*Make sure the horse is adequately sedated before giving butorphanol if detomidine has been given by IM route.

Table 8.2. Equine dosage chart for anaesthesia.

	Xylazine 100 mg/ml	OR	Detomidine 10 mg/ml	Followed in 2–5 minutes	Ketamine 100 mg/ml
Dose	1.1 mg/kg	OR	0.02 mg/kg	Followed in 2–5 minutes	2.2 mg/kg
Route	IV	OR	IV	Followed in 2–5 minutes	IV
Weight	ml	OR	ml	Followed in 2–5 minutes	ml
50 kg	0.55	OR	0.1	Followed in 2–5 minutes	1.1
100 kg	1.1	OR	0.2	Followed in 2–5 minutes	2.2
150 kg	1.65	OR	0.3	Followed in 2–5 minutes	3.3
200 kg	2.2	OR	0.4	Followed in 2–5 minutes	4.4
250 kg	2.75	OR	0.5	Followed in 2–5 minutes	5.5
300 kg	3.3	OR	0.6	Followed in 2–5 minutes	6.6
350 kg	3.85	OR	0.7	Followed in 2–5 minutes	7.7
400 kg	4.4	OR	0.8	Followed in 2–5 minutes	8.8
450 kg	4.95	OR	0.9	Followed in 2–5 minutes	9.9
500 kg	5.5	OR	1	Followed in 2–5 minutes	11
550 kg	6.05	OR	1.1	Followed in 2–5 minutes	12.1
600 kg	6.6	OR	1.2	Followed in 2–5 minutes	13.2
650 kg	7.15	OR	1.3	Followed in 2–5 minutes	14.4
700 kg	7.7	OR	1.4	Followed in 2–5 minutes	15.4

intravenous catheter is advisable, but with very experienced practitioners is not essential. Having all the equipment prepared in advance is vital because speed is required. The longer the animal is recumbent the greater the risk of anaesthetic problems.

8.18 Agents for Euthanasia

Somulose and triple-strength pentobarbitone must be used only for euthanasia and never for anaesthesia. Veterinary surgeons used to 'putting dogs to sleep' often say they are putting a horse to sleep. This terminology gives the wrong impression to owners and should not be used as horses often collapse violently to the ground. Veterinary surgeons should also be aware that when a horse dies its legs collapse under it. However, if the horse is being destroyed because it has tetanus, it will die in a tetanic spasm and lurch forward. The veterinary surgeon and the handler should *not* stand in front of a horse which is suffering from tetanus and which is being destroyed by chemicals or a gun.

Cinchocaine and quinalbarbitone

These two substances are combined as a proprietary product, prepared solely for euthanasia, and should never be used for any other purpose. In the UK and many other countries, it is classed as a dangerous drug and certain restrictions are applied on its storage and handling. It is very viscous and should not be stored below freezing ambient temperature. Premedication with any of the sedative regimes described above is worthwhile, unless the horse is recumbent. However, one authority has discovered problems with xylazine given immediately prior to cinchocaine, and some authorities avoid this combination. The author has used xylazine sedation followed by cinchocaine on numerous occasions without any problems. It is strongly recommended that a catheter be put in place following premedication. The dose is 50 ml for a horse and 25 ml for a pony. The injection is given slowly i/v over a 12 s period. The term 'putting to sleep' should not be used, as this will raise the owner's perceptions. The horse falls like a ton of bricks and does not sink down gently. Often there are some paddling movements, but these are minimal if premedication is used. The owner should be warned to lessen the shock. It is also prudent to warn of the possible Cheyne-Stokes reaction (abnormal breathing just prior to cardiac arrest), as this can be distressing. However, having pointed out all these possible problems, this is still the best drug available.

Pentobarbitone sodium

A barbiturate routinely used at 'triple strength' to euthanize small animals, it can cause problems in the horse. If possible, its use should be avoided. However, previous deep sedation with any of the combinations described above can lessen the dangers. Sedation should be followed by catheterization. Then, for a 500 kg horse three 60 ml syringes should be loaded with 'triple-strength' pentobarbitone sodium. This full dose should be injected as rapidly as possible. The horse should be held on a long lead rope, not wrapped around the hand. The handler should be told to hold on firmly, as often the horse will rear or go backwards before collapsing. If no cinchocaine is available a suitable alternative is to anaesthetize the horse with any of the combination of agents listed above and then to give pentobarbitone sodium in a controlled manner.

Thiopentone sodium

This is a barbiturate that can also be used for euthanasia. The horse should be anaesthetized with any of the combinations listed above, including thiopentone sodium. Once the horse is anaesthetized, a very large dose of thiopentone sodium can be rapidly injected i/v, but in a controlled manner. A suitable dose of thiopentone sodium for a 500 kg horse would be 20 g.

Other methods of euthanasia

Free bullet

The use of a 0.32 pistol placed against the head at the centre of a cross of two lines linking the ear to the opposite eye firing a free bullet is a straightforward method of euthanasia. This often causes haemorrhage (Fig. 8.1). It should not be used in a public place and in the UK, it has largely been replaced by chemical euthanasia. There is also a gun apply named a bell gun which also can be used and placed in the same position. It is shaped like a big handbell. This is a 0.310 calibre, and the ammunition is hard to obtain. The use of a weapon firing a free bullet has the disadvantage of requiring the user in the UK to have a firearms license and keeping the weapon in a locked gun safe secured to a building or in a locked gun safe secured to a vehicle. It is important that veterinary surgeons take care when using such weapons. It is acceptable to sedate the animal first if the veterinary surgeon is inexperienced.

Shotgun

If a pistol or bell-gun is not available, then a 12-bore shotgun may be used by a veterinary

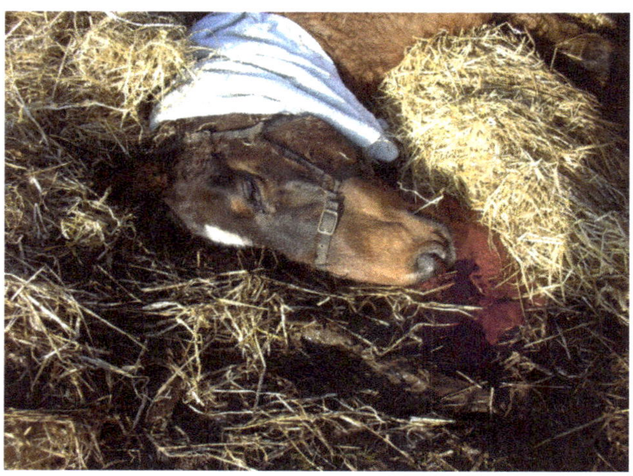

Fig. 8.1. Haemorrhage is standard with the use of a free bullet for euthanasia.

surgeon without a firearm licence or a shotgun licence, provided the owner has a shotgun license and gives his or her permission for its use. The gun should not be pressed against the head but should be fired 1–2 ft away, aimed at the same spot as previously described.

Captive-bolt pistol

In certain circumstances, e.g. in an aircraft, on a ship or in a trailer an experienced veterinary surgeon can use a captive bolt pistol aimed at the same point. The danger is that the pistol has to be held firmly, but must be dropped immediately on firing as the captive bolt may remain in the horse's head and break the wrist of the operator. The other problem is that the equid then has to be pithed to ensure that it is dead and not just stunned.

Scalpel

In old textbooks a method of euthanasia is described where the veterinary surgeon severs the dorsal aorta rostral to the bifurcation with a scalpel blade per rectum. The author has seen such a procedure carried out and strongly feels that it is non-humane.

Further Reading

Henston Large Animal and Equine Veterinary Vade Mecum. 24th edn. (2008) Henston Veterinary Publications, Peterborough, UK.

Petruccione, I. (2023) Equine sedation and anaesthesia: Right options at right time: Part 2. *Vet Times* 53(18), 9 May: 11–12.

Turner, A.S. (ed.) (1994) Emergency treatment in the adult horse. In: *The Veterinary Clinics of North America: Equine Practice*. W.B. Saunders, Philadelphia, Pennsylvania.

9

Nutrition

Abstract
In this chapter aspects of nutrition are discussed with particular relevance to working animals which, because they work for long proportions of their lives, require special considerations. From a welfare perspective it is vital that they receive adequate nutrition.

9.1 Normal Feeding Patterns

In the wild a horse will spend approximately 18–20 h/day foraging and feeding. Donkeys feed for slightly less, 14–16 h/day. This may be because donkeys are more efficient at digesting food. Working animals must be given sufficient time to feed as they also need time to rest. Unlike pleasure horses and donkeys in the developed world, which are often too fat, working equines are normally too thin (see Fig. 9.1).

9.2 The Role and Structure of the Equine Gut

The equine, unlike the ruminant, has a relatively small stomach, approximately 9% of the total gut capacity. On the other hand, it has a large hindgut, which consists of a colon and a caecum, representing 38% and 16% of total gut capacity, respectively. The equine rectum represents 7% of total gut capacity, and is extremely efficient at removing the water content of the droppings. The long small intestine represents 30% of total gut capacity, and it is rarely full; in fact, the total gut fill is usually less than one-third of total capacity.

All food has to be converted into a form that can be readily absorbed. First of all, it has to be physically ground down by the teeth. Although each bolus of food will be chewed several times before swallowing, the equine's food, unlike that of the ruminant, is allowed only one passage through the mouth. Forage needs to be chewed more than concentrated feeds. Not only is there more lateral excursion when long-fibred forage is chewed, but also the number of times it is chewed is greater. One kilogram of concentrated feed requires 1000 chews, while 1 kg of poor-quality roughage needs three times that number of chews. The condition of an equine's teeth is extremely important, and therefore it is very important that they are checked regularly. However, an equine has only a finite amount of tooth to last its lifetime, unlike a rodent, and therefore only the sharp enamel overgrowths should be removed by regular rasping. The occlusal surface, unless there are other problems, should not be touched.

DOI: 10.1079/9781800624283.0009

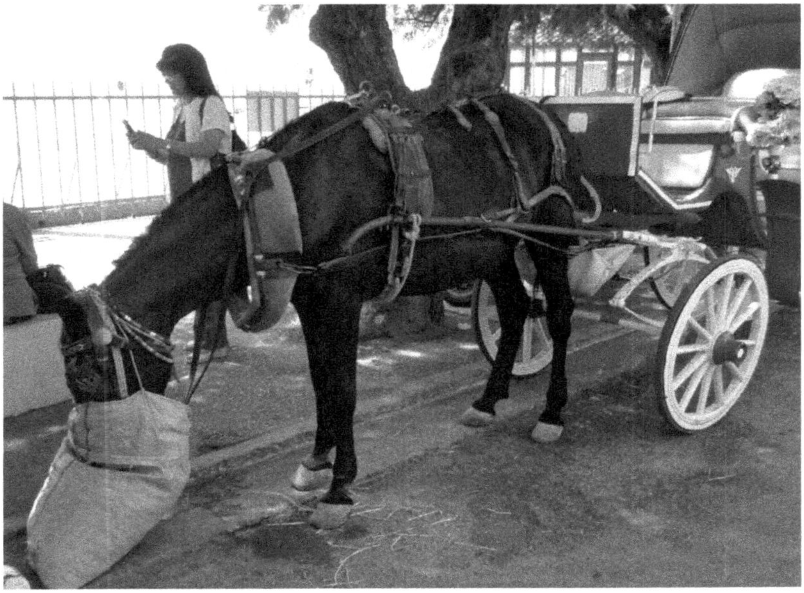

Fig. 9.1. Horses need to feed for 18 out of every 24 hours.

After the physical maceration of the food, the animal has to break it down chemically, initially in the stomach and small intestine. This is the process of digestion, when the enzymes produced by the glands in the intestinal wall break down the food. Further along the gut there is a process of fermentation, where the animal is assisted by enzymes produced by bacteria, protozoa and fungi to break down the fibrous food into nutrients that can be absorbed and utilized by the body. The fibre consists of hemicelluloses, cellulose and lignin. The latter cannot be broken down by the enzymes and is voided via the rectum. Hemicelluloses are digestible fibre, but cellulose requires fermentation by microorganisms before it can be absorbed and utilized by the animal.

9.3 Water

Over 60% of an equine's body is water. It is vital for life. Any deprivation is not only cruel, but will depress appetite and reduce the equine's ability to work. It is therefore the most important requirement. It should be clean and free from salts. In fact, equines, and particularly donkeys, are well adapted to an arid environment – they will absorb any water available in their diet. Donkeys are more thirst tolerant than horses and will maintain their appetites in conditions of water deprivation. Nevertheless, their overall requirements are the same. Water should be provided to all working equines regularly during their work and ad lib during their resting time.

9.4 Energy Requirements

Energy is required to live and to work. In the young animal extra energy is required to grow. In the adult animal energy is required for reproduction; this includes oestrus, mating, pregnancy and lactation.

The main energy requirement is going to be supplied by the ingestion of carbohydrate. However, some energy may be supplied from the ingestion of protein that is in excess of the animal's protein requirement. Energy can also be supplied from a limited ingestion of fat.

In developed countries horses are often fed large amounts of so-called non-structural carbohydrates, which are mainly starch. These short feeds include corn, which is usually either oats, barley, wheat or maize, which are quickly converted by the liver to glucose. Horses, and particularly ponies and donkeys, tend to be too fat. This is poor husbandry; it compromises the animal's welfare as it causes many easily avoidable diseases. On the other hand, working equines that would benefit from such a diet do not receive one in the developing world. The ideal diet for an equine is a high-roughage diet containing a large amount of structural carbohydrate. The problem with a high-roughage diet is that it takes time to chew, in the region of 18 h/day. Time is just what a working equine does not have. Therefore, ideally a working equine should receive a balanced diet containing a large amount of long fibre containing structural carbohydrate, with a supplement of short feed containing non-structural carbohydrate.

Obviously, grass contains both structural and non-structural carbohydrate, and is the most natural food for an equine, bearing in mind that it was originally a grazing animal. Grass is also good because it provides protein. Once again, there is a disparity between the developed and the developing world. In the developed world the grass is 'too rich' and animals have ample time to eat too much. In the developing world the grass is of poor quality and working equines do not have enough time to graze it.

The fact that grass can contain high levels of protein is good for growing and lactating animals. Nonetheless, animals requiring a maintenance diet will convert the protein into carbohydrate and then to body fat. Also, this conversion requires an increase in liver function, which is not beneficial in animals with liver disease.

Grass will grow only if conditions are right. In temperate climates, as it requires a certain temperature it will grow only in the warmer times of the year. In tropical and semi-tropical climates, it will grow throughout the year, but rain or irrigation will be the regulating factor. Because of the seasonality of grass, it will often be preserved as hay or haylage, or even silage. The quality of these preserved forages will vary enormously, depending on a range of factors such as the state of the grass when it was cut and the method of preservation. The storage conditions are also important. There are certain aspects of preserving forage that are hazardous to horses, which will be discussed in Chapter 19 (Poisons).

As stated earlier, energy is required by all horses for maintenance. Growing horses require more, and this should be supplied at a regular rate so growth is also maintained at a regular rate. In the foal's early life, the amount of energy supplied will be regulated to some extent by the mare. In turn, she will require a regular supply of energy to maintain her lactation. This is a difficult balance to attain. Obviously, the mare will require extra energy in late pregnancy to allow for the larger energy requirement of the fetus. However, in proportion to her maintenance diet, that increase is not large. On the other hand, lactation, particularly peak lactation at 4–6 weeks, requires a large increase in energy. There is a temptation to overfeed pregnant mares in late pregnancy. This should be avoided. Nevertheless, it is vital that the energy in the diet is increased at a rapid but steady rate immediately following parturition, so that the mare can maintain her body weight and supply milk in increasing quantities. It should be borne in mind that a breeding mare will also be required to exhibit oestrus and become pregnant at this time.

Obviously, water in food weighs heavily, so that direct comparison between foods is not realistic based simply on weight. To allow for this, foods are valued by their dry matter (DM) content. It is then easy to work out how much digestible energy there is in 1 kg of DM for an individual feed. A horse will consume approximately 1.5% of its body weight of DM daily. If a horse weighs 500 kg (or that is the weight it should weigh), then it will eat 7.5 kg of DM. If its daily requirement for digestible energy is 44 megajoules (MJ)/day, then the diet will require an energy density of 5.87 MJ/kg DM (44/7.5). Reasonable-quality hay would represent such a diet. If the horse was working or lactating, then the diet would have to contain a higher percentage of digestible energy.

9.5 Protein Requirements

As stated above, protein can be converted by the horse to energy. However, horses, like all animals, require protein in its own right. Most diets for horses, e.g. hay, contain sufficient protein so that, providing the energy requirements are met, there is sufficient protein and therefore it is not necessary to calculate special protein requirements. A diet of just barley straw would supply insufficient energy and protein. Cut grass would supply sufficient protein (Fig. 9.2). It is important to remember that this rule of thumb does not apply to young growing animals, lactating mares or hard-working animals; these animals will need a diet with a higher protein percentage. The actual weight that the working horse is required to carry is important. This horse in Cyprus (Fig. 9.3) was actually not carrying an excessive load. As a rule of thumb, a horse should not carry more than 15% of its own weight. Working horses are rarely fed adequate diets (Fig. 9.4) when pulling carts. There is no hard-and-fast rule for how heavy a cart and its load should be. In the developing world most working equines are ponies, mules or donkeys which pull carts as shown in Fig. 9.4. In many situations owners work in groups, so they have several animals which can be used in rotation. In the UK there are rules on the number of passengers that can be pulled in a carriage rather than its weight. On the flat, two horses weighing 500 kg each could be expected to pull a carriage weighing 5000 kg. Two heavy horses weighing 800 kg each could be expected to pull 8000 kg.

9.6 Fat Requirements

Horses do not have a requirement for fat in their food. Nevertheless, it is often present and can be utilized by the horse to fulfil some of its energy requirements. It can be used beneficially in the prevention of some of the myopathies described in Chapter 12; for example, when a horse requires a large amount of energy for work but when that energy is supplied as carbohydrate, leading to rhabdomyolysis. In such cases it can be added to the diet as liquid vegetable oil, up to 500 ml daily for a 500 kg horse. Foods that are the by-products of oil extraction from plants often contain quite large amounts of fat and can be usefully fed to horses. These often contain fat-soluble vitamins which are useful to the horse, as described in Section 9.7.

9.7 Vitamins

Vitamins can be divided into two groups: (i) the fat-soluble vitamins A, D and E; and (ii) the water-soluble vitamins B, C and K. On the whole, the water-soluble vitamins are synthesized in

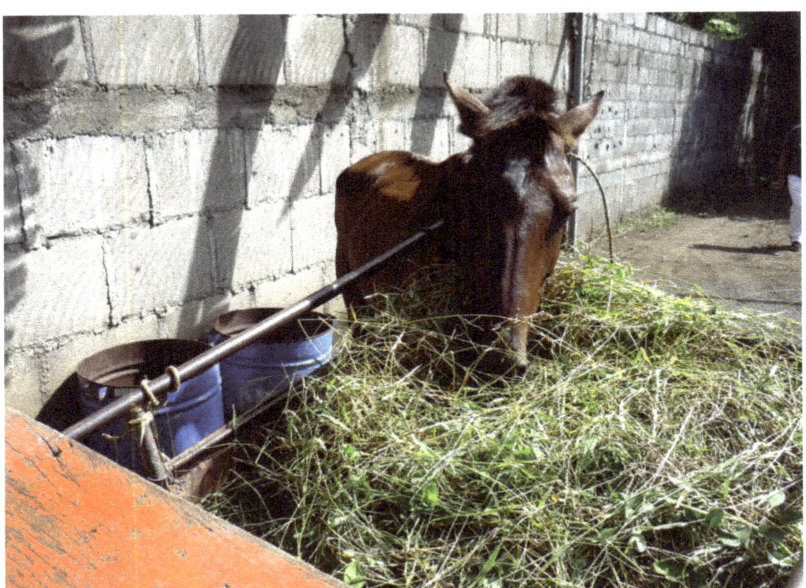

Fig. 9.2. A diet of cut grass would supply sufficient protein for this overworked, emaciated horse in Nicaragua.

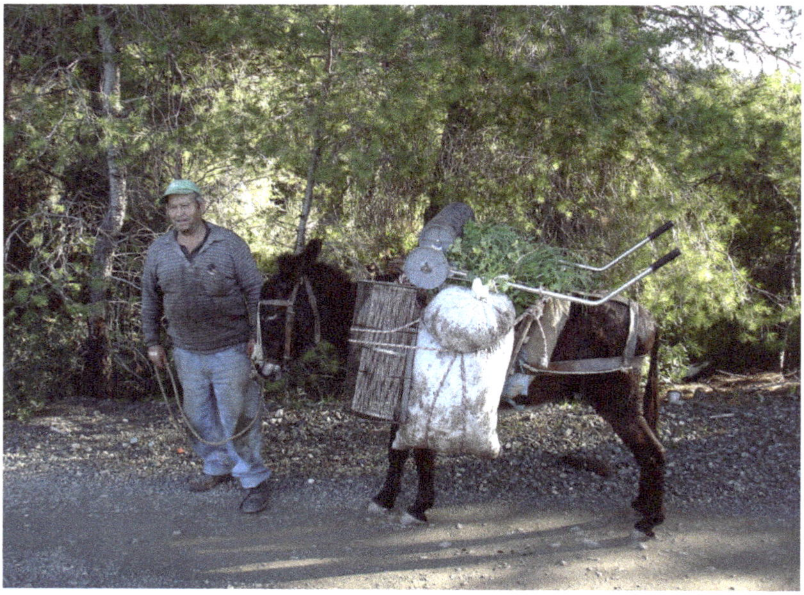

Fig. 9.3. Looks can be deceiving. The load was just bulky on this donkey in Cyprus.

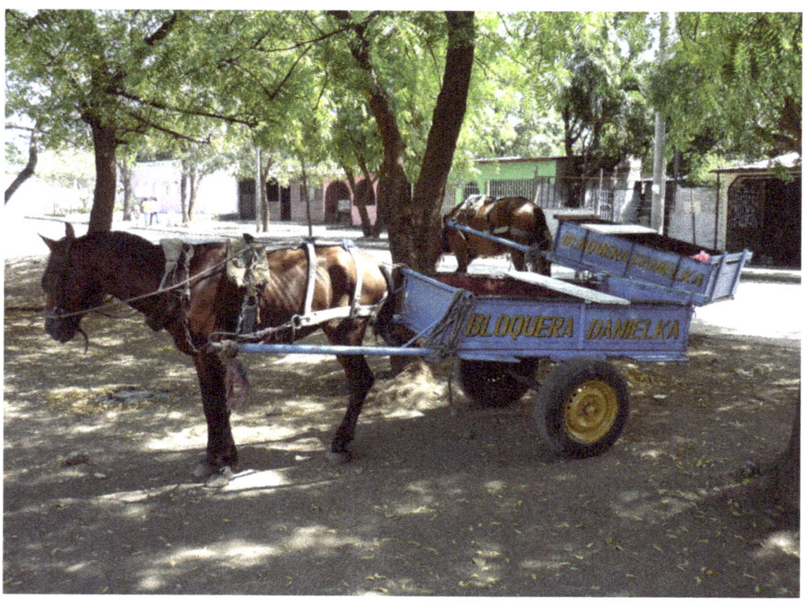

Fig. 9.4. The harness hides the emaciation of this pony in Nicaragua.

the large intestine of the horse. It is the fat-soluble vitamins that can be deficient in the horse.

The requirement for vitamin A is normally met by carotene, its precursor in plants. This is abundant in green grass and preserved forage. However, it is broken down by oxygen and sunlight and therefore may be lacking in old forage. As stated above, vegetable oils are a very good source. Deficiency can occur in young animals and pregnant and lactating mares. Vitamin D can also be deficient in this group of horses in temperate climates when there is little sunlight. This problem does not occur in the tropics or subtropics, except when horses are confined in buildings. Fat-soluble vitamins are stored in the liver, and so prolonged deficiency is required for deficiency signs to appear. The main sign seen in vitamin A deficiency is damage to the retina of the eye, causing irreversible blindness. Deficiency of vitamin D in young animals is manifest as rickets.

Vitamin E deficiency is not straightforward, as it is linked with the mineral selenium (see Section 9.8) in the prevention of nutritional muscular dystrophy. This condition is seen in selenium-deficient areas in hard-working horses and lactating mares. It is prevented by the addition of selenium to the diet or injections of vitamin E. Selenium should not be injected in the horse on account of the irritant nature of preparations.

The water-soluble vitamins become deficient only when certain plants are fed in excess to horses, e.g. bracken (causing thiamine, vitamin B_1 deficiency) or mouldy sweet clover hay (causing vitamin K deficiency). These diseases are described in Chapter 19.

9.8 Minerals

Small quantities of minerals are required by horses. Nonetheless excess of one mineral will cause problems with another. Supplementary feeding should be carried out with care.

Calcium and phosphorus

The need for these two minerals is much greater in young animals than in mature animals. Work does not increase the requirement, but pregnancy, lactation and age increase it by up to 50%. The ratio is important: ideally, it should be 1.5 parts calcium to 1 part phosphorus. However, provided there is sufficient overall phosphorus, the calcium portion of the ratio may be doubled. A horse fed mainly on roughage and little grain is likely to be low in phosphorus. On the other hand, a horse fed on a high-grain diet and low roughage is likely to be low in calcium.

Sodium and chlorine

Salt requirements are markedly influenced by losses in the sweat. A horse in moderate work in a temperate climate will lose 50–60 g of salt a day in sweat and 35–40 g of salt in the urine. This may be trebled in the tropics. Salt can be supplemented in the diet to about 1% of the total; it should also be offered ad lib. Salt poisoning is a danger only for a salt-starved animal not supplied with water.

Potassium

Deficiency is rarely a problem in healthy horses, as most roughages and protein supplements provide sufficient potassium. Only horses that are starved or receiving diuretics are at risk.

Magnesium

Unlike in ruminants, tetany caused by a lack of magnesium is extremely rare in horses, although it has been recorded. However, horses do require magnesium on a daily basis, at approximately 10 mg/kg body weight.

Iodine

Deficiency of iodine is rare as there is normally sufficient iodine in the salt. Excess is seen in horses fed large amounts of seaweed.

Copper, sulfur and molybdenum

These three minerals are linked. High sulfur or molybdenum levels may lead to a deficiency of copper. Primary copper deficiency is extremely rare, but secondary deficiency has been reported as causing anaemia in the foal.

Selenium

There is a link between selenium and vitamin E. Both are necessary, but the levels have not yet been determined.

Cobalt, iron, manganese, zinc and fluoride

These do not appear to cause deficiency or excess problems in equine nutrition.

9.9 Food Allergies

Food allergies are extremely rare, but will occur. They tend to be non-seasonal, unlike allergies to insects. Nevertheless, it should be remembered that certain foods are available only at specific times during the year. Owners often think allergies are caused by too high a dietary level of protein; this is not the case, but it is a specific protein in the diet that will trigger the allergic reaction, which is seen as urticaria. Certain intolerances to gluten, etc., seen in humans have not been demonstrated in the horse.

The clinician should always eliminate insect sensitivity and contact allergy before trying to test for food allergy. There are expensive blood tests available to test for food allergies, but these have not been verified in the horse. The only sure method of diagnosis and treatment is by removing certain items from the diet sequentially. Allergies can suddenly develop to a particular food, even if that food has been eaten by the horse for many years; that food should be removed from the diet for a minimum of 6 weeks. Assuming the condition improves, then the animal can be rechallenged, but it is a long-drawn-out procedure. Pruritus (skin irritation) is not normally a feature, unlike in atopy. This latter condition is an extremely rare condition in the horse. It is inherited and tends to be seen in young adult horses and becomes worse with age. Intradermal skin testing is the only realistic diagnostic test for atopy.

9.10 Consistency of the Diet

There are at least two important conditions which affect working equines which require the normal long fibre to be removed from the diet and be replaced by a completely pelleted diet or a mash. It is vital that the animal receives sufficient nutrients when it is suffering from colitis or severe dental problems. In both of these conditions appetite maybe reduced. Voluntary enteral nutrition is preferred, but horses that are not ingesting enough to meet the minimum recommended requirements should be fed via NGT. Naturally this should be carried out for as short a time as possible and be replaced by normal feeding. Dental problems can normally be solved very quickly. However, colitis may require a longer period of sympathetic nursing.

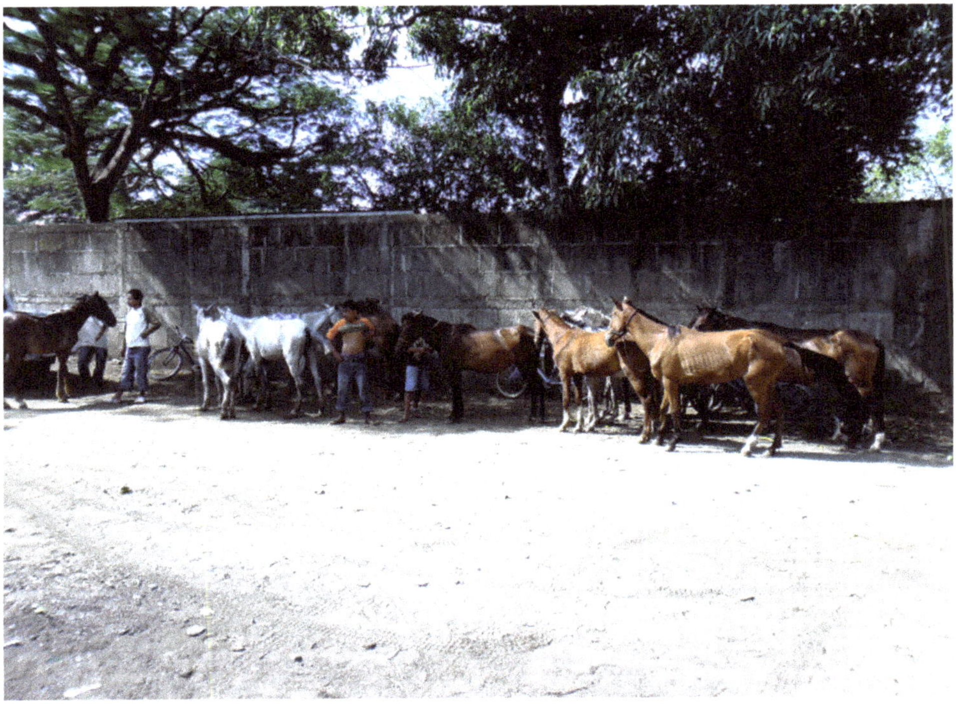

Fig. 9.5. A mixed bunch of equines awaiting dentistry in Nicaragua.

Further Reading

Hickman, J. (1987) *Horse Management*. Academic Press, Oxford, UK.

Svendsen, E.D. (1997) *The Professional Handbook of the Donkey*. Whittet Books, Linton, UK.

UK Government Code of Practice for Horse-drawn Vehicles (2000) https://www.gov.uk/government/publications/code-of-practice-for-horse-drawn-vehicles/code-of-practice-for-horse-drawn-vehicles.

10

Dentistry

Abstract

This chapter includes not only problems with teeth, but also conditions affecting the surrounding structures in the head. Tooth problems are in the main more important in working equines compared with animals in other disciplines, as working animals are rarely able to eat while they are working. It is important that owners are aware of this and that regular dental examinations and treatments as described in this chapter are adhered to.

10.1 The Reasons for Equine Dentistry

Equine dentistry is a major part of equine practice in the UK, accounting for an estimated 10–20% of practitioners' time. A survey of horse owners in the UK has shown that 84% of owners elect to have prophylactic dental treatment performed at set time intervals, and guidance on horse ownership suggests that dental examination and treatment should be performed on a 6-monthly basis. The importance of equine dentistry worldwide may not be so large. However, an understanding of the basic anatomy of the equine head is very important for the equine practitioner.

The horse evolved in the Americas *c.*55 million years ago. The dawn horse (*Hyracotherium*) was a rabbit-sized animal that browsed on soft leaves. It had short brachydont (low-crowned) teeth similar to human or canine teeth. There then occurred climatic changes and hence a change in vegetation. The evolving horse developed a large caecum and colon for microbial digestion of cellulose. The brachydont teeth of the dawn horse changed to long-crowned hypsodont teeth to cope with eating an abrasive grass diet containing high levels of silica, for up to 18 h/day. As the horse evolved there was a migration from South America up through North America, and across the Bering Strait to Asia. In Central Asia there was an evolutionary branching, with the southern branch going to the Middle East and Africa; the northern branch went to Europe. Humans first came into contact with horses at this period. There are drawings of wild horses in the Lascaux caves in south-west France dated *c.*15,000 BC. Horses were only a source of food then. However, the first evidence of equine domestication is bit-induced cheek teeth damage in a fossil equine skull dated *c.*4000 BC found near the Black Sea.

The Middle Eastern horses developed the small, delicate, often dish-shaped head of the modern Arab horse. These were the stock from which the thoroughbreds and Welsh ponies developed. The European branch produced the heavy horse breeds with their big head, the

DOI: 10.1079/9781800624283.0010

warmbloods and the traditional ponies. Man has crossed Middle Eastern-type horses with European-type horses; simplistically, we then get horses with a small head and large teeth and horses with a large head and small teeth. As you can imagine, this causes problems with dentition. Also, horses have evolved to eat a very abrasive long-fibre diet. Humans now provide soft long-fibre diets (rye grass is notoriously low in silicates) and soft short feeds, so that the natural abrasive quality of the diet has been removed. This also creates a need for equine dentistry.

There are structures other than the teeth that are important when considering equine dentistry, as described below. A list of equine dental equipment, and their respective functions, is given in Section 4.7.

10.2 Muscles of Mastication

The main muscles are the temporalis and the internal and external masseter. These should be palpated and examined for symmetry. Directly in front of a horse is not a very safe place to stand, but it is the only real way that the practitioner can examine the differences between the two sides and assess symmetry or, in the event of a problem, asymmetry.

10.3 The Temporo Mandibular Joint (TMJ)

This is a very functional joint. Equine dental technicians (EDTs) would have horse owners believe that joint problems are common. This is not the case. Arthritis of the TMJ is extremely rare and is normally a result of trauma and not the result of poor dental wear. The TMJs should be examined for lack of symmetry. If asymmetry is found then ultrasound is the best imaging modality for the TMJ. If using radiography, only skyline views are helpful. It should be stressed that major dental pathology might cause TMJ disease, but TMJ disease has not been shown to cause dental disease.

10.4 Equine Dentition

A horse has heterodont dentition. This means that it has different types of teeth. The canines and the first premolars are brachydont teeth; the incisors and cheek teeth are hypsodont teeth. Hypsodont teeth have a long reserve crown, which is slowly worn down by the grinding of the occlusal surface of the tooth. The rate of attrition for the cheek teeth is approximately 2.5 cm over 10 years. At one time it was thought that the teeth of the donkey were harder than those of the horse, but this has been shown to be incorrect. The tooth length is finite: no further tooth is formed, unlike in rodents. The horse is also diphyodont, having both deciduous and permanent teeth.

There is now a new system of nomenclature for equine teeth. It is not actually particularly new, but is new for equines. Invented by a Swiss human dentist, it is called the 'Tridan' system. Each tooth has two numbers. The first number shows which quadrant and the second number shows the exact tooth. The quadrants are numbered 1 to 4 by standing in front of the horse and starting at the top left (i.e. the horse's right side), then moving in a clockwise direction. The teeth are then numbered from the front. The central incisor is number 1, the lateral incisor is 2 and the corner incisor is 3; the canine, regardless of presence, is 4; the first premolar or 'wolf' tooth is 5, regardless of presence; the other three premolars are 6, 7 and 8 and the molars are 9, 10 and 11. To give you some examples: the right mandibular corner incisor would be 4/03, the left upper first premolar or 'wolf' tooth would be 2/05 and the third left mandibular molar would be 3/11.

It appears complicated, but with repeated usage it becomes much simpler. There is general confusion if you describe a tooth as e.g. the upper right second premolar. This is in fact the first cheek tooth in the cheek tooth row and may be the first premolar if the 'wolf' tooth is absent. If the practitioner is being very correct, the deciduous teeth should be numbered in quadrants of 5, 6, 7 and 8. Therefore, the central incisor in a yearling on the upper right-hand side would be 5/01. This would then be replaced by 1/01 at 2½ years of age. At the same stage another example would be the second premolar on the lower left arcade in a yearling, which would be 7/07; this would be replaced by 3/07 when the cap is shed.

10.5 Eruption Times of Equine Teeth

The eruption of deciduous teeth in foals is fairly consistent. At birth they have two cheek teeth in each cheek tooth row, i.e. 06 and 07. The 08s erupt within 1 month. They have their central incisors at birth. The laterals erupt within 1 week and the corners in 1 month. These incisors are replaced, starting with the centrals, at 2½ years, the laterals at 3½ years and the corners at 4½ years. The permanent premolars, starting rostrally, erupt at 2½, 3 and 4 years. There is good evidence that the maxillary cheek teeth shed their caps up to 6 months before the mandibular cheek teeth. There is also evidence that colts shed their caps earlier than fillies. The molars, which by definition are permanent, erupt at 1, 2 and 3½ years. It is worth remembering that the first molars, the 09s, are the oldest teeth in a horse's mouth. They are the most likely to give problems.

10.6 Prehension of Food

The 12 incisors, together with the lips and tongue, prehend the food. However, it should be remembered that horses can cope with significant incisor pathology without developing problems of 'dysprehension'. Weight loss in horses is extremely rarely associated with incisor problems. The incisors, like all teeth, have cementum on the outside, which attaches the tooth to the socket. This is soft and is worn away when exposed. Under the cementum is the enamel, which is the hardest substance in the body. It is composed of 96% inorganic salts. There are two types of enamel: type 1 is the hardest and the most brittle. This is found in the upper cheek teeth. Type 2 is slightly softer and less brittle. It is found in the incisors. The lower cheek teeth have a mixture of both types. The body of the incisor is formed by the dentine, which is 70% inorganic salts. It is softer and much less brittle than the enamel. Inside the dentine is the pulp cavity, which provides blood and nerves to the tooth. The pulp cavity lies rostral to the infundibulum. As the tooth wears it is replaced by secondary dentine, which takes on the colour of the food and forms the dental star.

10.7 Oral Examination

Like any veterinary examination, the oral examination should be preceded by the taking of history. The age and use of the horse are then recorded. Any signs of dental disease should be noted. These may be related to eating, *dysphagia*, or grinding of the food, *dysmastication*. The position and carriage of the head should be noted, particularly in relation to the horse's behaviour when being worked. Any problems with the bit should be noted.

A full examination of the outside of the head is the next stage. Particular attention should be given to any facial swellings, nasal discharge or smell. From a position in front of the horse the symmetry of the head is examined, with particular reference to the facial muscles, the masseters and temporalis and the temporomandibular joints.

The area of cheek over the cheek teeth should be pushed in towards the cheek teeth to gauge a pain reaction. If such a pain response is initiated, it is advisable to rasp the buccal aspects of the upper cheek teeth at this point, as application of a gag will be resented by the horse.

Next, the head is examined from both sides and the lips curled back to examine the incisors. The bars of the mouth are then examined and palpated. The movement of the jaw should be studied to estimate at what point the molar occlusal angle forces the incisors out of occlusion. At this stage it is useful to smell the horse's breath, before washing out the oral cavity with a dilute solution of chlorhexidine. The incisors should be examined before applying a gag (Fig. 10.1).

A Hausmann or similar gag should then be applied after warning the handler of the dangers (Fig. 10.2). Special arrangements need to be made if there are problems with the incisors. If examination reveals food matter still in the oral cavity it should be syringed out.

The commissures of the lips are then closely studied and the tongue reflected to examine the lingual aspect of the bars of the mouth. The tongue should be thoroughly examined and palpated.

The four cheek teeth rows should be palpated (Fig. 10.3) and then examined: a tongue retractor is useful here to perform a full examination. Next, the buccal aspect of the cheek teeth are examined with the aid of a cheek retractor.

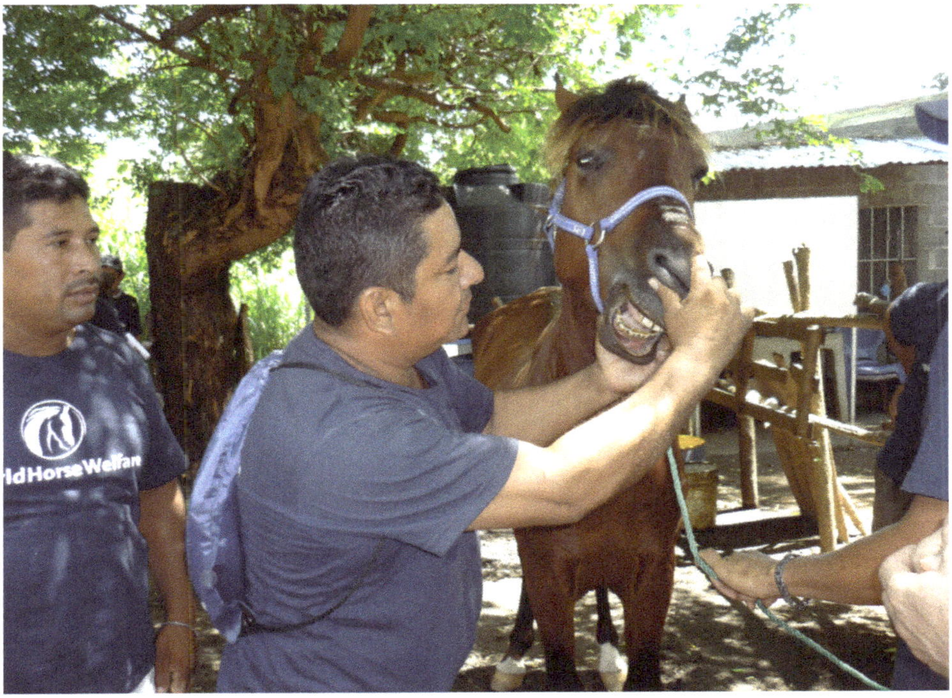

Fig. 10.1. The lower jaw has to be moved laterally to examine the incisor tables.

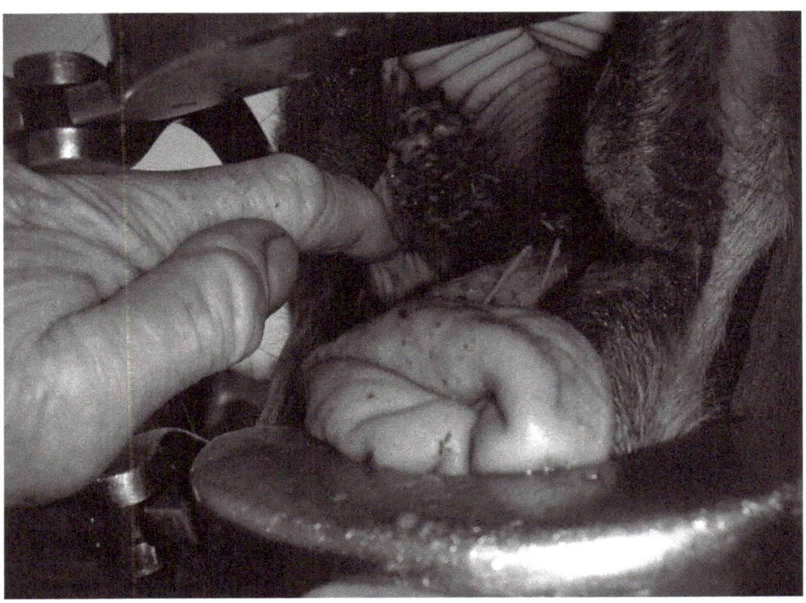

Fig. 10.2. Oral examination of the horse, with a gag inserted.

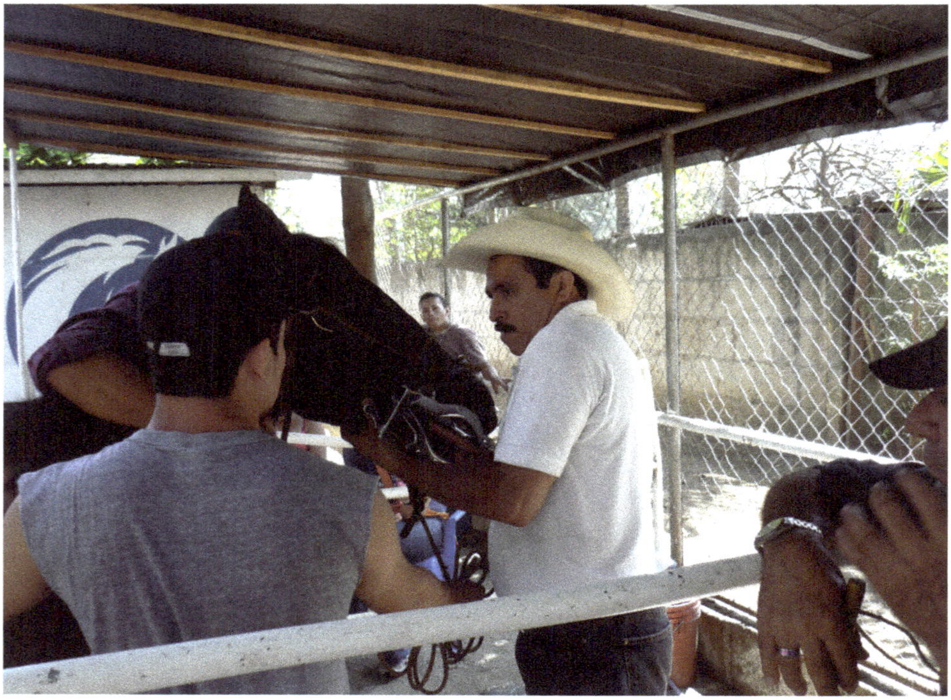

Fig. 10.3. Digital palpation is important.

Once each cheek tooth row has been examined as a whole to check for such abnormalities as wave mouth, shear mouth and diastema (see below), each individual tooth should be examined. The teeth are next checked for stability and the occlusal surface checked for any cavities. To accomplish this, a mirror and thin dental probe will be required. Naturally, the teeth should be counted to check for missing or extra teeth.

Last it is very important to record all the findings on a dental chart. The owner is then given one copy while the other is to be filed for your clinical records.

10.8 Ageing the Horse by Its Teeth

The eruption of the permanent incisors at 2½, 3½ and 4½ years of age is an accurate method of ageing a young horse. Examining the occlusal surfaces of the incisors for wear is also helpful, but less accurate. Numerous surveys have been conducted by veterinarians into ageing, and there is absolutely no doubt that as the horse gets older the accuracy diminishes. There is a definite reason for this. Some horses have deep infundibulae, others shallow. Some horses have pulp cavities near to the occlusal surface and others are deeper. So the effect of wear on the appearance of these two structures will vary enormously. Other means of ageing, e.g. hooks and grooves, are now known to be worthless. The take-home message is to record what you see but to put an exact figure only up to the age of 8 years. There is no doubt that as the incisors erupt with age they take on a more triangular shape and they appear to meet at an angle rather than in straight apposition.

The canines or tushes occur in male horses, regardless of castration. They can also occur in approximately 10% of mares, then appearing small or even 'blind' when they actually do not erupt through the gingiva. However, in the male they provide a useful clue in ageing, as they erupt at 4½–5 years. It is the 5-year-old horse with a full set of permanent incisors that may be confused with the 2-year-old with a full set of deciduous incisors. If the canine is seen, the horse must be 5 years or older, rather than 2. The canines are brachydont teeth, and they should not be confused with the first premolar or 'wolf' tooth, which is also a brachydont tooth. In the UK the first premolars are commonly seen in the upper jaw, but are extremely rare in the lower. However, in Australia and the USA they are seen more commonly in Standardbreds in the lower jaw.

10.9 Dental Problems Associated with the Incisors

The deciduous incisors are replaced by the permanent incisors from a rostral direction, i.e. the central incisors are replaced first, followed by the laterals and then the corners. Occasionally, the deciduous teeth will remain in situ, and such a horse should be examined carefully; if the retained deciduous tooth is changing the direction of the permanent tooth, the former should be removed (in reality it may be that the permanent tooth is not erupting in quite the correct direction and so is not pushing out the deciduous tooth). Very rarely there are supernumerary incisors present, and these are often extremely difficult to remove. Therefore, unless these are causing problems, they should be left alone. If incisors are fractured, then the loose fragment should be removed. If both fragments are loose, then they should both be removed. If food becomes packed between two incisors it should be regularly cleaned away from a caudal direction with a toothbrush. If the food has become tightly lodged, it should be removed with a dental pick and the diastema (gap between teeth, see below) should be widened with a hacksaw blade. Rarely, the incisors will have become covered by tartar, which should be removed with a small pair of extractors.

If an incisor has become excessively long it should be rasped down carefully, so that as soon as the pink stain of the pulp cavity is seen on the occlusal surface the rasping can stop. More rasping can be carried out in 3 months' time. In cases of shear mouth (described below) the incisors will show a marked slant, if the condition is unilateral. Should gradual correction of shear mouth be carried out then the incisor slant will correct itself. If the condition is bilateral then the incisors will take on the shape of a smile, with the corners of the upper incisors shorter than the central incisors and the lateral incisors being of intermediate length. The lower incisors will show a mirror image. This configuration is often seen in the normal donkey.

In the last 25 years, there has been a steep rise in the number of articles on equine odontoclastic tooth resorption and hypercementosis (EOTRH). This is primarily seen in incisors, but it is also seen in canines. It is extremely rare in cheek teeth. Early diagnosis is difficult to achieve (Albers *et al.*, 2023). The radiographic appearance of subtle pathological changes has not been described in detail and might be confused with age-related changes.

The disease is progressive, and the only realistic treatment is extraction of badly affected teeth. The cause is as yet unknown. Individuals should be monitored as there is every indication that the condition is painful.

10.10 Dental Problems Associated with the Canines

The canines are brachydont teeth covered in an enamel layer. They are always present in male horses regardless of when castration has been performed. They erupt at 4½–5 years of age. They can cause problems on eruption, as the mucosa may be tender just before penetration of the tooth, but this is a short-lived phenomenon. They also appear in 5–10% of mares. They can cause problems if they do not perforate the mucosa, when they are termed 'blind canines'. Owners often think they are a problem, but in reality they are not; they are often alleged to be a cause of headshaking, but this can be refuted by covering the mucosa with local anaesthetic gel. If the horse continues with its problems, then these are unlikely to be due to the canines.

The canines have long, curved roots which make extraction impossible except by using a buccostomy technique. However, there is actually no good reason to extract them. Owners complain sometimes that they are too long, but this does not actually cause any problems. They should not be clipped, cut or rasped as the enamel layer will be destroyed and the pulp may become infected. It is common for them to become covered in tartar, which should be removed regularly with a small pair of extractors to prevent gingivitis.

10.11 'Wolf' Teeth

The task of removal should be viewed with caution. Sadly, there is often little evidence that the 'wolf' tooth is causing the problem. It is often extracted on the whim of the owner. The most frightening complication of removal is severance of the palatine artery, which runs palatally to the upper cheek teeth. If the palatine artery is accidentally severed, there will be a large amount of haemorrhage; it is alarming to the owner but not life threatening. The vessel is impossible to pick up with artery forceps and ligate, so this should not be attempted. Haemorrhage can be controlled by digital pressure. However, as soon as the finger is removed haemorrhage recommences. The horse should then be sedated. A towel, not cotton wool, which is always messy, should be rolled up into a tight roll, and this should be put in the mouth behind the incisors in between the cheek teeth. The jaws should then be clamped shut with a head collar that is a size too small for the horse, and this should then be left in place for at least 45 min. Next, the mess in the stable should be cleared up, and the horse led out into a paddock before the towel is carefully removed. There still may be some haemorrhage, but it will not be so noticeable.

'Wolf' teeth very rarely interfere with the bit or the noseband. If these teeth are not closely aligned to the 1/06 or 2/06, they are more likely to cause problems, and this is particularly so if they stick out at an angle buccally. If there is any doubt as to whether they are 'wolf' teeth or canines, radiographs should be taken. If they are loose, they may affect head carriage. If they occur in the mandibles, as seen in Standardbreds, they might well interfere with the bit. The most common reason for removing them, however, is because they obstruct the clinician from rasping the 1/06 and 2/06 into a smooth outline.

Good sedation is vital for 'wolf' tooth removal. Gel containing local anaesthetic should be rubbed into the gingiva surrounding the tooth, then 2 ml local anaesthetic locally infiltrated around the tooth. Some practitioners find it easier to use a butterfly catheter to do this. The tooth then needs to be elevated, and it is easier to do this without a gag. The elevators need to be concave so they do not slip off the tooth; you can use the corer-type elevators, either Burgess or Musgrave. These come with an offset handle and a set of different-sized circular elevators. The main thing to remember when pushing up with these instruments is to keep one hand on the horse's nose to warn you if the horse is about to move. The lower hand doing the pushing must not only push up but also push the handle in medially. This will ensure that, should the instrument slip, the head of the instrument will be directed buccally and not towards the palate. Once the tooth feels loose it should be grasped with forceps for extraction. Antibiotics and pain relief must be given. Tetanus cover, as with all extractions, is mandatory. There is a little haemorrhage, but rarely much.

'Wolf' teeth are very easy to extract in young animals; they normally erupt at about 6 months. Many fall out naturally at 2½ years of age, when the 5/06 and 6/06 are shed as caps.

If the 'wolf' tooth breaks off above the gingiva, then it is important to extract it. If there is very little crown left, it can be removed with Rongeur forceps (see Section 4.7). If broken off below the gingiva, it can be left as this will rarely cause any harm, but the owner should be informed. After removal it is worth checking that there is not a sharp buccal point on the first cheek tooth or, worse, a focal overgrowth. If there is, the first cheek teeth should be rasped smooth.

10.12 Dental Problems Associated with the Cheek Teeth

Introduction

As mentioned above, cheek teeth are hypsodont teeth with a long reserve crown and short roots. Each of the four rows has six teeth – three premolars and three molars, which act together as a single grinding unit. There is an angulation of the 6 and the 11 so that there is a compression force keeping them together. This prevents the formation of gaps between the teeth, called diastema. As this is a Greek word, the plural is diastemata. A diastema, if formed, will allow food packing into the periodontal pocket and a resulting gingivitis, which is the most painful equine dental disease. Elephants avoid diastema, having evolved a single, large cheek tooth in wear, which lasts approximately 10 years and is replaced up to seven times, which is one of the reasons that the elephant lives so much longer than the horse.

The equine cheek teeth lie caudal to the bars of the mouth, which is the normal position for the bit. Some horsemen erroneously call the bars of the mouth the diastema. The bit lies up against the commissures of the lips, but does not lie anywhere near the normal position of the first premolar. As stated above, the first premolars are vestigial teeth, called 'wolf' teeth, with short, tapered roots, unlike the canines, which have long, curved roots.

There is another interesting adaptation of the cheek teeth, when a horse is said to be anisognathic. This means that the upper cheek teeth are approximately 25% wider than the lower cheek teeth, with the occlusal surfaces of the cheek teeth being at an angle of 10–35° – the molar table angle. When the incisor teeth are in occlusion the cheek teeth are not in occlusion. This occurs when the horse is prehending food or when the head is held by the handler 'in collection' (the head is held up, with the chin tucked in towards the neck). However, as the incisors move laterally, one cheek tooth row comes into occlusion. Due to the molar table angle the incisors then move apart as the arcade grinds. The incisors then move to the other side and the other cheek tooth row occludes. This movement is large when long fibre is being chewed but is shorter with short feed.

Therefore, in a normal horse fed principally on long fibre the cheek teeth are ground down straight across the occlusal surface at the normal molar table angle, but if the horse is not fed long fibre it eats with a chopping motion. The buccal sides of the upper cheek teeth develop sharp enamel points and the lingual sides of the narrower lower cheek teeth also develop enamel points. These sharp points cause trauma to the cheeks and the tongue (see below). If these are not corrected they are self-perpetuating, as they restrict the movement of the teeth still further. This then makes the molar table angle more acute. If this becomes >45°, it is said to be a shear mouth (see below). The sharp enamel points are formed from the lateral vertical ridges of the upper cheek teeth and the medial vertical ridges of the lower cheek teeth. The sharp buccal points on the front maxillary cheek teeth will interfere with the bit and cause the horse at best discomfort, and at the worst severe pain.

The upper cheek teeth have infundibulae. If you imagine a tooth in the middle of an arcade in profile from a rostral perspective, there are two infundibulae formed from the occlusal surface up into the body of the tooth. If you then imagine a cross-section of the tooth, these infundibulae will look like two eyes of cementum and enamel. The bulk of the tooth is dentine, but nature, however, has not created the tooth and the infundibulae round and square but has made the enamel layer crinkle-shaped. This allows for a larger amount of enamel on the occlusal surface. The lower cheek teeth do not have infundibulae; they have an irregular arrangement of enamel. Because of this and the fact that there is a mixture of types 1 and 2 of enamel, there are fewer fractures in the mandibular cheek teeth.

When you look into a horse's mouth you will see ridges on both the hard palate and cheek teeth. The ridges on the hard palate allow the horse to move the bolus of food between each side slowly backwards before it is swallowed. It is therefore ground many times. The ridges on the teeth are called transverse ridges, and these increase the grinding surface area. They are locked in a pattern with the ridges on the lower cheek tooth row. If these transverse ridges become excessive, they will form a diastema in the opposite arcade. The clinician must be aware that transverse ridges are normal: the horse has evolved over 40,000 years and these ridges are a useful adaptation to give the horse more grinding surface. They should be rasped only if they are really excessive (Fig. 10.4).

Shedding of the deciduous premolars

The deciduous premolars slowly become ground down until they are like little hats over the permanent premolars underneath them. These are called dental caps. Starting rostrally, they are

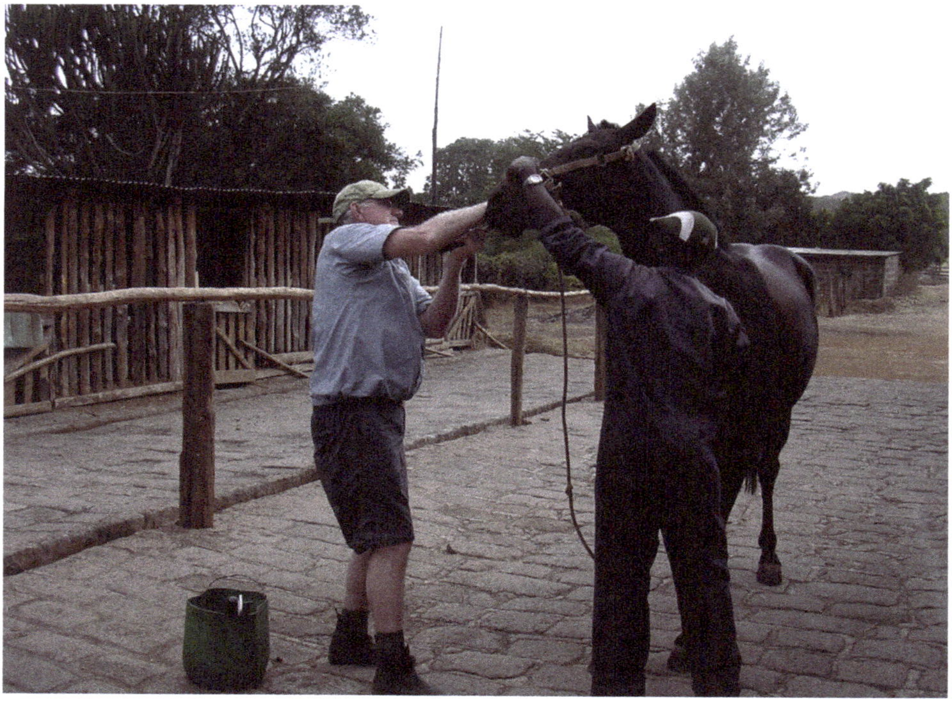

Fig. 10.4. Rasping can be performed without a gag.

shed at 2½, 3 and 4 years. They are therefore not really a problem in the horse that is not bitted at this stage; however, they are a real problem in the young horse required to be bitted. There is now a great deal of pressure put on veterinarians to remove these caps prematurely: this should be resisted. Caps should be removed only if loose or the cap in the opposite jaw has been lost. Otherwise, there may be damage to the underlying permanent tooth.

Swellings may be seen on the mandibles of the young horse. If these are equal on both mandibles they are not a problem. They are particularly common in young thoroughbreds and are often called 3-year-old bumps. The reason for their formation is that there is not sufficient space in the mandible to accommodate the 8 cm of a cheek tooth. If the swellings are not mirrored on the opposite side, they should be monitored carefully. If they burst they are likely to be a tooth root or apical abscess. As the tooth is worn down the tooth will erupt and the bone in the mandible will thicken with age.

Wearing of the cheek teeth

Slowly, the cheek teeth become worn away at roughly 2.5 mm/year. Eventually, most of the enamel surrounding the tooth will have disappeared, leaving just the less hard dentine. This becomes smooth, like a pebble on the beach. Americans actually state that these animals have 'smooth mouths'. Great care is needed when rasping the odd tiny remaining enamel points, as the roots now are very short and it is easy to loosen the tooth. Eventually these teeth will drop out on their own, a condition called oligodontia that is common in older animals. It can also occur in the younger animal that does not develop the correct number of teeth, but this situation is very rare. Oligodontia results in a super-eruption of the opposing tooth. Also, because of pressure of the number 6 teeth caudally and the number 11 teeth rostrally, the cheek teeth tend to move and the spaces between become smaller. The opposite condition is called polyodontia, where there are supernumerary

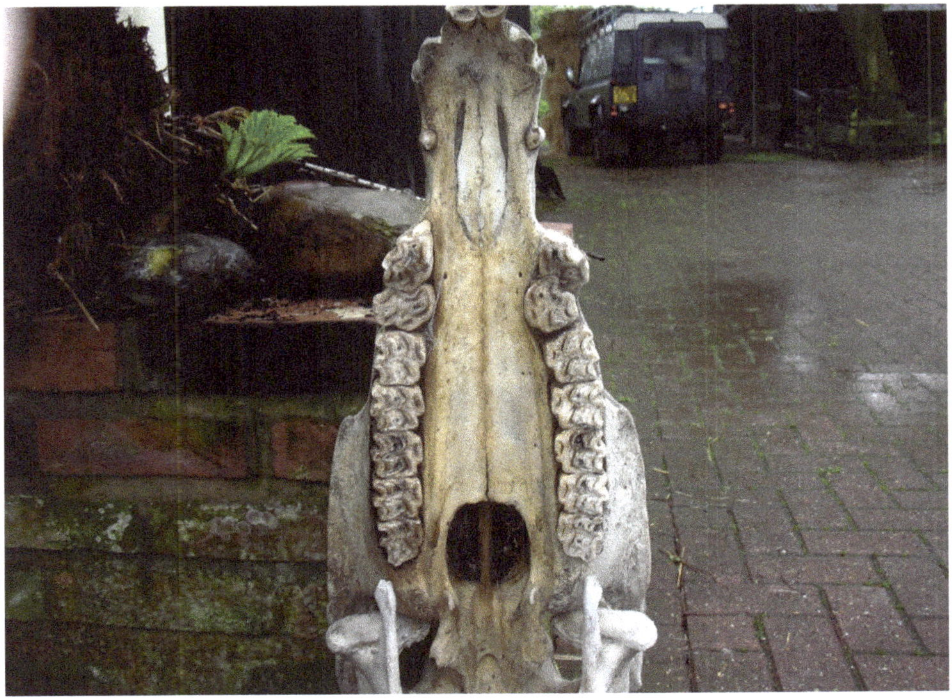

Fig. 10.5. Polyodontia.

cheek teeth, an extra caudal cheek tooth being the most common. Figure 10.5 shows the skull of a Suffolk Punch with an extra 1/12 and 2/12. These extra teeth may be connated (i.e. double teeth).

Parrot mouth

The correct terminology for this condition is 'relative rostral displacement of the maxillary teeth'. This may simply be a lengthening of the maxillary bone rostrally to the cheek teeth, i.e. the maxillary teeth are in normal apposition but the upper incisors are rostrally displaced with regard to the lower incisors: this is a true parrot mouth. Raising the jaw to pull hay out of a hay net can increase the visual effect. Horses are grazing animals, so any horse with a parrot mouth should be fed on the floor, when the effect is then lessened. If the whole maxillary bone is lengthened, then the cheek teeth will be rostrally displaced. Overgrowths will form on the rostral aspect of the front upper cheek teeth and another two overgrowths will form on the caudal aspect of the most caudal lower cheek teeth. Care must be taken when deciding whether there are lower caudal focal overgrowths in small-headed horses. Such horses, e.g. Arabs, have an upward curve of their lower caudal cheek teeth called the curve of Spee. The level of the lower caudal cheek tooth may be normal for that horse and not a lower caudal focal overgrowth.

The opposite condition is often called 'sow mouth', or in the USA it is called 'monkey mouth'. It is very much rarer than parrot mouth, and really should be termed 'relative rostral displacement of the mandibular cheek teeth'. This condition is seen only in the smaller pony, where an overgrowth on the rostral aspect of the lower cheek teeth and the caudal aspect of the upper cheek teeth occurs.

Sharp enamel overgrowths

Likely to be found on the buccal aspect of the maxillary cheek teeth and on the lingual aspect of the mandibular cheek teeth, these should be removed by rasping, keeping the rasp at an angle of 45° to the overgrowths. It is important that the occlusal surface is not rasped. The clinician may find it easier to carry out this procedure on the maxillary cheek teeth if the gag is not in position. In some smaller horses and donkeys the upper cheek teeth rows may curve palatally, caudally. In this case a long, flat rasp with an offset will be required. If a solid carbide blade is used it will need to be set 'on the pull'. Some clinicians prefer to rasp the sharp enamel overgrowths on 1/11 and 2/11 with the gag in position, across the mouth, using an upturned rasp. If this has a solid carbide blade it should be set 'on the pull'. Often, there is a sharp enamel overgrowth on the lingual aspect of the 3/10 and 4/10 teeth. The use of a Gledhill rasp will greatly improve the ease of rasping.

Focal enamel overgrowths

As described above, these will tend to be present on 1/06 and 2/06 in the upper jaw, and on 3/11 and 4/11 in the lower jaw in cases of parrot mouth. In cases of sow mouth, they will tend to be on 1/11 and 2/11 in the upper jaw and on 3/06 and 4/06 in the lower jaw. These are often called hooks, beaks or ramps by the layman, but clinicians should stick to the term focal enamel overgrowths to avoid confusion.

These overgrowths will need to be rasped to reduce them to the same level as the rest of the cheek tooth row. Care needs to be taken when rasping the number 6 teeth that the pulp cavity is not entered by excessive rasping. If a small area of pink dentine is seen, rasping should be halted and further work then rescheduled for 3 months' time. If actual blood is seen then calcium hydroxide powder should be applied, which will hopefully seal the pulp cavity and prevent infection. The clinician will find it very difficult checking the pulp cavity of the number 11 teeth, although a mirror may be helpful. However, it is very rare for the pulp cavity to be that close to the occlusal surface. The clinician must also take care that focal enamel overgrowths on 3/11 and 4/11 are real overgrowths and not just imagined on account of the angle of Spee.

Focal overgrowths can be checked by examining the depth of the exposed crown relative to the mucosa. If the level is the same but the caudal border is raised, then there is a focal overgrowth that needs rasping. Rasping of cranial focal overgrowths is carried out by placing the rasp between the gag and the jaw. Care must be taken that the horse does not move its head violently, as the rasp will be difficult to withdraw quickly. The type of rasp used needs to be short, with a downturned angle to the head; alternatively, an offset short rasp can be used, often termed a 'molar roller'. If a solid tungsten carbide blade is used, this needs to be set to cut 'on the push'. To rasp focal overgrowths on the caudal cheek teeth the rasp needs to be very slim so that it can be slipped slowly down the cheek tooth row, then placed firmly on the caudal overgrowth and moved sharply forward. If a solid tungsten carbide blade is used it must be set 'on the pull'. As this procedure is very laborious the clinician may need motorized dental equipment; obviously, with the use of such equipment, the horse will need to be sedated.

Excessive transverse ridges (ETRs)

Transverse ridges are normal and are vital for the horse to enlarge its cheek teeth area to increase the cheek teeth's grinding ability. However, occasionally the transverse ridges become excessive. They then tend to form a diastema between the opposing cheek teeth. In these cases, with the gag in place the excessive ridge is rasped down to the level of the rest of the cheek tooth row. It is important to maintain the correct molar table angle.

Wave mouth

A wave mouth is said to be present when the occlusal surface of the cheek tooth row is undulating. Normally, a mirror-image wave is seen on the opposing cheek tooth row. These waves may have started with ETRs, but this has not been proved. The clinician has a dilemma: excess tooth must not be removed from the occlusal surface; equally, it would be beneficial to the horse if the wave is smoothed out. Therefore, with care the clinician should rasp down the high points of the exposed crown in both the upper and lower cheek tooth rows. The aim is to lessen the wave and not totally obliterate it. This procedure can be repeated at 3-monthly intervals.

Step mouth

In some ways step mouth can be a more advanced case of wave mouth. However, the former does not normally develop in the same manner, but instead from loss of cheek teeth; opposing teeth then super-erupt. In rare cases there are extra cheek teeth – polyodontia (see above). The clinician has to use judgement as to the merits of rasping the overgrown teeth, leaving them alone or extracting them.

Missing cheek teeth

This is a condition called oligodontia, normally occurring with age (see above). Nonetheless, a few individuals will not develop teeth, either as an inherited defect or from trauma to the dental bud during development. Without dental management these cases will develop into step mouth, as the teeth opposite the missing teeth will super-erupt.

Over-erupted cheek teeth

These occur opposite missing teeth. The problem of super-eruption tends to occur in younger animals. These teeth need to be rasped down in stages, as the pulp cavity will not be very far below the occlusal surface. They should never be cut with shears, as there is a danger that the tooth will split in a vertical direction. Equally, they should not be sawn with embryotomy wire – either the pulp cavity will be entered or the heat generated will cause the death of the tooth.

Shear mouth

It is normal for a horse to have a molar table angle, with the buccal sides of the maxillary cheek teeth higher than the palatal sides. This is mirrored by the mandibular cheek teeth, where the lingual sides are higher than the buccal sides. The molar table angle used to be considered to be 10–15°, but it is now known that it can be as great as 30° and still be considered normal. Exact measurement is difficult, but any angle >45° is considered abnormal and is called a shear mouth. This can occur bilaterally, but is much more common unilaterally. Authors in Newmarket (Grant and Barnett, 2019) report a case secondary to temporohyoid osteoarthropathy on the left-hand side of a 20-year-old horse which had cheek teeth rows abnormally steep (50° from horizontal). This was diagnosed by CT examination. Normally, the clinician will be alerted to the condition as the incisors will have a slant on their occlusal surface. The best way of dealing with this is to rasp the long side of the cheek teeth slowly, i.e. taking off a centimetre or so every 3 months. There is little need to rasp the incisors, as they will correct themselves.

Motorized rasping of teeth

The use of high-speed motorized equipment has now become the norm in the UK, Europe and North America. The author is convinced that it's use will become more widespread in working equines in the developing world. There are dangers, particularly of over rasping. It should be stressed that entry into the pulp cavity should be avoided *at all costs*. Even the hint of pink in the dentine is dangerous. The other danger is thermal injury, as pointed out by one author (Pascoe, 2018). He concludes that research clearly indicates that there is a likelihood of uncooled motorized instruments causing significant heating of dental tissues during their use. The consequences of this heating remain unestablished in the clinical situation, although it is clear that temperature increases to the levels likely to cause thermal trauma to the pulp in other species are possible with inappropriate use. His final conclusion is that using water-cooled instruments can eliminate temperature increases.

Loose cheek teeth

Whenever the mouth is examined, the clinician should feel all the teeth individually to check for loose ones. If any are loose these need to be extracted, as they will cause pain when the horse is chewing. Sometimes they are so loose they can be removed with the fingers without any sedation, but in most cases sedation will be required. The tooth can then be grasped by a pair of molar extraction forceps. The tooth should be rocked from side to side and will eventually come free and may be removed. There is no need to pack the hole, as granulation tissue will rapidly fill the cavity.

Diastema

This is the term used for a gap in between two teeth. Normally, food will become packed into this gap, then will ferment and cause halitosis; the next stage will be gingivitis, the most painful equine dental disease. The horse will demonstrate this pain by quidding (dropping) its food. The initial course of action should be to clean out all the food from the teeth with a dental pick. If there are several diastemata (plural), a water pick is useful. The ETR above or below the diastema should then be rasped.

Often, with a week's course of antibiotics and NSAIDs the mouth will settle down and no further action need be taken. Slowly, the rostral caudal drift will bring the cheek teeth together and the mucosa will regenerate. If this does not resolve the quidding problem, then the diastema should be widened with a diastema burr in a 'Powerfloat', a fairly expensive piece of equipment that may not be available; it is battery-powered with a set of three diastema burrs. It is very important not to enter the pulp cavity of either tooth. The clinician should start burring with the smallest conical burr. This is then followed by the bigger conical burr, and finally the larger round-headed burr. This is a much less invasive technique than extraction. Also, as no real gap will be left in the arcade, there will be no ensuing super-eruption of the opposing tooth.

Infundibular caries in cheek teeth

These have been recognized for over a century. However, the author found no evidence of them in a post-mortem study of 50 equine skulls published in *Equine Veterinary Education* (Brigham and Duncanson, 2000). Their clinical significance has recently gained renewed interest (du Toit, 2017). This author found them highly prevalent in the UK equine population, particularly in older animals. They were most commonly seen in cheek tooth 09, with the rostral infundibular most commonly affected. They commonly resulted in endodontic infections or fractured teeth. Early identification with disease progression is required with treatment to prevent painful dental disease. Workers in Edinburgh (Borkent *et al.*, 2017) found infundibular caries to be common but they found no specific diet to be the cause.

Peripheral caries

Infundibular caries, particularly of the maxillary cheek teeth, have received considerable attention in the literature. More recently, there has been closer scrutiny of caries located on the buccal, lingual and palatal aspect of cheek teeth; so-called peripheral caries (Barnett, 2019). The aetiopathogenesis dental caries in most species is similar, with microorganisms in the oral cavity metabolizing dietary carbohydrates and producing acid that dissolves the mineralized tissues of the teeth. Of the three structural dental tissues of the teeth; cementum, dentin and enamel, it is the cementum that has the lowest mineral content and is thus the most readily demineralized in less acid conditions. Cementum lines the infundibulae of the maxillary cheek teeth and the periphery of all equine teeth, and thus is one of the reasons these locations are particularly prone.

From scanning the literature, it would appear that the incidence of peripheral caries has risen dramatically. It has been postulated that this is because clinicians are better equipped to diagnose them. The author does not agree with this hypothesis but considers the feeding of fermented forages and concentrates is a more likely causation.

Fissure fractures

These fractures have been reported in many studies and yet their clinical relevance is not known. It is certainly possible that they may allow bacteria to reach the pulp. They may also lead to slab fractures. At the present time, the author agrees with most practitioners that their recording on dental charts would be too onerous to be widely carried out.

Apical abscessation of the cheek teeth

The cause of apical abscesses is debatable. It certainly can be caused by damage to the pulp on the occlusal surface of the tooth, but it can also be caused by infection tracking down beside the tooth from damage to the gingiva and the alveolar socket. Dental caries is rare, but may provide an entry port for infection. The apex of the mandibular teeth may be damaged by trauma, again leading to infection. Last, infection may be blood-borne.

The main sign of an abscess in the mandibular cheek teeth is a swelling below the tooth that may then fistulate. Clinicians should be aware that bilateral mandibular swellings in 2- or 3-year-old horses are normal (see above); these are formed because there is not sufficient room in the bone for the tooth. Swellings are considered diseased only if they are fistulated or unilateral. If there is a unilateral swelling, or indeed a fistula, the horse should be given antibiotics for 1 month to see whether the abscess will disappear; if it does not then extraction is indicated. The roots of the number 6, 7 and sometimes 8 maxillary cheek teeth lie in the maxillary bone. The sign of an apical abscess will be a swelling and/or fistula. Once again 1 month of antibiotics should be tried in hope of medical resolution. If the fistula remains, extraction will be required. Normally, the apices of the number 8 and 9 maxillary cheek teeth lie in the rostral maxillary sinus; the apices of the number 10 and 11 teeth lie in the caudal maxillary sinus; these two sinuses are interconnected. Any apical abscess will be manifest as a unilateral, foul-smelling nasal discharge. A month's course of antibiotics should be tried but is rarely successful in controlling the discharge, and so extraction is the only course of action.

10.13 Nerve Blocks

Introduction

Perineural nerve blocks are often used in equine practice, especially since the use of diagnostic and surgical procedures in the standing sedated horse have expanded over recent decades. Normally, blind approaches are used and these will be fully discussed. In human medicine, the role of guided techniques, such as ultrasound guidance, advanced imaging guidance and nerve stimulator guided techniques are described. They are mainly too advanced for this publication. However, they are mentioned for further reading (Hermans *et al.*, 2019).

Local anaesthetic agents

Table 10.1 lists anaesthetic agents commonly used in horses.

Mental nerve block

A mental nerve block desensitizes the mental branch of the mandibular nerve (the mandibular branch of the trigeminal nerve (CN V). It is used for:

- surgery of the lower lip;
- incisor extraction;
- lower incisor endodontic and restorative procedures;
- lower wolf tooth removal; and
- lower canine treatments.

Technique

The mental foramen is located on the lateral aspect of the mandible in the interdental space (Fig. 10.6) and can be palpated externally. A vein emerges from the foramen alongside the nerve. A 21G × 40 mm needle with its hub bent at a slight angle is introduced into the skin approximately 1 cm rostral to the foramen and directed caudal using a digit to guide the point into the foramen (Fig. 10.6).

Infraorbital nerve block

An infraorbital nerve block desensitizes the infraorbital (IO) branch of the maxillary branch of the CN V. It is used for:

Table 10.1. Anaesthetic agents commonly used in horses. Used with permission from Tremaine (2019).

Drug	Trade name	Lipid solubility (Potency compared to procaine)	Time to onset (min)	Estimated duration (min)	Use
Lignocaine (lidocaine)	Lignol 2% w/v solution for injection (Dechra) Wilcain solution for injection (Dechra)	Low toxicity, rapid onset (2x)	5–15	30–60 (>180 with adrenaline)	Infiltration nerve block
Prilocaine	Citanest (Dentsply)	Low toxicity, rapid onset	5–15	30–60	Infiltration nerve block
Mepivacaine	Intra-epicaine 20 mg/ml solution for injection for horses (Dechra)	More effective in low pH and hence inflamed tissues (2x)	5–30	>90	Infiltration nerve block
Bupivacaine	Marcain (AstraZeneca)	High, long duration, poor penetration in inflamed tissues, higher toxicity (8x)	15–30	>240	Long-acting nerve block, epidural analgesia
Amethocaine (tetracaine)	Minims (Bausch + Lomb)	High, long duration			Topical corneal or gingival analgesia
Benzocaine	Orajet (Dentsply Sirona)	Good penetration of skin and mucous membranes	2–5		Topical gingival analgesia

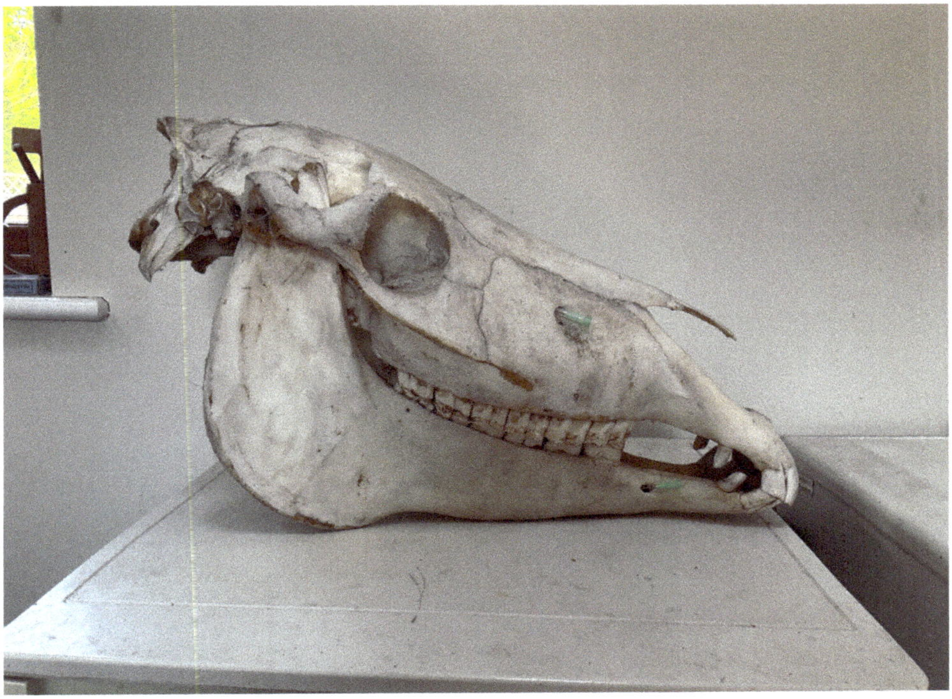

Fig. 10.6. The infraorbital foramen on the maxilla and the mental foramen on the mandible.

- desensitization of the upper lip and nostrils; and
- dental procedures to the upper incisors, canines, wolf teeth, incisive bone and rostral premolars.

Technique

The horse should be sedated before performing this nerve block as patients can respond violently to it. A 21G × 40 mm needle that has been bent to facilitate syringe attachment should be used. The IO foramen, from where the IO nerve emerges from the maxillary bone (Fig. 10.6), is obscured by the musculus levator nasolabialis but can be located by displacing the muscle dorsally. It lies 1 cm dorsal to an imaginary line joining the rostral facial crest to the nasoincisive notch. The direction of the canal is worth noting, as the needle should ideally be introduced parallel to it. The foramen is approached from 1 cm rostral. Ideally, the needle is placed at the foramen and 1 ml of local anaesthetic is introduced subcutaneously before advancing the needle further. If the needle is advanced into the foramen at its ventral aspect, the risk of trauma to the nerve is minimized and, when in position, 4 to 5 ml of local anaesthetic can be injected slowly. This then flows along the canal, desensitizing branches to maxillary premolars. The IO nerve is extremely sensitive and even in heavily sedated horses a sudden vertical movement of the head can be evoked when the nerve is stimulated or contacted. The location of the foramen and nerve can also be determined accurately using ultrasound guidance (Hermans *et al.*, 2019) (Fig. 10.7).

Maxillary nerve block

The maxillary branch of the CN V is desensitized when using a maxillary nerve block. This block is used for:

- maxillary sinus surgery;
- maxillary dental procedures;
- nasum septal surgery;

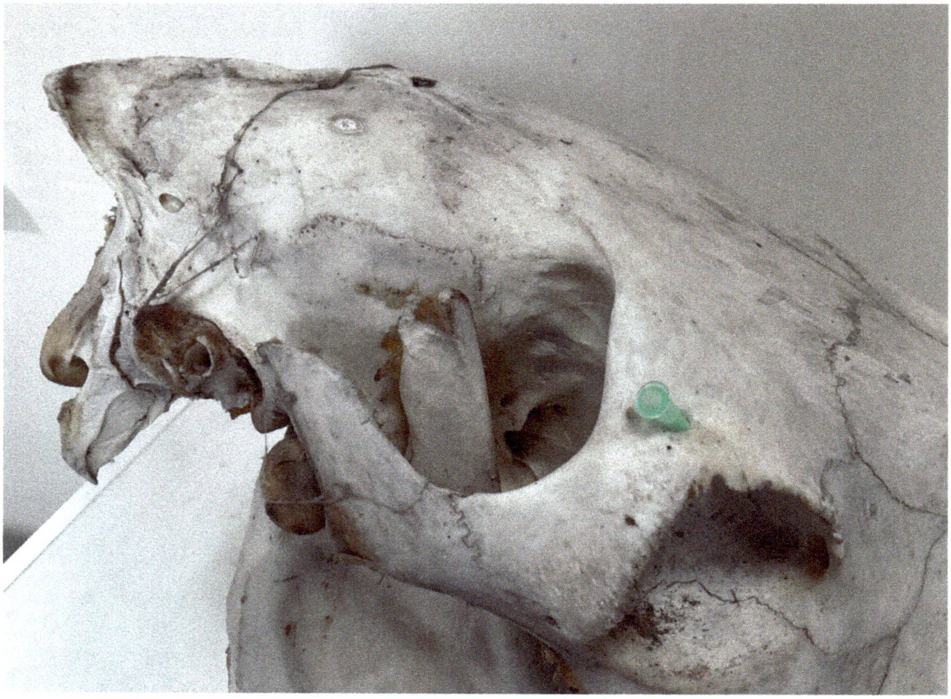

Fig. 10.7. The supraorbital foramen.

- incisive bone repair; and
- desensitization of the maxillary nerve in the diagnosis of trigeminal neuropathic pain (headshaking syndrome).

Technique

There are four approaches in common use for performing a maxillary nerve block: caudal, lateral, lateral periorbital and dorsal. The author is only familiar with the first two approaches (Tremaine, 2007). To avoid confusion the author will only describe these approaches which aim to deposit 4–6 ml local anaesthetic at the entrance to the pterygopalatine fossa adjacent to the maxillary nerve (Fig. 10.8). The site is clipped and prepared aseptically just below the zygomatic arch and a skin bleb is injected just vertically to this structure. A 22G × 9 cm spinal needle is directed at 45 degrees to the skin caudodorsally and parallel to the facial crest, and advanced until it contacts the palatine bone immediately dorsal to the nerve entering the palatine foramen (the direction is approximately towards a point imagined on the rostral contralateral facial crest) (Fig. 10.7).

Side effects

The side effects of the maxillary nerve block include haematoma formation after inadvertent articular puncture (the haematoma is usually self-limiting and resolves within 24 h), globe prolapse due to inadvertent extraocculomotor muscle paralysis, Horner's syndrome and a failure to sensitize the nerve, nostril self-trauma if the horse experiences an unpleasant sensation as the block recedes and a painful cellulitis in the pterygopalatine fossa if infection is introduced. These side effects can be avoided by:

- asepsis;
- accurate needle placement;
- use of narrow 19 to 22G spinal needles;
- avoiding excessive volumes of local anaesthetic (5–10 ml is sufficient if accurately placed); and
- appropriate restraint of the horse.

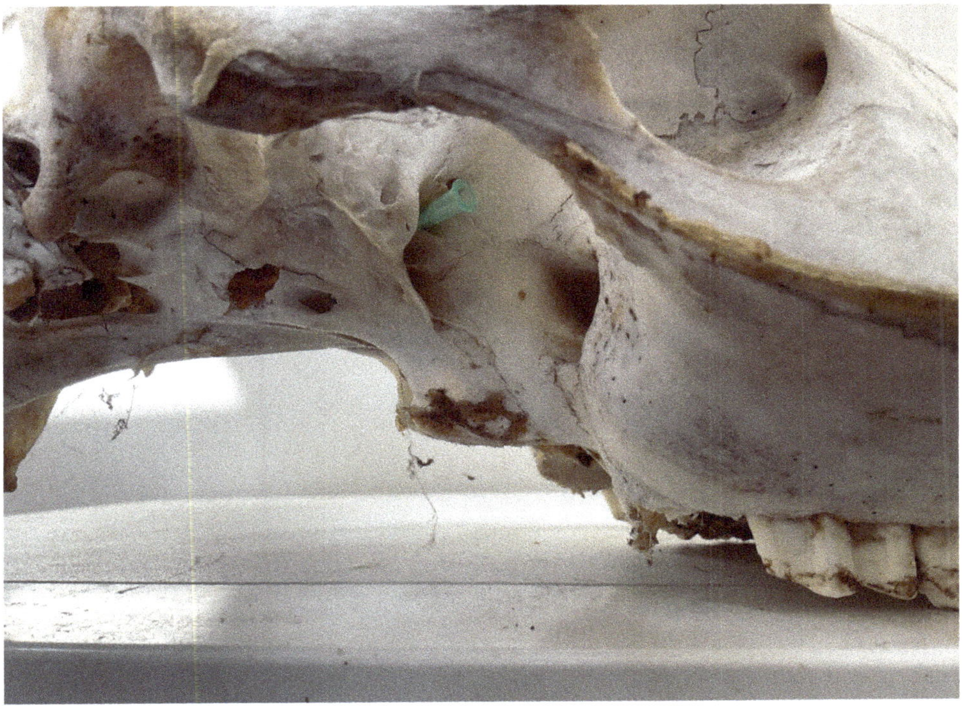

Fig. 10.8. The entrance to the pterygopalatine fossa.

Intraligamental dental nerve block

An intraligamental dental nerve block is highly effective for analgesia of the gingiva and coronal periodontium, and is useful for:

- dental extractions; and
- peridontal procedures.

Technique

Prilocaine gel can be injected intraligamentally into the periodontal ligament of a tooth using a 21G intraligamental needle to desensitize this structure effectively.

Submucosal infiltration

Submucosal infiltration of lignocaine using a butterfly catheter for desensitization of the gingiva and mucosa in the caudal oral cavity is useful for dental extraction and standing soft palate treatments. A dental syringe and a fine 25G or 27G needle can be useful for this during removal of wolf teeth (vestigial first premolar) in a field situation when local anaesthetic is deposited palatally and buccally to the tooth to be removed. The groove in which the greater palatine artery lies should be appreciated and intra-articular injection should be avoided.

10.14 Cheek Tooth Extraction

Introduction

There are three methods available to the clinician – buccostomy, repulsion and oral extraction. For repulsion and buccostomy a general anaesthetic is required. For repulsion, a small circle of skin is removed over the offending tooth or over the sinus above the offending tooth. The periosteum is scraped, then a hole is made in the bone with a trephine and the piece of bone removed. A punch is applied to the apical end of the tooth, which is then hit hard with a mallet until the tooth comes out. The hole remaining is left to granulate. Professor Lane at Bristol Veterinary School, UK, felt that this butcher-like technique could be bettered. An excellent surgeon, he developed a buccostomy technique having fewer post-operative complications. However, this technique is not advised, as the nearby salivary gland ducts and important nerves are very vulnerable.

Oral extraction

The best method for cheek tooth extraction is oral extraction performed under sedation and possibly local nerve blocks. This, in fact, is an old method revisited; it is not a difficult technique except in certain circumstances. It does, however, require a variety of quite expensive instruments. It is not for all practitioners, but certainly it is a method that can be used outside of a referral centre.

Historically, before the advent of routine general anaesthesia in the horse, oral extraction was the only method available to the practitioner. It was succeeded by dental repulsion and lateral buccotomy techniques under general anaesthesia. These resulted in a high percentage of post-operative complications, so now, with good standing sedation strategies available, oral extraction is the preferred method for cheek tooth removal. Post-operative complications are rare. The author recorded none in a series of 125 extractions published in *Equine Veterinary Education* (Duncanson, 2004).

In some horses the loose tooth can be removed manually without pain relief or sedation; however, sedation is normally required, with some local anaesthesia injected into the gingiva with a dental syringe. Many surgeons now give regional nerve blocks (see Section 10.13). Periapical infection is by far the most common indication for extraction of teeth, especially in younger horses. Periapical infections have a variety of aetiologies, including periodontal disease, fractures, infundibular caries of the maxillary cheek teeth (it should be noted that mandibular cheek teeth do not have infundibulae), iatrogenic pulpar exposure and anachoretic infection of the pulp tissues. The clinical signs of a periapical infection depend on which tooth is infected. The roots of teeth 1/06, 2/06, 1/07, 2/07, and the rostral roots of 1/08 and 2/08 lie in the maxillary bone and so if they are infected they cause facial swellings and even fistulae. The roots of the remaining maxillary cheek teeth lie in the maxillary sinus and so if they are infected, there is a unilateral malodorous nasal discharge.

Idiopathic cheek tooth fractures are relatively common, and patients may present with clinical signs of quidding and halitosis, as well as biting and behaviour problems. A number of fracture configurations can be observed, but lateral slab fractures are the most common. Often the smaller slab can be removed relatively easily. The remaining part of the tooth can then be left in situ but monitored regularly. In the author's experience wear on these teeth will continue and in a few years the tooth will be seen as normal.

Supernumerary, misaligned, dysplastic and impacted teeth may need to be extracted if they show clinical signs.

Almost all tooth extractions are performed in the standing horse. The gingival margins of the tooth are elevated both lingually and buccally with dental picks to expose as much of the tooth as possible. Molar spreaders are then applied between the tooth to be extracted and the tooth in front for 3 min; this procedure is repeated behind the tooth. Ideally, this procedure should be carried out several times using a series of wider and wider spreaders.

The use of a series of spreaders is excellent, but they are expensive instruments. Most clinicians can manage with just one pair and a wide dental pick, which serves the purpose well. This procedure should not be carried out between the first and second cheek teeth if the second cheek tooth is to be extracted, because of the danger of loosening the first cheek tooth. Similarly, spreaders should not be placed between the fifth and sixth cheek teeth if the fifth tooth is to be extracted.

The correct size of molar extractors are placed in position on the tooth as near to the apex as possible. The correct size is important, and as many as six separate pairs may be required. It is vital that the extractors are tight enough on the tooth so that they do not slip and cause burring of the tooth. Equally, they must not be applied too tightly to the tooth or there is a danger of fracturing the tooth. Once the extractors are in place a piece of bicycle tyre inner tube is placed around the end of the extractors so that the hands of the operator can relax. Then the hard part starts. The operator moves the extractors with a slow, rocking movement from side to side. It is vital that excessive force is not used or the exposed crown will be shattered. Ideally, there should be three operatives, one to hold each side of the head of the horse, and one to rock the extractors; they should regularly change round, as the procedure is very tiring. The worst-case scenario is in the young horse. The rocking motion may have to be continued for up to 3 h. However, in the old horse even multiple extractions may be accomplished in 20 min.

There are dangers in having the gag open for long periods; the use of a kitchen timer is helpful, so that the horse can have a rest every 20 min. The gag is not taken off completely, but just lowered to relax the temporomandibular joint. There are not normally any complications with this joint. The extractors are not removed every 20 min because once they are in a good position it is better for them to remain in place; to constantly reapply the extractors may damage the tooth.

The horse is controlled during long periods of extraction, initially with a mixture of detomidine hydrochloride (1 mg/100 kg) combined with butorphanol tartrate (2 mg/100 kg) in the same syringe i/v (see Sections 8.5 and 8.7). This can be topped up as required with half-doses; a 2 h extraction may require three top-ups. Ideally, the horse should be in stocks that have a front extension, with the head held at the right height with a dental halter. Most horses tolerate this arrangement very well; they tend to hang back, resting their rear on the tailgate of the stocks. The top-ups can be managed by a drip arrangement, which gives a steady infusion of detomidine and butorphanol. Diazepam (10 mg for a horse, 5 mg for a pony) can be added to the mixture at the start. This relaxes the tongue and allows easier placement of the molar spreaders and extractors.

Obviously, 3 h is an extreme duration. Normally, even teeth in younger horses can be removed more quickly than that. The clinician has to continue rocking until a squelching noise is heard. The molar forceps, still in place, are elevated with a piece of hard wood taped to them to act as a fulcrum. In the young horse with very long teeth the forceps will need to be rotated lingually to achieve extraction. The roots are small but the crown is very long. In some animals complications may arise because the small roots splay out at an angle, which impedes extraction. If teeth have been diseased or loose for a long time, hypercementosis may have occurred; this makes the teeth wider at the apical end. Extraction is therefore extremely difficult, particularly if the tooth is caudal.

If X-ray facilities are available, it is useful to take preoperative radiographs; radiography of a horse's head is very helpful (see Section 10.15). Sedation is vital, and the use of a rope halter rather than a headcollar with buckles is mandatory. It is best to use a large cassette in order to include the whole cheek tooth row. This makes orienting the teeth much easier. It is easier to have the chin of the horse resting on something soft and elevated, so that the cheek teeth rows are parallel to the floor, which makes obtaining the oblique angle easier. However, this is difficult with a really big horse. An oblique angle is necessary to highlight the apical aspect of the teeth.

For maxillary cheek teeth the plate needs to be against the affected side and the beam needs to come from higher on the opposite side, at roughly 30° to the horizontal. On the other hand, to highlight apical aspects of the mandibular cheek teeth, the beam needs to come from 30° below the horizontal. If there is any facial swelling a marker should be applied there to help orientation. It is useful to use a probe in any fistula.

The problem with interpretation comes with the caudal maxillary cheek teeth, i.e. numbers 8 to 11, which lie in the maxillary sinus. Obviously, it is vital to extract the correct tooth. Normally, the clinician can get correlation between the radiographic evidence and visual evidence from very careful examination of the teeth with a fine dental probe. If there is any doubt, the radiographs should be referred to a more experienced veterinary colleague or even a human dentist, as these experts often examine several radiographs daily.

Post-operative radiographs can be useful with fractured teeth. With this intra-oral extraction technique, the old adage 'remove the tooth, the whole tooth and nothing but the tooth' does not have to be applied so rigorously. Where teeth are fractured at an angle it is more prudent to remove the smaller fragment, which normally is easy, and leave the body of the tooth in situ. Over time the reserve crown will erupt and the whole occlusal surface will become normal. On the other hand, if the fracture line runs down into the pulp cavity, it is likely that you will get an apical infection, then or in the future, and both fragments should be removed.

With this intra-oral approach, it is better to allow the socket to granulate on its own. This occurs very rapidly and will, without infection, occur within 3 weeks. If there is a suppurating sinus, the owner should flush out the hole with very dilute chlorhexidine solution daily. A sinus will take longer to heal, normally 6–8 weeks. If a buccostomy or repulsion technique has been used, then the socket will need packing with dental impression compound.

On the day of the extraction phenylbutazone (see Section 6.8) should be given i/v for longer-term pain relief following the butorphanol; the owner should continue this by mouth for 6 days. This can be supplied in paste form in case the horse is inappetent, although horses are rarely inappetent. Antibiotics should be given for 2 days before extraction by mouth and continued for 5 days after the operation. It is not safe to give TMS i/v injection at the time of the extraction because of the danger of conflict between TMS and alpha-2 sedatives. The author considers that most patients justify the use of peri- and post-operative antibiotic therapy.

It is not advisable to feed long fibre for 2 weeks after the extraction. Ideally, the horse should be kept out at grass. One of the benefits of intra-oral extraction is that there is no external wound, and so flies are not a problem. After approximately 2 weeks the mouth should be examined to make sure the socket is granulating. The owners should be warned that there will be a smell from the mouth for some time. In the longer term, clinicians should stress to the owners that regular dentistry, particularly rasping of the occlusal surface of the opposing tooth, is vital.

10.15 Radiography of the Equine Head

Introduction

Most portable X-ray machines are quite adequate for imaging of the horse's head, although the task is not easy. Part of the problem is that the majority of us do not take sufficient numbers of radiographs to perfect the technique. Sedation is vital. A rope halter is helpful, as the buckles on a headcollar are invariably in the wrong place. A minimum of two operatives is required, and they must be adequately protected against radiation.

A padded table or headstand is required so that the rostral mandible can be rested. Ideally, the cheek teeth rows should be parallel to the floor (unless visualization of a fluid line is required). If there is a sinus tract present, it is important to insert a radiopaque probe as far into it as possible. If there is a swelling on the maxilla this should be marked with a radiopaque marker.

Lateral view

A straight lateral view is rarely useful, since the two arcades of teeth are superimposed on each other. However, it is important to have the *whole* cheek tooth row on the image, and so the plate should be large enough to accommodate this. The centre of the beam should be focused on the rostral end of the facial crest. It is also important to take a true lateral view and not a caudal–rostral oblique.

Oblique lateral view

This is a much more useful view, as the roots can be skylined (see below). Recommendations are as for the lateral view. If the main purpose is to obtain an image of one side of the upper cheek teeth rows, the plate should be on that side; the X-ray beam then should be above the head, at 30° to the horizontal. On the other hand, if the roots of a mandibular cheek tooth row are to be visualized, the camera should be below the horse's head and pointing upwards at 30°.

Open-mouthed views

These are used to visualize the crowns of the teeth. The incisor teeth will need to be kept about 25 mm apart, with a piece of wood or a Butler gag. The lateral view will be the same as above, but the oblique views will be the exact opposite, i.e. the beam for the upper cheek teeth rows will be pointing upwards from below the horse's head, while the beam for the lower cheek teeth rows will be pointing downwards from above the head.

Dorso-ventral view

The plate should be placed below the mandible and the beam should be above the horse's head, pointing directly downwards. It is very important that the head is in a true dorso-ventral plane and the beam is pointing directly downwards.

Intra-oral views

These are very useful to visualize the roots of the incisors. However, sophisticated equipment is required for intra-oral views of the cheek teeth.

Skyline view of the TMJ

Workers in the UK at both Edinburgh and Newmarket have described these. The camera can be placed above the head and the plate below or totally opposite. The actual area of the joint visualized is small. If ultrasonography is available, the clinician will find it more useful for this joint.

Gamma scintigraphy

Some authorities maintain that this modality can reveal apical abscessation earlier in the course of the disease than can routine radiography. Nonetheless, it is accurate only very early on in the course of the disease.

Computed tomography (CT)

This is available at some referral centres and is the gold standard, but sadly is unlikely to be affordable in most cases.

Reasons for radiography

The main reasons are:

- differentiation of different types of teeth, e.g. to ensure that we are attempting to remove a 'wolf' tooth and not a canine;
- differentiation between deciduous and permanent teeth, e.g. to ensure we are attempting to remove a deciduous and not a permanent incisor;
- location of tooth root abscessation so that we remove the correct maxillary cheek tooth that is actually causing the unilateral nasal discharge, or the correct tooth associated with a discharging sinus or facial swelling;
- location of a fractured tooth and making a decision as to whether both parts of the fracture need to be removed;
- location of extra bone laid down on the bars of the mouth by excessive use of the bit;
- aiding in the diagnosis of facial swellings, e.g. dentigerous cysts or facial tumours; and
- location of post-operative dental or alveolar sequestra.

References and Further Reading

Albers, L., Albers, J., Dullin, C. and Staszyk, C. (2023) Early incisor lesions and equine odontoclastic tooth resorption and hypercementosis: Reliability of radiographic findings. *Equine Veterinary Journal* 55: 261–269.

Allen, T. (2003) *Manual of Equine Dentistry*. Mosby Elsevier Science, Melbourne, Australia.

Baker, G.J. and Easley, J. (2005) *Equine Dentistry*, 2nd edn. Elsevier Saunders, Maryland Heights, Missouri.

Barnett, T. (2019) *Equine Veterinary Journal* 51: 277–279.

Barnett, T. (2020) Modern equine cheek tooth extraction. *Veterinary Practice*, 17 January.

Borkent, D., Reardon, R. and Dixon, P.M. (2017) Epidemiological survey on equine cheek tooth infundibular caries in the United Kingdom. *Veterinary Record* 181: 235.

Brigham, E.J. and Duncanson, G. (2000) An equine *postmortem* dental study: 50 cases. *Equine Veterinary Education* 12(2): 59–62.

du Toit, N. (2017) Clinical significance of equine cheek teeth infundibular caries. *Veterinary Record* 181: 233.

Duncanson, G.R. (2004) A case study of 125 horses presented to a general practitioner in the UK for cheek tooth removal. *Equine Veterinary Education* 16: 166–168.

Grant, M.J. and Barnett, T.P. (2019) Shear mouth secondary to temporohyoid osteoarthropathy. *Equine Veterinary Education* 31(2): 93.

Hermans, H., Veraa, S., Wolschrijn, C.F. and van Loon, J.P.A.M. (2019) Local anaesthetic techniques for the equine head, towards guided techniques and new applications. *Equine Veterinary Education* 31(8): 432–440.

Klugh, D.O. (2010) *Principles of Equine Dentistry*. Manson Publishing, London.

Pascoe, R.J. (2018) Does thermal injury affect teeth during dentistry? *Equine Veterinary Education* 30(11): 623–625.

Pence, P. (2002) *Equine Dentistry*. Lippincott Williams & Wilkins, Philadelphia, Pennsylvania.

Rahmani, V., Hayrinen, L., Kareinen, I. and Ruohoniemi, M. (2019) History, clinical findings and outcome of horses with radiographic signs of equine odontoclastic tooth resorption and hypercementosis. *Veterinary Record* 185: 729.

Tremaine, W.H. (2007) Local analgesic techniques for the equine head. *Equine Veterinary Education* 19: 495–503.

Tremaine, H. (2019) Local analgesia techniques for dental and head procedures in horses. *In Practice* 41: 165–176.

11

Hoof Conditions and Problems within the Hoof Capsule

Abstract

All the pathological problems which have been recorded in the equine foot are discussed in this chapter. Where differences are marked in the donkey the problems in that species are discussed separately. Working equines do not suffer as much with laminitis as equines in other disciplines. However, because the disease is so painful and the welfare considerations are so immense it is discussed in detail.

11.1 Hoof Balance

To assess hoof balance, each foot needs to be examined from several different perspectives. First, looking from a lateral view the hoof pastern axis can be evaluated. The angle of the dorsal wall of the hoof should be the same as the angle of the first and second phalanges. If the dorsal wall has too low an angle the axis is said to be broken back; the reverse, when the dorsal wall is too steep, is said to be broken forward. This condition is so commonly seen in donkeys that it may even be considered to be normal. The coronary band should be examined from the lateral aspect; it should form a very gradual downward slope from the dorsal point to the bulb of the heel. Second the foot should be examined from behind; the distance from the coronary band to the ground should be equal between the lateral and bulbs of the heel. Third the foot should be examined from the front; a line through the foreleg should bisect the hoof and the coronary band should be parallel to the ground. Last the bottom of the foot is examined; the weight-bearing surface should be symmetrical and the sole slightly concave. Practitioners should note that as many as 25% of horses will not have symmetrical feet, comparing left and right. This is not an unsoundness as such but should always be noted. Fig. 11.1 demonstrates poor hoof balance.

11.2 Puncture Wounds of the Foot

These may be trivial but should never be treated in a cavalier fashion, for if deep tissues are involved these wounds can be life threatening (see Fig. 11.2). Clinicians need to be careful what they say; it is all too easy to let the owner think that the farrier is to blame, but it can be very difficult for the farrier if there is little hoof wall in which to place nails well clear of sensitive tissues.

If the nails are too close to the sensitive tissue but not penetrating it the result is 'nail bind'; the horse will show mild lameness within a few hours of shoeing and there will be pain

DOI: 10.1079/9781800624283.0011

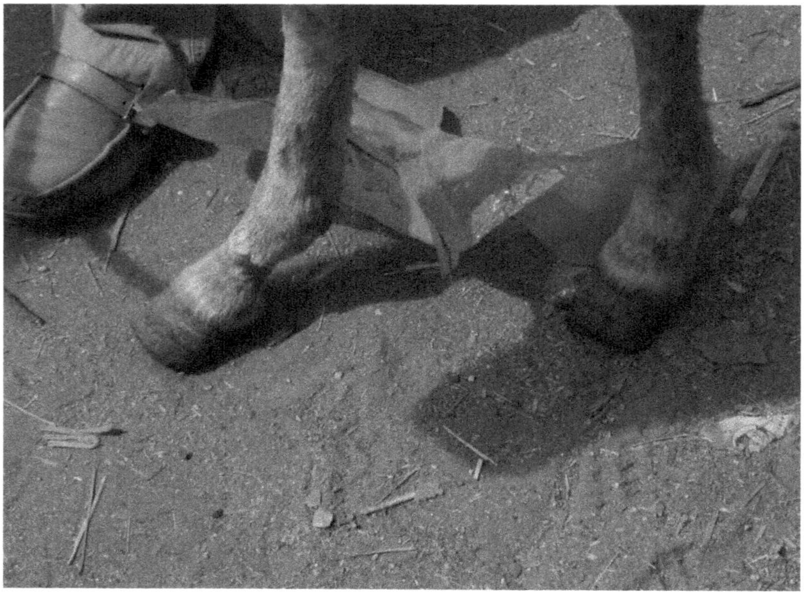

Fig. 11.1. Poor hoof balance.

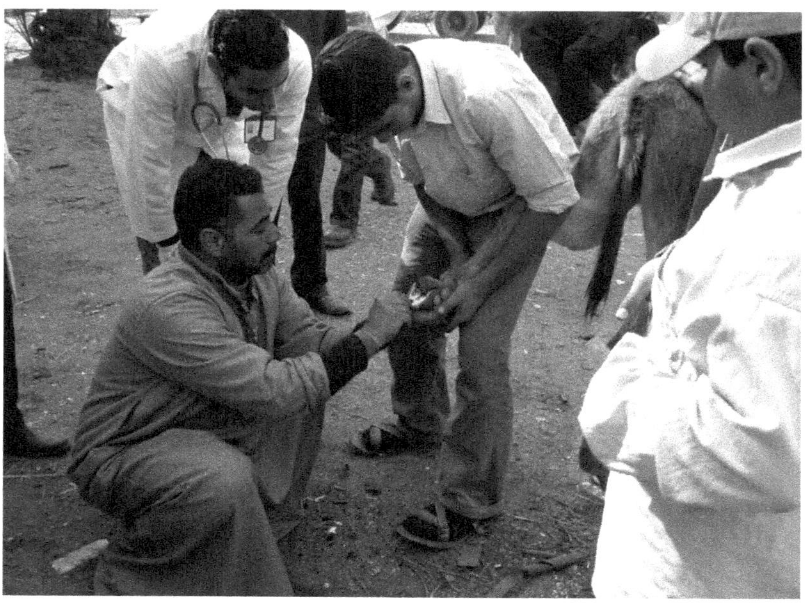

Fig. 11.2. Careful examination of the foot.

around the offending nail when hoof testers are applied. The offending nail should be removed. Normally, the condition will settle down with a relatively low dose of NSAIDs. Clinicians must remember to determine the tetanus immunity status of the horse.

If there has actually been a shoeing prick there will be immediate pain, and there may be haemorrhage. If this occurs, actual sepsis is less likely to occur but, if it does occur, the degree of lameness will get worse over 48 h until in many cases the horse appears to be fracture lame. The shoe should be removed and the foot poulticed. If possible, the point where the sepsis has built up should be cut open carefully with a hoof knife to allow the pus to be released (see Fig. 11.3). Timing may be difficult, as from a welfare point of view the clinician wants to open the hoof as soon as possible. However, it is difficult to visualize the purulent tract if the approach is made too early. Obviously, NSAIDs will be helpful in this situation. The horse must be covered for tetanus. Pressure may be put on the clinician by the owner to administer antibiotics, but these are rarely helpful unless the infection has spread up the leg, resulting in a painful swelling. This is not the case in the donkey, where an i/m injection of procaine penicillin is helpful.

The third problem associated with shoeing is when the shoe is too short, so that the end or ends of the shoe lie not on the wall but on the sole. A corn develops in the angle between the wall and the bars of the foot; this position is called the 'seat of corn'. Lameness may be mild unless there is actual sepsis, and then it will be pronounced. Treatment for an infected corn is similar to that for a foot abscess, as described following shoe prick. It should be remembered that drainage is vital. Corns do not occur in the unshod horse.

Most abscesses in the foot are not related to shoeing, and in fact are more common in the unshod horse. The initial penetration often goes unrecorded, or the infection may be from haematogenous spread. Pus builds up between either the wall or the sole of the hard hoof and the underlying soft tissue. The pain is intense and is relieved only by releasing it with a hoof knife or by the pus breaking out above the coronary band. A classic history of an untreated horse would be lameness progressing in severity over 72 h and then suddenly improving. If the point where the pus is escaping can be found, then the point of penetration will be directly below it. Ideally, a hole should be made in the sole. Sterile saline can then be irrigated into one hole and will flow out of the other. Both holes should be kept open to allow the soft tissue to heal within. If pus is allowed to build up again, pain will return and the degree of lameness will increase.

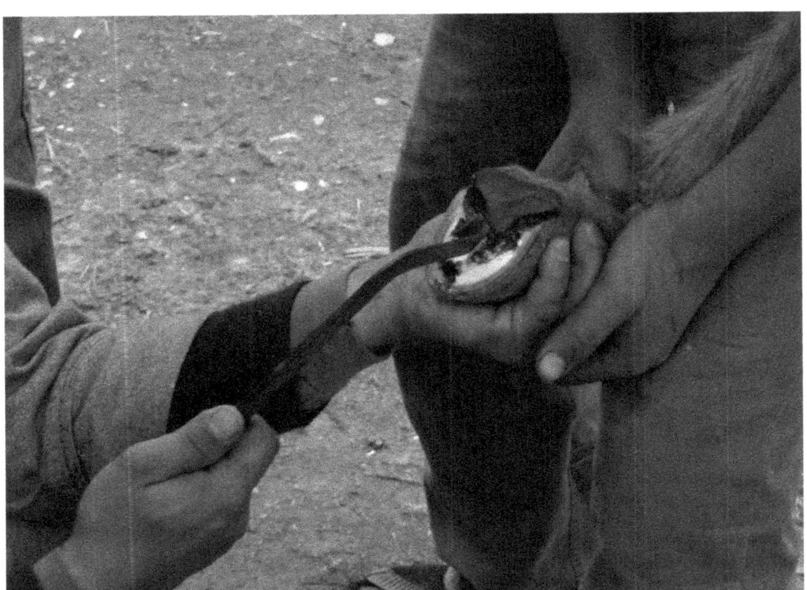

Fig. 11.3. Pus being drained from the foot with a hoof knife.

Therefore, it is advisable that a poultice is applied until healing is completed. The horse can be shod when the infection has dried up. NSAIDs can be given to reduce the pain. Once again, the horse must be protected against tetanus.

Clinicians should always be on their guard to detect serious foot penetrations. These may cause articular sepsis of the navicular bursa or the distal interphalangeal joint or involve the deep digital flexor tendon sheath. If the penetration is in the frog or the sulci, the path of the penetration will be very difficult to follow. The whole foot will be very painful, so hoof testers are not very helpful. Because of the pain, strong sedation will be required, or even an abaxial sesamoid block. In the chronic situation, it is important to debride all the affected tissue and then poultice the foot to allow continual drainage. This will occur for several weeks if there has been damage to the pedal bone. If there has been synovial penetration, radical debridement is required. This can be performed with a general anaesthetic and an arthroscope. However, in field conditions a cure can be effected eventually by radical drainage. This operation is called a 'street nail' procedure. Welfare here is very important; high doses of NSAIDs will be necessary.

In temperate climates it has been found that abscesses found in the summer were treated for 9.4 times as long as those diagnosed in winter (Cole *et al.*, 2019). It is reasonable to extrapolate that in tropical climates treatment of foot abscesses would be more prolonged in the dry season. These authors also found that abscesses at the coronary band were treated for 3.2 times as long as those at the toe. They also recorded that animals with a lameness score >3 at presentation resulted in a shorter treatment time.

11.3 Thrush

Thrush is a degenerative condition of the horn of the sole and frog caused by anaerobic bacteria. It is made worse by poor hygiene, i.e. the horse continually standing in faeces and urine. Nonetheless, thrush is not caused by bad conditions alone and so the practitioner should not be too quick to blame the owner. The condition will be recognized by the smell and the black, crumbling horn tissue. Rarely does the condition cause lameness unless the sensitive tissue is involved. If there is tracking of pus up in the middle of the frog, pain may be found in this area under digital pressure, and the horse will be seen to be lame when trotted up. Radical removal of the abnormal horn tissue is required. Hydrogen peroxide, as a cleansing agent, is useful on account of the anaerobic bacteria present. Formalin, vinegar, zinc and copper sulfate have all been used for treatment in this condition. It should be remembered that in all foot pain it is unlikely that the degree of lameness will be altered by flexion tests.

11.4 Keratoma

A benign but locally invasive tumour, keratoma is rare. Its initial manifestation will be seen as 'pus in the foot'. The observant clinician will notice the white disc of abnormal horn. Once the pressure of the pus has been relieved the lameness will stop, although it will soon recur. Radical treatment is required to remove the wall of the hoof lying over the fat, worm-shaped tumour running up towards the coronary band. This has to be removed in total or recurrence will occur. The hole in the hoof must be packed with gauze soaked in iodine. The hole regenerates very quickly. The condition following radical removal carries a good prognosis.

11.5 Laminitis in the Horse and Pony

Laminitis is extremely complex, not only in its aetiology but also in its pathology. Endocrinopathic laminitis is the most common form of the clinical syndrome and encompasses laminitis associated with insulin dysregulation which is defined as abnormal insulin metabolism in response to a normal physiologic process such as eating (Menzies-Gow, 2023). In horses and ponies, it manifests in three forms: basal hyperinsulinemia, in which circulating insulin concentrations are consistently high; an excessive insulin response to carbohydrate, in which ingestion of sugar or starch results in abnormally high circulating insulin concentration peaks; and tissue insulin resistance, in which the resistance is at the level of the tissues. Any combination of these three forms can exist in an individual animal. It is well established that hyperinsulinemia induces laminitis in horses and ponies; however, the exact mechanism remains to be determined. The mechanism underlying insulin dysregulation in equine metabolic syndrome is also unclear, but evidence exists for a role for genetics, epigenetics, the microbiome, obesity, diet and endo-disrupting chemicals. Similarly, the mechanism by which pituitary *pars intermedia* dysfunction is associated with insulin dysregulation has yet to be determined; however, it is postulated that some *pars intermedia* hormones antagonize insulin. Alternatively, in some cases, the animal has both equine metabolic syndrome and pituitary *pars intermedia* dysfunction, and so the insulin dysregulation preceded the pituitary *pars intermedia* dysfunction and might not have been recognized. Management of endocrinopathic laminitis should focus on identifying and treating the underlying endocrinopathy and providing appropriate analgesia and foot support. The classic cause in horses – and more commonly in ponies – is too much rich, green grass. Grass that is itself under stress, i.e. when the nights are cold but the days are hot, is more likely to bring on an attack of laminitis. There will be a higher level of fructans in the grass. Animals become overweight, with a rock-hard crest of fat, and suddenly become acutely lame. This can occur in all four legs, but much more commonly in only the front legs. The animal will adopt a classical laminitic stance, leaning backwards and trying to take as much weight on its hind legs as possible. It will be very reluctant to move. However, if it is on soft ground, it will move better once it has got started. This accounts for the old-fashioned treatment, which was to make the animal work. This should not be done, however, as it is not only cruel but also it bruises the feet and makes the condition worse. Having stated this, if the owner thinks that the pony or horse is about to get laminitis then exercise on soft ground is beneficial; animals being worked consistently rarely get laminitis. Therefore, it is a rare condition in working horses and ponies. If a case is suspected, the animal should immediately be taken away from any access to grass. In severe cases of laminitis, the animal may well lie down; this is good and should be encouraged.

Diagnosis should not be a problem, though inexperienced clinicians must beware of mistaking the recumbent laminitic with the recumbent colic. Animals with laminitis will continue to eat, but obviously, apart from a measured quantity of good-quality hay, that should be discouraged. The animal with laminitis will have marked bounding digital pulses, whether felt in the palmar digital position or in the abaxial sesamoid position. The laminitic will be reluctant to have a front foot picked up, as this puts a higher load on the already painful opposite front foot. If the clinician is able to hold a front foot up, it will be found that the foot in the area of the sole halfway between the toe and the point of the frog will be extremely sore on hoof testing. In very severe cases of laminitis the sole of the hoof will be painful even simply on thumb pressure.

Sadly, in neglected cases clinicians will observe that the pedal bone has penetrated the sole. In these cases prompt euthanasia is advised. In other cases, particularly in heavy horses or cob types, the pedal bone will sink within the hoof capsule. This can be perceived by pushing a finger into the groove that will have appeared at the coronary band: this action will be acutely painful for the horse.

Acute laminitic cases should be treated as an emergency. As stated above, the diet must immediately be adjusted to avoid hard food and grass. The surface on which the animal is standing is also very important. Sand or a very deep bed of shavings are both recommended; straw is less suitable, since not only will the horse eat it and may then get an impaction, but also the straw may be scraped round by the horse until it is then standing on bare concrete. Deep manure might be considered, but it should be avoided as it tends to soften the feet excessively and may bring on other conditions (see thrush, Section 11.3). Concrete or very compact earth are the worst possible surfaces: these should be covered with rubber matting. If this is not possible the feet should be covered with a clog of thick polystyrene. Another action which might be suggested is to apply 'lily pads', which are pieces of hard rubber approximately the same size as the frog. They should be taped on to the frog with gutter tape to apply 'frog pressure'.

There is still an ongoing debate on what to do about shoes. One school of thought suggests that you leave the shoes in place, as they are at least providing some support. It is certain that removing shoes will be very painful for an acute laminitic. It is also certain that it will be impossible to replace the shoes. Another school of thought suggests you remove the shoes so that the animal can be more comfortable taking weight on its soles rather than on the walls of the feet. When the animal has become more stabilized, heart bar shoes may be fitted to apply frog pressure. These may be either solid-fixed heart bar shoes or more sophisticated adjustable shoes, the latter being capable of having more pressure applied by being tightened up twice a week. There are also modern malleable materials which can be fashioned to the shape of the hoof to give the horse more comfort. Obviously, once the initial acute pain is controlled, the feet will need to be trimmed by a skilled farrier. The toes should be radically shortened to try to make the angle of the hoof conform to the angle of the pedal bone. A skilled farrier will probably be able to do this by eye. However, a lateral radiograph will be very helpful here.

Apart from these husbandry aspects, the main treatment is focused on providing pain relief and reducing the inflammation; NSAIDs will play a very pivotal role, the most commonly used being phenylbutazone, but others described in Section 6.8 all have their followers. The author has found that paracetamol can be given at the same time as phenylbutazone at the dose rate of 20 mg/kg twice daily. This is a safer treatment than raising the dose level of the phenylbutazone. Clinicians should pay strict attention to the weight of the animal and dose accordingly. They should remember that, with the husbandry advised above, the weight should be reducing rapidly, and doses thus must be reduced accordingly. Clinicians must remember that the dose rate of phenylbutazone for the donkey is twice that for the horse.

The other treatment aspect which may be considered is lowering the blood pressure by the use of acetylpromazine (see Section 8.4). This medicine is also a tranquillizer and will have the added benefit that it will help encourage the animal to lie down. Owners should be told of this other effect so that they are not concerned if the animal appears sedated. Obviously, this medicine should only be used for a limited length of time, i.e. for a maximum of 3 days.

There is evidence that cryotherapy aids the treatment of laminitis, particularly if it has been induced by sepsis. Using ice and cold water, the hoof and pastern should be maintained at a temperature below 10°C. An old-fashioned treatment of standing the animal in a stream with a sandy bottom seems to be helpful.

Laminitis is not only caused by overfeeding of green grass, it can also be caused by overfeeding of concentrates. The classic example is the horse which has broken into the feed shed and gorged itself overnight. The first task in treatment is to try to move the ingesta rapidly through the intestine to cut down adsorption. This can be achieved by giving magnesium sulfate (Epsom salts: 0.5 kg for a 500 kg horse) dissolved in water, by nasogastric tube. Sodium bicarbonate can be added to this to act as an antacid, as well as bismuth and charcoal to act as adsorbents for the toxaemia. It is not only the excess carbohydrate that will cause the laminitis but also the toxaemia. The NSAID flunixin meglumate should be injected i/v to help counteract the endotoxaemia.

Toxins from other sources will also cause laminitis. Metritis from a retained fetal membrane, if not treated aggressively, will cause a toxaemia and laminitis. Equally, a mastitis, if not treated with antibiotics and NSAIDs, will cause a toxic laminitis. Any poison that causes a toxaemia may result in laminitis, e.g. acorn poisoning causing an impaction may well cause a bowel toxaemia by delaying ingesta transport time.

Severe pedal concussion, e.g. a pony galloping several miles on a tarmac road, will result in laminitis in all four feet. A horse with a fracture, if not fully supported by slings, may well develop laminitis in the opposite leg to the fracture on account of the excess weight load on that foot.

All these causes must obviously be avoided. However, in the event of laminitis the condition should be treated in a similar way as described above.

One other cause of laminitis is high levels of circulating corticosteroids. This may occur in Cushing's disease (see Fig. 11.4), as described in Section 20.16, or it may occur iatrogenically by veterinarians injecting corticosteroids. These injections, e.g. for joint medication, should be limited to a very few at any one time. Steroids should not be injected to treat conditions such as urticaria in the overweight animal, which is a likely candidate for developing laminitis.

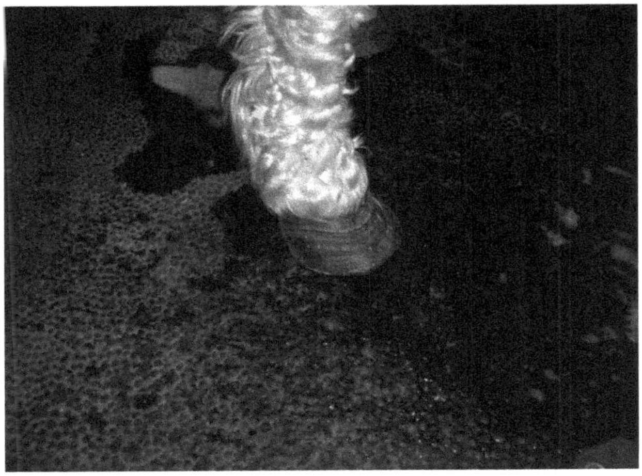

Fig. 11.4. Cushing's disease resulting in laminitis.

It is vital that underlying endocrinopathies, which are common, are treated at the same time. The first treatment for pituitary *pars intermedia* dysfunction (PPID), commonly called Cushing's disease, is the dopamine agonist pergolide. The initial dose is 2 mg per os once a day for 4–6 weeks.

11.6 Laminitis in the Donkey

Donkeys, like horses may become laminitic for a variety of reasons, but the most common are either too much lush grass or grain overload. Donkeys will also suffer laminitis as a result of Cushing's disease. It is very important that donkeys are not starved, as this may result in hyperlipaemia, which should be avoided at all costs.

11.7 Treating the Lame Donkey as a Result of Infection in the Foot

Many equine clinicians struggle with the lame donkey. The donkey's stoicism means that it does not react in the same manner to pain or injury as a horse or pony. You get the occasional very bad-tempered individual that seems to be able to kick out with all four feet at all angles, often with two legs at the same time. Nevertheless, most donkeys are good-natured and ready to do their work, but are equally happy to be left alone.

The most common cause of lameness in the horse is in the foot, but if you consider the donkey, 'pus in the foot' is far and away the most common cause of lameness. It is a very painful condition and we owe it to donkeys not only to ameliorate the condition but also to give them pain relief. However, diagnosis is not easy. Rarely will a donkey show pain on hoof testers. Paring away the hoof may reveal the source of infection but, sadly, many black tracts seem to peter out and not reward the clinician with the pus he or she seeks. In the horse, parenteral antibiotics are rarely helpful unless the infection has spread up the leg; on the other hand, antibiotics seem to be helpful in the donkey: an injection of 5 ml of a penicillin/streptomycin mixture does seem to help some individuals. An Animalintex® poultice (Robinson Healthcare, Worksop, UK) with extra magnesium sulfate paste held in place with black gutter tape will help to draw the pus to the coronary band or soften the foot to allow drainage.

Oral pain relief can be given disguised in a piece of apple. *The donkey is very susceptible to tetanus, so remember to check the vaccination status.* If there is any doubt, administer a full horse dose of 7500 IU (7.5 ml of most preparations) tetanus antitoxin. It is important to try to encourage donkey owners to keep their donkeys fully covered for tetanus. The first vaccination of a course can be carried out at this time.

11.8 Problems with the Navicular Bone

The most acute problem with the navicular bone is a vertical fracture. This is extremely rare in the front foot but is seen more commonly in the hind foot, particularly in the young animal. The normal cause is the young horse kicking out really hard at a very solid object, e.g. a reinforced concrete post. There will be a sudden onset of acute lameness. The severity of the lameness will pass in a few days, leaving a horse 4/10 lame. The lameness will not be affected by flexion tests. Diagnosis can be suggested by the history and a response to a palmar digital nerve block, but a definitive diagnosis will be achieved only by radiography.

Normally, fusion of the bone will occur, but this will take up to 12 months. It has been suggested that surgery be carried out, by placing a long screw horizontally through the navicular bone. However, healing rates with surgical intervention do not appear to be better or quicker than with conservative treatment. Arthritis is not normally a problem, as fractured navicular bone is a condition seen mainly in the young horse; if it occurs in an old horse the prognosis is very poor.

There is a multi-factorial condition called 'navicular disease', a condition normally associated with large jumping horses. Nevertheless, it may also be seen in big carriage horses, the main clinical sign being a shifting bilateral foreleg lameness. The condition will improve with rest but will return with work. It will mainly be seen in the 8–12-year-old range. No improvement will be seen after treatment with NSAIDs, but pain will be alleviated by a palmar digital nerve block. If the principal lame leg is blocked first, the lameness in the other leg will become more apparent. Radiographs will reveal radiolucent areas in the navicular bone. On post-mortem, the navicular bone will appear to be aerated. Over the past 50 years there have been a variety of treatments, both surgical and medical, advocated for this condition; some have recorded successes, but these have never been sustained. The bisphosphonate tiludronate, recently recommended, may well be helpful; this drug is said to reduce bone resorption without affecting bone formation. It has to be administered over a 60 min period as an i/v drip at a dosage rate of 0.1 mg/kg.

The most radical treatment for 'navicular disease' is neurectomy of the palmar digital nerve, but this is not recommended. Often there is incomplete desensitization of the heel area and so there is no improvement; sensation will return in around 4 months. Far more serious consequences are also possible, e.g. rupture of the deep digital flexor tendon or loss of hoof wall.

The treatment of choice for the clinician in the field would be the fitting of round shoes. Farriers are always reluctant to fit these shoes as they are rather easily pulled off by the hind feet. However, lameness will often appear to be alleviated by their use.

11.9 Fracture of the Third Phalanx

This is a condition that can catch out the unwary practitioner. The horse will have a swinging leg lameness; it will show positive pain on hoof testers and therefore will look like 'pus in the foot'. However, no black pus track will be found when searching the sole. A poultice should be applied to the foot and left in place for a week. On removal, still no pus will be found and the lameness will be as bad. There will be no swelling further up the leg, which you would expect if there had been pus in the foot for a week. An abaxial sesamoid nerve block will lessen the lameness, but not totally remove it. However, this would also be seen if there was 'pus in the foot'. The only definitive method of diagnosis is radiography. Most fractures will heal eventually in 6–9 months, and lameness will slowly improve. The fracture line will still be visible long after the lameness disappears. In a few cases the lameness will persist, and in these cases the fracture line will be found to have entered the distal phalangeal joint.

11.10 Pedal Osteitis

Pedal osteitis is a very contentious condition. Literally, it means an inflammation of the pedal bone. Indeed, in some lame animals inflammation can be seen on a good radiograph of the foot. However, inflammatory changes can also be seen in the pedal bones of non-lame horses. The majority of clinicians agree that there is a clinical condition of chronic mild lameness shown by cob-type horses carrying out long hours of work on hard ground. The lame foot can be blocked out by an abaxial sesamoid block. These horses improve with rest and NSAIDs. They can be brought back into limited work but can never do as much work as before without the lameness recurring.

11.11 Bruised Sole

Corns, as discussed in Section 11.2, are a type of bruising caused by ill-fitting shoes. However, the sole can become bruised from direct trauma caused by an uneven surface; this is less likely if the horse is shod, but it can occur even in a shod horse. The lameness will not be very marked on soft surfaces, but on stony ground it will be noticeable. Careful examination of the sole will reveal the blood-stained area. If there is no further trauma the bruising will grow out and the lameness will disappear. However, the bruised area may become infected if the sole is cut by a sharp object, e.g. a flint; alternatively, the bruised area may become infected by haematogenous spread. In either case there will be secondary sepsis and the clinician will have to treat the hoof as if there had been a puncture wound of the sole.

11.12 Problems with the Sidebones

Problems with the sidebones are very rare but are often given prominence in textbooks. Pus in the heel is common and can cause diagnostic difficulties. However, for the infection to involve either the bony or cartilaginous parts of the sidebone is very rare; if this does occur it is called quitter. The traditional treatment was to curette out the infected bone and cartilage using a specially designed knife with a spoon-like cutting end, called a 'quitter knife'. It is important to remove diseased tissue, and it is safer to allow adequate drainage by making a hole below the sepsis. Saline and antibiotics can then be instilled at the top end above the bone to flush out the infection. Healing will eventually occur by granulation from within. Fracture of the sidebone is reported but is extremely rare. Healing will take place with time, with the hoof acting as its own splint.

11.13 Damage to the Wall of the Hoof

The most common damage to the wall of the hoof is a vertical crack, often called a sand crack. This, if beginning on the distal part of the hoof wall, is caused by lack of foot trimming and subsequent trauma. If sand crack is treated promptly, by careful trimming and even shoeing, it will not cause a problem. If a shoe is applied it is useful to have two toe clips so that the single toe clip, which is normally on a front shoe, does not aggravate the crack. The hoof wall is replaced proximally from the coronary band and so the damaged wall will be replaced by good horn. This can be speeded up by a good diet and a supplement containing zinc, biotin and methionine. Sand crack may become infected if neglected, and there will then be acute lameness. In these cases, radical trimming is required to allow good drainage; any exposed sensitive tissue must be protected from further infection while the hoof wall grows out. If shoeing is not possible the hoof should be dressed with gauze and bandaged with gutter tape; this bandage should be replaced regularly.

A more serious type of vertical crack originates from the coronary band; this is particularly critical if there is a horn deficit, as the sand crack will be permanent. Hopefully, however, the deficit will not be permanent. In this case the sand crack will grow out provided the crack can be stabilized. After correct trimming, the sides of the crack can be brought together with carefully positioned staples, or by fixing two screws, one at each side of the crack, and joining them with wire. It is wise to bandage the whole hoof with waterproof gutter tape. The hoof must be regularly trimmed, and extra fixing devices may have to be applied.

Horizontal cracks may appear in the hoof. These occur when the horse has suffered some generalized debilitating condition such as laminitis. This latter condition will form a ring around the hoof, and as this grows distally a crack may appear. Lameness may not occur unless the sensitive tissue underneath becomes infected, and drainage then has to be accomplished. However, as the horizontal crack nears the distal end of the wall its attachments will be less stable, so that it may break off. If this occurs prematurely it will expose sensitive tissue. The horse will then be acutely lame. The sensitive tissue needs to be protected until hard hoof horn overgrows it.

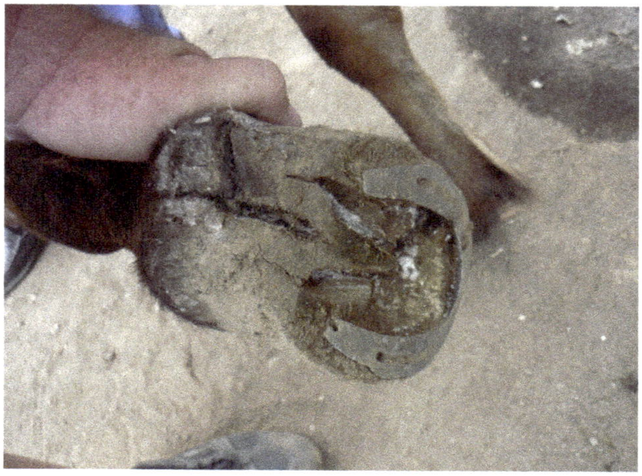

Fig. 11.5. Infection in an overgrown hoof with a shoe which is terribly worn and needs replacement.

11.14 Proud Flesh Protruding through the Sole

We have described several times in the foregoing the need to obtain adequate drainage when there is infection within the hoof. Clinicians should be aware that on occasions they may enlarge a hole in the sole through which proud flesh from the sensitive tissue underneath will then protrude. The sole should then be poulticed to make 100% certain that there is no more infection. When the clinician is satisfied that there is no remaining infection, the proud flesh should be removed with a very sharp knife. There are no nerves in this flesh, so the horse will feel no pain, but it is very vascular so haemorrhage will be copious. The foot should then be bandaged to allow the sole to heal. If the proud flesh is extensive this procedure may have to be repeated until the sole is totally closed.

References and Further Reading

Cole, S.D., Stefanovski, D., Towl, S. and Boyle, A.G. (2019) Factors associated with long treatment days, increased veterinary visits and complications in horses with subsolar abscesses. *Vet Record* 184(8): 251. Available at: https://doi.org/10.1136/vr.104138 (accessed 1 September 2023).

Menzies-Gow, N. (2023) Endocrine laminitis: Causes and management. *Vet Times* 53(16), 2 May: 6–10.

Pollitt, C. (2001) *Equine Laminitis*. Rural Industries Research and Development Corporation, Kingston, Australia.

van Nassau, R. (2007) *Hoof Problems*. Kenilworth Press, Shrewsbury, UK.

12

Orthopaedics

Abstract

This chapter covers common causes of lameness associated with both fore and hind legs. It focuses on simple diagnostic techniques. However, as equine practice and veterinary treatments in working horses have become more sophisticated this chapter has been enlarged.

12.1 Advances in Imaging of the Equine Distal Limb

Injuries and diseases of the distal limb constitute the commonest causes of lameness in horses, and diagnostic imaging plays a central role in their diagnosis. There have been tremendous advances in the development and application of diagnostic imaging techniques used to evaluate the distal limbs in the past 15–20 years, with advanced cross-sectional imaging modalities, such as magnetic resonance imaging (MRI) and computed tomography (CT), being increasingly utilized to provide diagnostic information, in combination with the more 'traditional' techniques of radiography and ultrasonography. These new imaging techniques do not replace radiography and ultrasonography but complement them – indeed each technique has its own advantages and limitations. They can all be used in the standing horse, thereby increasing their practicality and availability in equine practice. The arrival of positron emission tomography (PET) will undoubtedly add to and refine our diagnostic capabilities for conditions of the distal limb in the next five years.

12.2 Sedation and Pain Relief Used during the Diagnostic Procedure

Historically, no systemic drugs were used when local diagnostic injections were used to try to isolate areas of pain experienced by the animal. However, workers from Bristol (Termansen and Meehan, 2021) have answered the question of whether sedation with alpha2-adrenergic agonist alone or alpha2-adrenergic agonists in combination with butorphanol tartrate effect the degree of lameness. They concluded that, in general, sedating a horse with an alpha2-adrenergic agonist alone or in combination with butorphanol tartrate does not change the baseline of lameness. Due to the large variation in the measurements, the small magnitude of few significant effects and inconsistency of these findings, there is insufficient evidence to recommend avoiding the use of sedation in cases where it would increase the safety of those involved. However, regardless of protocol used, clinicians must appreciate the possibility of individual horse variation.

Practitioners are advised that they should take into account multiple factors, not limited to

DOI: 10.1079/9781800624283.0012

individual clinical expertise, patient's circumstances and owners' values, country, location or clinic where they work, the individual case in front of them and the availability of therapies and resources.

12.3 Treating the Lame Horse

As with all treatments, the clinician needs a history, followed by an examination, in order to make a diagnosis. The treatment plan can then be designed.

History

Any history should obviously include the age of the animal and the work it is doing. Enquires should be made into any previous lameness or injury. The length of the current lameness and whether it had a sudden onset should also be discussed. Was the onset injury related? The leg that the owner considers to be the problem should be recorded.

Examination

A general examination should be made, which need not be prolonged. However, it is vital that the general health status of the animal and its general demeanour is assessed. Its stance and any muscle wasting should be noted. The animal should be checked for any wounds or infected areas, and any swellings noted.

The animal should be walked in a straight line away from and back towards the clinician, and any change in gait discussed with the owner. The animal is then led round in a 5-m circle to both the left and the right. If no severe lameness is noted the animal should be trotted in a straight line. Hopefully, agreement will be reached between the clinician and the owner as to which leg the animal is actually lame on. Great care should be taken to make sure that the animal is lame on only one leg, and that two or more legs are not involved.

Once the affected leg or legs have been identified, they must then be checked carefully for any swelling, which is discussed with the owner to determine its duration. Any swelling is palpated carefully to assess texture and pain. The hoof is next for examination, after having been picked out and squeezed with hoof testers. Each joint should be flexed and extended to check for both the degree of movement and any pain. Flexion tests are then carried out; ideally, the leg opposite to the lame leg is tested first. Starting with the front legs, the leg is picked up and the fetlock flexed firmly. Obviously, the carpus and the other joints higher up will be partially flexed; flexion should be maintained for 1 min, after which the horse is trotted away in a straight line for at least 12 m; any aggravated lameness should be noted. This should then be repeated after flexing the carpus more severely. It is important not to hold the leg by the metacarpus, as the resulting pressure on the tendons may confuse the result. Flexion tests are next performed on the hind legs, starting by flexing the fetlock and hock. In the repeat test the hock must be as straight as possible, while flexing both the stifle and hip. When these examinations have been completed, the results should be evaluated and then discussed with the owner; a further plan of action may then be devised.

It may be decided to carry out these flexion tests again with the horse lunged in a circle; perhaps the horse may be examined on different surfaces and lunged on various surfaces. It may be decided to canter the horse as well as just trotting it. It may even be decided to have the horse pull a vehicle to further evaluate the lameness. It should be remembered that this careful examination does not require any sophisticated equipment and can be carried out in nearly all circumstances. However, there can be problems; some horses, particularly very small ponies, will not trot. Other horses, e.g. pacers and Icelandic horses, have a fifth gait and may also be reluctant to trot.

Preliminary diagnosis

Practitioners need always to keep an open mind, but should concentrate initially on the common conditions. A large percentage of lameness cases are related to the foot, the most common being the so-called 'pus in the foot'. It is rare in cases of 'pus in the foot' that some pain is not seen on hoof testing. Conditions affecting the foot of the horse are described in detail in Chapter 11.

If a preliminary diagnosis is made there is a large benefit to the animal on welfare grounds if treatment can be initiated immediately. To give an example, a horse may have pastern dermatitis, a condition described fully in Section 20.19. If this condition is even moderately severe it will cause lameness. Equally, the clinician may be concerned that there is an underlying cause of the lameness as well as pastern dermatitis, which may be on several limbs. It is therefore logical to treat the pastern dermatitis and cure, if possible, that condition before going on with a more intensive lameness investigation.

If joint pain is suspected, it is quite reasonable to treat the animal with NSAIDs immediately on welfare grounds. However, it must be remembered that this may interfere with a more detailed lameness investigation, although it may cure the condition and render a more detailed examination only an academic exercise. It is paramount for practitioners to remember that their role is centred on relieving pain and helping the horse before making a definitive diagnosis. It might be argued that only through a really accurate diagnosis can the pain be relieved, but with joint pain this is rarely the case.

Simple treatment options available to the clinician

1. Non-steroidal anti-inflammatory drugs (NSAIDs; see Section 6.8). These must be injected i/v. Those used in equines are phenylbutazone (PBZ), flunixin, ketoprofen, meloxicam and carprofen. This can then be followed up in oral form, either as an oral paste in the case of PBZ and flunixin or as a powder for them all. Aspirin, the oldest known NSAID, is available as a powder. Large doses of aspirin, e.g. up to 100 mg/kg, are often required before any effect is seen.

2. Chondroprotection nutrichemicals. There are very few double-blind trials for these chemicals. They are expensive and have exaggerated claims for their efficacy but, having said that, it is likely that they do have some effect. The clinician should be aware that the ingredients are often not actually what is stated on the label and that many are not actually available to the horse in the form in which they are supplied.

3. Management. Under this heading should be included foot balancing and farriery, very valuable adjuncts to treatment that are described in Section 11.1. The main management tool, however, is rest. The ultimate is when the animal is cross-tied and in slings. However, so-called 'box rest', when an animal is confined to a stall or very small outside area, is very useful. It is very important in many conditions when higher doses of NSAIDs are being given that the animal is confined so that it cannot overuse the damaged joint. Many damaged joints, tendons and ligaments will heal if they can be rested. This is very difficult to achieve with certain horses that do not settle well when confined, but there are some tricks available to help the clinician: (i) having another quiet horse confined in the next box; (ii) having a mirror in the stable; or (iii) using various devices that oblige the horse to take a considerable time in obtaining its food. Advice should always be given with care. It is obviously counter-productive to have a horse that constantly 'box-walks' confined to a box; it would be better to have such a horse confined to a very small paddock.

It is very important that management does not bring on some other condition, e.g. having the horse confined on manure and it then developing 'thrush', or not allowing a horse to move that then develops laminitis. All management tools should be discussed with the owner and, if the clinician is in any doubt, a follow-up visit should be arranged.

4. Glycosaminoglycans. Intramuscularly, these may be effective in certain conditions. Their use will be more likely to be worthwhile if several joints are involved, but it is expensive.

5. Sodium hyaluronate. An i/v injectable, this is even more expensive, so the cost–benefit balance needs to be considered with care.

6. Tiludronic acid. This treatment is even more expensive than the foregoing, as not only is the medicine expensive but it also has to be given as a drip under veterinary supervision. The main claims for success involve spavin (see Section 12.7) and navicular damage (see Section 12.10). However, any joint condition requiring bone remodelling should benefit.

12.4 Fore Limb Lameness in the Donkey not Associated with the Foot

It is not sensible here to make a long list of all possible lameness problems in the donkey, as many conditions will be covered in the sections below on the horse (Sections 12.6 and 12.7). However, it should always be remembered that the donkey is an extremely stoical beast. Fractures should always be considered with even moderate lameness; obviously, any swelling will direct the clinician to the source of lameness. However, in the absence of clues it is important to work up the leg methodically once foot lameness has been eliminated. Radial paralysis may mislead the clinician: the donkey initially appears fracture lame, but careful observation will reveal that the animal is able to bear weight when the leg is placed in the correct position. Normally, there is a lack of skin sensation on the dorsal aspect of the pastern. Prognosis in these cases is good, as the animal rapidly learns to flick the foot forward when walking. Normally, the animal will appear sound in 3 months, but full sensation may not return for over 12 months.

Osteoarthritis causing lameness is common in the elderly donkey, the carpus being the most commonly affected joint. Joint effusion is marked. A joint block (see Section 12.10) can be performed to confirm the diagnosis, but with experience this may be unnecessary. Draining the fluid and injecting intra-articular steroid may be all that is required. This procedure gives considerable relief to the donkey and will often remain so for more than 18 months. Naturally, it can be repeated, but the effective relief is much shorter following second and subsequent injections.

12.5 Hind Limb Lameness in the Donkey not Associated with the Foot

Upward fixation of the patella is not uncommon in the young, poorly developed donkey, and so the need for median ligament desmotomy is rare. Most of these cases will cure with time provided that nutrition and exercise are improved. A short course of phenylbutazone is worthwhile.

A much less common condition, which may confuse the practitioner, is rupture of the peroneus tertius muscle, part of the reciprocal apparatus. In this condition the stifle will flex but the hock remains in extension. This condition may be seen in the old, debilitated donkey, but it has also been reported to occur in the overworked animal. The prognosis is not good in the older animal, but normal function will return within 2–3 months if the debilitated donkey is rested and fed well.

The third condition in this group is when the Achilles tendon slips off the point of the hock. This condition will alarm the donkey, which will try to move and then may even bolt, as the leg feels strange. However, I do not think this condition is actually acutely painful. The prognosis is good and normal function returns within 2 months.

12.6 Fore Limb Lameness in the Horse not Associated with the Foot

Sweeny

Sweeny is atrophy of any group of muscles. However, when considering the horse, it is normally associated with atrophy of the supraspinatus and infraspinatus muscles of the shoulder. This is seen as complete wasting of these muscles, revealing the spine of the scapula. The cause is trauma to the suprascapular nerve by a blow to the point of the shoulder, which may be from a kick, hitting a gatepost or striking the shafts of a cart. Nevertheless, rarely is the cause of the trauma discovered as muscle atrophy takes time to occur. There is no treatment. Rarely do the muscles regenerate. However, the horse is seldom lame and can be used as normal.

Inflammation of the bicipital bursa

Again, this is caused by trauma to the cranial aspect of the shoulder, and lameness is marked. There will be pain in the area of the shoulder, particularly when the joint is flexed. A standard flexion test will make the degree of lameness worse. Treatment is usually by parenteral NSAIDs, or even topically. Normally, box rest is not required provided the horse is not allowed violent exercise. The horse should become sound within 12 weeks.

Arthritis of the shoulder joint

A rare condition, it is associated with either: (i) violent movement of the joint, causing a small fracture of the tuber scapulae; or (ii) a kick, causing a small fracture of the lateral tuberosity of the humerus. There is no instability of the joint, but the horse will become progressively more lame, particularly after flexion. There is rarely any swelling – or indeed pain – associated with the area. A definitive diagnosis could be made with a shoulder joint nerve block (see Section 12.10). Radiography may be helpful, but often the fracture is hard to visualize. Joint medication with a long-acting steroid is helpful and may be effective for 12 months. However, repeated medication will not last nearly as long, and NSAIDs will be palliative only initially. The long-term prognosis is poor.

Fracture of the scapula

This fracture will present a confusing picture. The horse is going to be very lame, with sudden onset. With a severe fracture of the neck of the scapula there will be crepitus and abnormal movement, and so the diagnosis will be straightforward; prompt euthanasia is the only course of action. However, there may be less obvious fractures that, if they do not involve the shoulder joint, will eventually fuse and the horse will become sound; this process may take 9–12 months. There is no need to box-rest the horse provided no violent exercise is permitted.

Paralysis of the radial nerve on its own or associated with a fracture of the humerus

The horse will appear fracture lame. Indeed, there may be a fracture of the humerus, which is often the cause of radial paralysis as the nerve runs around the humerus in the musculospiral groove. In this case there will be crepitus and abnormal movement of the upper leg. Immediate euthanasia is indicated. However, it is vital that clinicians recognize when the radial nerve is paralysed without fracture of the humerus. The prognosis without a fracture is good. The radial nerve may be crushed or badly damaged by a fall on concrete or by having the leg crushed high up. Radial paralysis can also be caused by long recumbency on a hard surface, and this should be avoided at all costs during a long surgical operation.

As the radial nerve supplies all the extensor muscles of the fore limb, radial paralysis means that the horse cannot extend either its knee or fetlock, so it will drag the hoof along the ground. However, if the foot is placed on the ground the horse can bear weight without any problem. Remarkably quickly, the horse will learn to flick its foot forward, so that the problem will only be obvious to an astute observer. Obviously, the clinician hopes that the radial paralysis is only temporary but, even if the radial nerve is permanently damaged, the horse can still be worked as there is no pain involved.

Fracture of the olecranon

Ulnar fractures can be successfully repaired using plate fixation while sedated and restrained in stocks in the standing position. The plate should be removed in 3 months.

Capped elbow

Normally a self-inflicted problem, this is a bursitis on the point of the olecranon caused by repeated trauma from the hind shoe as the horse gets up. It rarely occurs in horses outside, but usually in the stabled horse. The hind shoes should be removed and the toes of the hind hooves shortened. A soft floor, ideally rubber matting, should be provided, or the horse should be turned out. Injecting corticosteroids into the bursa should be avoided on account of the danger of sepsis. The prognosis is good, except there is always likely to be some scarring. If the elbow develops an open wound, then the prognosis is very guarded; topical NSAIDs may speed recovery if the wound heals.

Fracture of the radius

Normally disastrous, this may be either compound, severely commuted or involving a joint.

Nevertheless, in extremely rare cases healing can be accomplished with a massive nursing input. For surgical repair a general anaesthetic is required. Four holes are drilled into the toe of the hoof, then two wire loops threaded through these holes and attached to a rope. Traction must then be applied with the horse anchored by another rope around the axilla. When the surgeon is satisfied that the ends of the fracture are in apposition, a cast covering the whole leg, including the foot, is applied as far towards the axilla as possible. The horse is given an assisted recovery and kept in slings. The cast will need to be removed and replaced in 3 weeks; in a further 3 weeks the cast can be removed and the leg splinted in a full Robert Jones, with a lateral wooden extension. The horse needs to be kept in slings for a total of 12 weeks. Hopefully, by then union will have been accomplished.

Problems associated with the carpus

Clinicians should remember that most conditions associated with the carpus are associated with swelling, and so diagnosis of the joint involved is straightforward. However, a specific diagnosis will often not be so easy.

Problems with the carpus are commonly seen in the foal soon after birth. There may be lateral or medial deviation, which must be differentiated from: (i) valgus, a deviation of the third metacarpal bone laterally; and (ii) varus, the less common medial deviation. These latter two conditions can be corrected surgically by reducing the growth of one side of the metacarpal bone. Surgery involves either the use of staples or stripping the periosteum. This must be carried out before 6 months of age, ideally at 3–4 months so that there is still ample growth left in the metacarpal bone.

The problem of deviation affecting the carpus cannot be corrected; if it is severe euthanasia is indicated. Casting the leg is recommended by some authorities, but this is extremely hazardous on account of the danger of pressure sores. Conservative treatment should be tried; the mare and foal should be kept on a small paddock and glue-on lateral or medial extension shoes applied.

There may also be seen a condition of the carpus involving anterior deviation, sometimes called 'bucked knees'. When standing, the horse will have one or both knees slightly flexed; if this is seen in a foal the condition will resolve in most cases without treatment. However, if it is severe, casting for a maximum of 10 days should be tried. Normally, the legs will then straighten after the cast is removed and the flexor tendons relax. Historically, the foal with this condition was treated with large doses of oxytetracycline: it was believed that the antibiotic reduced the uptake of calcium, but this is now known to be false. This condition can also occur in the adult following injury, resulting in overcompensation of the flexor apparatus; it is very unlikely to respond to casting or any other treatment.

Another problem seen in the foal affects not only the carpus but the entirety of both forelegs – they are both bowed in the same direction, the 'windswept foal'. The cause is thought to be when there is too little space in the mare's abdomen for the developing foal in the uterus. Normally this condition, provided the foal can feed, will correct itself.

Clinicians will commonly see, in the adult horse, a swelling on the anterior aspect of the carpus; this is called a hygroma and is a bursitis cranial to the carpal joint. It is normally caused by trauma. The horse is rarely lame, and the swelling should be left alone. If the horse is lame and the lameness is made worse by carpal flexion, treatment should be tried. First, the joint is surgically prepared; under sterile conditions the practitioner should draw off as much of the fluid as possible. The joint should be injected with a long-acting corticosteroid; a full Robert Jones splint is then applied for 10 days. The condition is likely to recur in 1–2 years, although the treatment can be repeated.

Horses can develop a true carpitis, which is osteoarthritis of the carpal joint and normally follows trauma. It will be seen as lameness, but this should diminish unless there is a fracture of one of the carpal bones. However, even without a fracture, new bone is likely to be laid down and will cause permanent lameness in the long term. Initial treatment with NSAIDs will be helpful, and permanent glucosamine treatment may be tried.

The most common fracture in the carpus is fracture of the radial carpal bone. However, fractures of other carpal bones will occur, resulting in acute lameness. Ideally, the joint should be radiographed and then the chip fragment of the fracture removed surgically. If this is not possible, conservative treatment involving box rest and NSAIDs should be tried. If no improvement is then noticed within 3 months, the horse should be destroyed to prevent further suffering.

There is one specific fracture, however, that is not uncommon, which is fracture of the accessory carpal bone. Obviously, this could be due to external trauma, but it may also fracture from the force of the flexor tendons, which run in a groove on its palmar surface; the fragments are pulled apart by the tendons. Interestingly, there is rarely severe lameness and the horse will bear weight; crepitus can be felt only in the early stages. The horse will show pain on flexion of the carpus and there will be marked swelling of the carpal sheath. The fracture will be clearly seen on a lateral radiograph. No internal fixation should be attempted and outside casting is not needed. A Robert Jones bandage is useful to lessen the pain and inflammation for the first 2 weeks, and NSAIDs should be given. The bone will heal by fibrous union within 6 months, and the horse may then be brought back into light work. However, there has been recent publication of osteosynthesis being performed in the standing horse which is worth recording (Aßmann *et al.*, 2023).

Damage to the extensor tendons

The signs of this condition will vary depending on the extent of the damage to the tendon or tendons involved; there will be swelling and pain on palpation. Trauma is the normal cause. Initially, the horse will stumble as it will be reluctant to extend its carpus and fetlock. As these tendons are not weight bearing, lameness normally regresses rapidly. Horses can manage well without one of these tendons, even if totally severed by a sharp object.

Contraction of the flexor tendons

This is normally a condition of the neonatal foal. The foal will have problems if the contraction is so severe that it cannot extend its leg sufficiently to bear weight and takes its weight on its fetlock, or worse, on its carpus. If the foal can bear weight, its own weight will stretch the flexor tendons and cure the condition. If it cannot bear weight, action has to be taken. The leg should be well padded and then bandaged into a piece of guttering that reaches just below its toe and above the carpus; this type of splint may have to be applied to both front legs. It should be checked every 3 days to ensure there are no pressure sores. As soon as the toe can bear weight the splint should be removed to allow the foal's own weight to stretch the tendons.

In rare cases this condition will be acquired in the first few months of life; the tendons will slowly contract, forming a box-shaped foot. The condition should be very closely monitored. If it becomes too severe, tenotomy should be performed; this will require a general anaesthetic and full surgical precautions. Antibiotics should be given pre- and post-operatively and tetanus antitoxin given. Initially, the superficially digital flexor tendon should be cut with the tendon under tension. If a bistoury (long, narrow-bladed knife) is used the incision can be small. If the condition is very severe the deep digital flexor tendon needs to be cut. This should be performed at a different site to limit the adhesions formed. A gutter splint should be applied for 10 days post-operatively.

Damage to the flexor tendons

This is the most common injury sustained by the racehorse, but is seen much less commonly in the working horse. It is mainly a condition of the foreleg, but occasionally will be seen in the hind leg. Normally, just the superficial digital flexor tendon is involved; rarely, the deep digital flexor tendon is involved and extremely rarely the suspensory ligament, as described below, is involved. Damage can occur high up, just below the carpus, at mid-cannon or just above the fetlock joint. When it occurs low down the annular ligament may be involved. There will be swelling and acute lameness, with pain felt over the site of the damage.

Immediate support with bandaging should be carried out, together with NSAIDs. There have been a large number of treatments advised in the past, but these have been shown not to be helpful. Rest is the most essential treatment. A very recent form of treatment, involving the injection of previously harvested stem cells, may well be the treatment option in years to come. However, most cases will recover in time, although severe cases may well require 9 months. Clinicians should be aware that in rare cases the severely damaged tendon will become infected by haematogenous spread. In these cases the pain and swelling will not subside as expected. The pus will then break out through the skin, just above the fetlock on the palmar aspect. Antibiotics and NSAIDs should be given. Provided there is good drainage the prognosis is similar to that of an uninfected tendonitis.

Metacarpal periostitis

A condition of young horses, it is often called 'sore shins'. Its cause is thought to be concussion, and it is seen only on the forelegs. It occurs in the young horse coming into work. There will be bilateral lameness, although one leg may be worse than the other. Pain will be elicited by palpating the dorsal surface of the metacarpal bone. All manner of treatments have been suggested, but time is the main healer. The prognosis is good.

Splints

Splints are very common in the young horse between 3 and 5 years of age. They are a disturbance of the interosseous ligament, which binds the second and the fourth metacarpal bones to the third metacarpal bone. They are much less common in the hind leg. Often, they will appear without the handler being aware of them. However, the horse will usually show a 2/10 lameness for 2 weeks, and a hard lump will become apparent; then the lameness will recover. Treatment is unnecessary.

Fracture of the splint bone

Damage here can occur in any age of horse, and is normally caused by trauma associated with a kick from another horse. There will be a swelling over the area and the horse will be 3/10–4/10 lame. The clinician should beware of dismissing this lameness, as in many cases it will continue. Misdiagnosis is most common in the young horse. Without radiography a definitive diagnosis is difficult. If the lameness persists for more than 4 weeks a fracture should be suspected. Local anaesthetic should be instilled into the area, and if the lameness is reduced thereby a fracture should be suspected. Many fractures will heal given time, but the correct procedure is to remove the lower fractured part of the bone. This should be done under general anaesthetic, with full surgical precautions. The clinician will find the lower fragment is not very ossified but closely attached to the third metacarpal bone; it should then be stripped off with a bone chisel. The subcuticular fascia is then brought together with absorbable suture material and the skin closed with interrupted monofilament nylon sutures. The leg should be bandaged for 10 days and the horse kept in a box. Antibiotics and NSAIDs are useful. Obviously, the horse must be covered against tetanus. The prognosis is good.

Damage to the suspensory ligament

The suspensory ligament is the most important part of the stay apparatus. Damage called desmitis normally occurs as a result of overextension of the fetlock joint when the horse is travelling at speed. The ligament bifurcates at the lower end of the metacarpal bone, a common position for damage. The actual ligament can be palpated and pain may be elicited. Once again, a long period of rest is required. The prognosis is guarded. Suspensory desmitis will be found in the hind leg. Lameness will be of low grade and diagnosis is difficult. Prognosis is very guarded, as often rest will not cure the condition.

Fracture of the metacarpal or metatarsal bone

An extremely serious fracture in either front or hind leg (Fig. 12.1), it is often compound and requires immediate euthanasia. Hairline fractures will be very difficult to diagnose without radiography. A full fracture will show crepitus

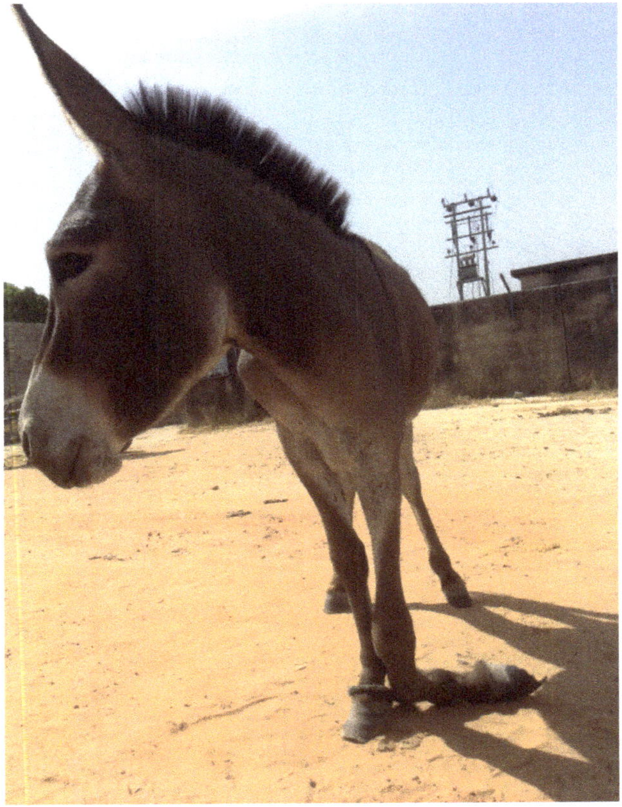

Fig. 12.1. A long-standing metacarpal fracture. A severe welfare problem.

and 10/10 lameness. The prognosis is very grave, but casting of the whole leg proximal to the carpus may be attempted, with the cast being replaced after 3 weeks. At the 6-week point a Robert Jones splint is applied for a further 6 weeks. Keeping the horse in slings will be very beneficial.

Fracture of the proximal sesamoid bone or bones

This is an acute injury seen mainly in the racing horse at the end of a race, but it may also be seen in the very tired working horse. Normally it occurs in a front leg, but it can also occur in a hind leg. There will be very severe lameness and very marked swelling. Obviously, the horse should not be moved. Ideally, radiographs should be taken and internal fixation attempted. However, the clinician in the field needs to use careful judgement. A good approach would be to apply a low Robert Jones splint and move the horse to a place of safety. If the clinician is very confident of the diagnosis a splint can be applied using a 10 cm plank of wood secured to the bottom of the foot and then strapped to the cannon. The joint is then in flexion and is taking the strain off the sesamoids. The horse is confined for 3 days on large doses of NSAIDs. The swelling will subside and casting can be attempted. The prognosis must be grave.

Fracture of the first phalanx

This injury is normally a disaster as there are often multiple fragments, and this is the so-called 'bag of ice fracture': immediate euthanasia is mandatory. If there is a single fracture line it will normally involve either the metacarpophalangeal or the proximal phalangeal joint. Lameness will persist, even with the fracture healing after long immobilization. Welfare must be considered. Casting should be carried out only in the young horse. Obviously, radiography is very helpful.

Sesamoiditis

The signs of this condition are similar to a sesamoid fracture, as described above; there is marked swelling of the fetlock, and pain particularly over the palmar aspect. The horse will be reluctant to extend the fetlock. Without radiography diagnosis is not possible, and therefore the clinician should treat the condition as if there was a fracture and hope that healing will occur with time. Certainly, the prognosis is better than for sesamoid fracture, but still very guarded.

Arthritis of the fetlock

Unlike ringbone as described below, the extra bone laid down with chronic arthritis cannot be palpated. Confirmation of the diagnosis can really be made only by intra-joint local anaesthesia. However, the clinician in the field can be fairly certain of the diagnosis by the response to flexion tests of that leg. Joint medication can be used for treatment or NSAIDs will be effective for some months, but eventually with either treatment lameness will not be controlled and euthanasia must be carried out.

Fracture of the second phalanx

A fracture less common than fracture of the first phalanx, but the advice is the same.

Fractures of the distal phalanx

These are even more uncommon that the fracture of the second phalanx. They can be treated conservatively by reduced limb loading and provision of adequate analgesia. There are considerable welfare considerations.

Ringbone

A very old term and perhaps one that should not really be used by the veterinary practitioner, it describes extra bone growth on the first and second phalanges. A high ringbone is extra bone at the distal end of the first phalanx and the proximal end of the second phalanx, and this can be felt; a low ringbone is extra bone at the distal end of the second phalanx, and this can only be diagnosed on radiographs. Neither condition causes lameness until the joints become involved. As the condition is progressive it is likely to cause lameness eventually. Ringbone is caused by concussion and is common in the cob but rare in the thoroughbred. Long-term NSAIDs will help, but eventually the lameness will be unresponsive, and euthanasia should be advised.

Pyramidal disease

This condition should be termed an exostosis of the extensor process of the third phalanx. Initial lameness will be slight, but the condition will be progressive. The clinician may think there is sepsis involved, but no purulent tract will be found in the toe and no pus will break out at the swelling on the coronary band. There is no treatment, and therefore euthanasia is indicated.

Fracture of the extensor process of the third phalanx

This is a condition similar to pyramidal disease, but it will have a sudden onset and will look even more like sepsis. Radiography would be useful, but the practitioner will be able to make the diagnosis clinically given time and the inability to draw out pus with a poultice. The swelling on the dorsal coronary band will remain large. There is no treatment, and therefore euthanasia is indicated.

12.7 Hind Limb Lameness in the Horse not Associated with the Foot

Fracture of the pelvis

Normally, this condition will have a sudden onset during fast work. The expected pathology is a partial fracture of the wing of the ilium, so crepitus will not be felt. However, there will be pain on pressure and with movement. If the neck of the ilium is fractured there will be crepitus and really severe pain. There is no treatment and immediate euthanasia should be carried out. In the partial fracture, however, healing will take place provided the animal is kept in a box for 6 weeks and then in a very small paddock for a further 4 months; the horse should then be able to return to work. There will be very little muscle wastage on the affected side.

Dislocation of the hip

Normally a condition in the pony, this will also occur in the horse that has been trapped in the harness and has struggled violently to retrieve a hind leg. The head of the femur is displaced upward and forward. A rectal examination should be carried out to confirm that there is no fracture of the acetabulum. The affected limb will appear shorter and on movement the hock will turn outwards, but the toe and stifle will turn inwards. Replacement under general anaesthetic is unlikely to be successful. Radical surgery has been suggested, but this is not to be recommended. If the pony is a mare and is young it might be possible for it to be kept for breeding, as young ponies have been documented as forming a false joint. However, euthanasia is the likely outcome.

Rupture of the round ligament of the hip without dislocation

Again, this is mainly a condition seen in the pony, the signs being very similar to those of dislocation of the hip; however, the legs will be of equal length. The toe of the affected leg, like the stifle, will be held outwards with the hock held inwards. Crepitus may be felt per rectum. The prognosis is very poor, although box rest and NSAIDs may be tried for 4 weeks. Euthanasia should be carried out if there is no improvement.

Bursitis of the greater trochanter

A condition resulting from trauma after a fall, this is an inflammation of the bursal sheath below the middle gluteus muscle. Pain will be felt from pressure over the greater trochanter. There is no crepitus, which would normally be felt with a fracture of the acetabulum. The horse will not track up normally and muscle wastage will occur quite rapidly. The prognosis is poor as there is no treatment, apart from high doses of NSAIDs. If normal movement is not established within 6 weeks, euthanasia should be carried out.

Femoral nerve paralysis

Resulting from trauma when a horse has had its leg caught in the harness and violently tries to pull it out, the horse will not bear weight and the leg will be held in a flexed position; the horse will be unable to bring its leg forward. There will be no crepitus, which would be felt with a fracture of the tibia. The horse should receive NSAIDs but not be confined, as the clinician hopes that the nerve supply has not been totally destroyed. There will be muscle wastage on the front and the sides of the femur. If there is no improvement after 1 month euthanasia should be carried out.

Upward fixation of the patella

A common condition, it is seen in the young, heavy yearling, the 2-year-old and also in the young pony, but also in older, debilitated animals. The clinical signs are diagnostic: the horse will move off dragging a hind leg, which it will normally then snatch forward and walk normally. In some cases, the leg will not come into flexion without really frightening the horse. In a very few cases the leg cannot be brought into flexion by any means, including the use of a sideline from the neck of the horse round the affected leg below the pastern and pulled strongly cranially. This type of case will require immediate surgery, but in the other cases the clinician has a dilemma: conservative treatment involving improvement in the diet, good exercise and NSAIDs will often cure many cases, particularly in the young horse. These horses go on doing very well and never have further problems with their stifles. On the other hand, a few cases will develop problems with arthritis of the stifle later in life, and the clinician might wish that surgery had been done previously. Surgery is relatively simple, but once again a few cases later in life will develop arthritis. Therefore, as a rule of thumb, give the young horse a chance but if it continues to lock up after 2 months, surgery should be performed.

The surgical technique required is sectioning of the median patellar ligament, which must be done standing. It is very difficult under general anaesthetic as the ligaments are not under tension. The horse should be sedated and the area around the median ligament clipped and prepared for surgery. Local anaesthetic is then instilled under the skin and around and under the median ligament. The area should be re-cleaned. With full surgical asepsis a 5 cm incision is made vertically along the median ligament, with the horse bearing weight on that leg. With blunt dissection a small pair of blunt-ended artery forceps is inserted from the dorsal aspect under the ligament to emerge on the caudal aspect. A bistoury is inserted beside the artery forceps and the ligament is sectioned in its entirety. The surgeon will perceive the full sectioning as the ligament retracts. The reason that the bistoury is not used on its own is because if the horse moves while it is being inserted, some of the ligament will be sectioned but the surgeon may not be 100% sure that the whole ligament has been. Three interrupted skin sutures of monofilament nylon are required to close the wound. There is no need to dress the wound, but it is prudent to keep the animal confined for 10 days before the sutures are removed. Antibiotics should be given. Only if there is marked swelling should NSAIDs be given. The tetanus status of the horse must be checked.

Inflammation of the stifle joint

As discussed above, the stifle joint may become inflamed from constant upward fixation of the patella. Equally, it may become inflamed as a result of sectioning of the median patellar ligament, but this latter condition is extremely rare.

The horse may also damage its stifle by trying to jump over doors, gates, fences, etc. Inflammation of the stifle is termed gonitis. The stifle is a very complicated joint and there are many parts that may become damaged, e.g. the medial and lateral collateral ligaments, the anterior and posterior cruciate ligaments, the menisci and the joint capsule itself. Normally, there is swelling and, in many instances, pain on palpation. Certainly there will be lameness, which will be worse on flexion test. Accurate diagnosis is very difficult without radiography, ultrasonography and even arthroscopy. The practitioner in the field should try confining the horse to a very small paddock and giving a prolonged course of NSAIDs. If lameness persists joint medication can be attempted, but the prognosis is likely to be poor.

Rupture of the peroneal tendon

Discussion of this condition in the donkey will be found in Section 12.5. The peroneal tendon is part of the reciprocal apparatus, and in this condition the stifle will flex but the hock will remain in extension. A problem seen in the overworked horse, the prognosis is not good in older animals, but normal function will return in 2–3 months in young horses that are rested and fed well.

Rupture of the gastrocnemius muscle and the superficial flexor tendon

The cause of these two conditions is always trauma. Normally, rupture of the gastrocnemius muscle precedes rupture of the superficial flexor tendon. The condition can occur in both legs at the same time. It normally occurs when a horse is trying to stop a heavy cart on a hill when the brakes have failed. The principal sign of the condition is a dropping of the hock, so that there is an excessive angle in the joint. The horse will appear to be squatting and unable to straighten its hind legs. If the Achilles tendon is totally ruptured the horse cannot bear any weight and should be destroyed immediately. If only the gastrocnemius muscle is partially ruptured on one side, healing may occur if the horse can be kept in a Thompson splint for 3 months.

Occasionally the Achilles tendon is not ruptured but slips off the point of the hock. This condition is alarming for the horse; it will try to move and then may even bolt, as the leg feels strange. However, I do not think this condition is acutely painful. The prognosis is good and normal function returns within 2 months.

Fibrotic myopathy of the semitendinosus muscle

Again, a condition of the overworked old horse, the semitendinosus muscle is damaged due to continual braking while hauling a cart. Adhesions are then formed with the semimembranosus and the biceps femoris muscles. Initially, there will be an alteration of the gait, which will then turn into a lameness that will not be altered by a flexion test. As the adhesions become ossified the lameness will become more pronounced. The action is pathognomonic in that as the foot is about to be placed on the ground it will jerk back 10 or so centimetres. There have been heroic attempts at surgery but these are rarely successful; euthanasia is the kindest action.

Stringhalt

This condition, which is an involuntary flexion of the hock during forward movement, is disastrous in driving horses as the high movement may involve the tack. However, it is a condition that can be tolerated in the riding horse. The aetiology is unknown, but there are plenty of theories. There is no treatment. Diagnosis can be made by making the handler push the horse backwards and then snatch it forward – the condition is more likely to be more obvious in these circumstances. Sadly there is no effective reliable treatment. Sectioning of the lateral digital extensor as it passes over the hock has been suggested, but the results are not reliable.

Shivering

A strange condition of involuntary movement of the hind limbs and tail, it is usually more pronounced when the horse is pushed backwards. The aetiology is unknown and there is no treatment. Unfortunately, the condition does seem to be progressive. It makes farriery very difficult, especially on the hind feet. NSAIDs should be given for 2 days before farriery is attempted, as low-grade arthritis will increase difficulties for the farrier.

Spavin

Other than conditions of the feet, this is the most common condition affecting the hind limb of the horse. It is often bilateral, with one leg being worse than the other. If the better leg has a flexion test it may appear to make the bad leg worse, but when the bad leg is tested a very marked lameness will be seen. A spavin is actually an osteitis affecting the medial aspect of the proximal end of the third metatarsal bone and the medial aspect of the third and central tarsal bones. Classically, in very advanced cases this bony swelling could be felt on the medial aspect of the hock. If it is very pronounced it is called a 'Jack spavin'; if it cannot be felt but the clinician is certain that it is present it is called a 'blind spavin'. There are two other swellings in that area that may cause confusion for laypeople. The first is a fluid swelling caused by joint effusion; this may indicate that a spavin is forming or, like a windgall on the fetlock, be of no relevance, and is called a 'bog spavin'. The second is an enlargement of a superficial vein, the saphenous, which is of no relevance but is called a 'blood spavin'.

Joint nerve blocks will establish a diagnosis, which can be reinforced by radiography. If a bony swelling is felt it is likely that joint medication will not be effective. In these instances, the horse should be medicated with suitable NSAIDs until sound, and then worked. Slowly, the medication can be reduced. It is hoped that the affected joint will ankylose and render movement of the hock, which will be reduced, pain free.

Thoroughpin

The familiar name for tenosynovitis of the tarsal sheath, which is a fluid-filled swelling that can be pushed from one side of the deep digital flexor tendon to the other in a position level with, or just below, the point of the hock. It does not affect the horse, and in fact it does not indicate the likelihood of any other problems and should therefore be ignored.

Curb

An enlargement of the posterior aspect of the fibular tarsal bone usually seen in the young animal, e.g. the yearling with poor conformation of the hock. When it is forming and there is inflammation there will be transitory lameness, but this will disappear to leave a small bony swelling, which should cause no further problems.

Capped hock

A condition of the stabled horse that repeatedly traumatizes the point of the hock when rising. Obviously, a good bed and rubber matting will prevent the condition. However, once it has occurred it is not so easy to treat, particularly if the skin has been broken and there is infection. The horse should be given antibiotics and NSAIDs. Oily cream should be applied to the wound and the horse turned out. Some cases are the result of a horse continually kicking a trailer ramp, and in these cases either the horse should be allowed to travel free or the tail ramp should be well cushioned.

12.8 Back Problems

Fractured ribs

A very painful condition, this normally results from an accident within the shafts of a cart. The clinician should be aware of the danger of pneumonia and pleural effusion, as described in Section 14.5. Antibiotics and NSAIDs should be given as soon after the accident as possible. The horse should be rested for 6 weeks before bringing it slowly back into work.

Myositis of the psoas and longissimus dorsi muscles

Often used as a blanket diagnosis for conditions of pain in the back, these cases can either be simply rested or given a course of NSAIDs. These NSAIDs may be given parenterally or may be rubbed in daily, as they are now available in a skin-penetrating form. Naturally, it is vital that these are applied with gloved hands.

Fistulous withers

This is a term used to describe supraspinus bursitis. Historically, it was thought to be caused by local infection of *Brucella abortus*. This is now thought to be unlikely even in countries where this organism is endemic. The more likely cause is chronic wounding from ill-fitting tack. The normal course of the disease is a painful swelling over the area of the withers which progresses to a fistula. Removing the root cause is vital. Skyline radiography is useful to confirm that there are no foreign bodies (the author has found an airgun pellet and a sewing needle in two cases) or fracture fragments of bone. Treatment is problematic and often not successful. Long-term antibiotics are rarely curative. A better course of action is total excision of all the necrotic tissue and allowing healing by secondary intention.

Kissing spines

A difficult condition to diagnose accurately, the underlying theory behind this condition is that on account of the mobility of the horse's back, the vertical spinal processes in the thoracic region touch and set up an inflammation, resulting in pain in that area. Skyline radiography will confirm that the spines do actually meet. If the pain is nullified by injecting local anaesthetic into the area around the spines the condition is thought to be confirmed. The spines may then be shortened by radical surgery under general anaesthetic, but there is some doubt on the usefulness of this operation. Obviously, a long rest period is required after such radical surgery. It is possible that the inflammation may have resolved in that same length of time.

12.9 Neck Problems

Vertebral fractures

Spinal fractures can occur in the back as well as in the neck; however, as radiography is very difficult for the large bulk of the back but is much easier in the neck region, fractures tend to be diagnosed more readily in the neck. Pain may be felt in the area of the fracture, and in severe fractures crepitus may be felt. There will be a reluctance for the horse to move its neck, and this can be demonstrated by the 'carrot test'. A carrot is shown to the horse and then moved round to the shoulder region. A normal horse should be able to reach around and bite the carrot on both sides. The carrot is then passed up the horse's brisket so that it projects just in front of its fore legs; once again, a normal horse should be able to reach the carrot. The clinician is going to have at least some idea that there is a problem with the neck if the movement shown by the carrot test is impaired. Also, the whole area of the neck should be tested for sensitivity by pinching small pieces of skin with a pair of artery forceps, and if there is any sensitivity deficit it should be noted.

The clinician without radiography will have difficulty with diagnosis, and in these cases the horse should be rested, given a course of NSAIDs and re-examined at 2-weekly intervals. If the neck pain diminishes, then obviously the horse should be given more time, but if the pain is just as bad after two months, then euthanasia is justified.

Poll evil

The correct term for this condition is cranial nuchal bursitis. Workers in Belgium (Corraretti *et al.*, 2023) describe successful treatment in two horses with complete surgical resection. This now rare condition was thought to be caused by *Brucella abortus*. This is not now thought to be the case. Blunt trauma is a possible cause. Before radical surgery, skyline and lateral radiographs are advised.

Wobbler syndrome

Mainly a condition of the young thoroughbred, it is rarely seen in other breeds and therefore might be seen in the young carriage horse. The age range would be 2–8 years, but most are in the younger range. The pathology occurs in the cervical region and involves a narrowing of the bony canal containing the spinal cord. The main sign is a progressive ataxia of the hind legs. There is no resistance to a tail pull as the horse is walking. The horse will have difficulties when turning in a tight circle and will fall when the condition has progressed. The progressive nature of the condition is important, as this will help the clinician to differentiate it from an injury to the spinal cord in the cervical region: the latter is likely to have a sudden onset. There is no treatment. Euthanasia is indicated before the horse becomes a danger to itself and its handler.

12.10 Nerve Blocks

Introduction

Nerve blocks are described earlier in the text as an aid to diagnosis. This book has been written for the practitioner in the field who has not got access to sophisticated imaging equipment; nor in most cases is a really accurate diagnosis required. Therefore, few nerve blocks are described below. The working horse is normally well trained and well behaved. However, having large numbers of injections into their legs quickly makes them unhandleable. The diagnosis may be very laudable from an academic point of view, but the horse has been ruined for performing its work. The clinician may choose instead to make a clinical judgement and inject joint medication into a suspected diseased joint under sedation, rather than make a definitive diagnosis.

The positions for injection as described below are called blocks. Obviously, nerve blocks cannot be medicated. However, joint blocks are the same for blocking and medication. All procedures should follow aseptic precautions, but these must be particularly strict for the joint blocks. Opinions vary as to the wisdom of instilling antibiotics into the joint at the same time as other medication; on the whole, it is better to give the antibiotics parenterally and instil as little foreign matter into the joint as possible. It should be remembered when consulting other textbooks that the location of the nerve block is described for the thin-skinned thoroughbred horse; most working horses have thick skin and often scarred legs, which makes the location of underlying structures difficult. Only the useful nerve and joint blocks for the field practitioner are described here, and the list is by no means exhaustive.

Palmar digital nerve block

A simple nerve block for use in the field, this will help the clinician decide whether there is pus in the heel, an infected corn or problems with the navicular bone. It can be bypassed if these are not suspected. Following preparation, the leg is held up by the practitioner and 3 ml local anaesthetic injected at both sides over the palmar digital nerve at the distal end of the first phalanx, using a 25G needle 16 mm in length; it is advisable to inject the medial branch first. To locate the nerve in the thick-skinned horse, the clinician should feel for the beating palmar digital artery – the nerve will run just caudal to the artery. A thin, fibrous structure may be felt caudally to the nerve – this is the ligament of the ergot. The local anaesthetic must be injected dorsally into this ligament. Allowing a minimum of 10 min, the block can be tested by pushing a ballpoint pen into the bulb of each heel: the horse should not react. In the event of failure, the clinician should wait a further 10 min, then the block should be repeated.

Abaxial sesamoid nerve block

Considered the most useful nerve block for the field practitioner, this will block out the foot. Clinicians should be aware that in acute sepsis of the hoof only partial function will be restored. This block can not only be used for direct diagnostic purposes but also to anaesthetize the foot for surgical procedures, e.g. digging out an abscess or removing a keratoma. It should not be used to lessen pain in the acutely laminitic animal, as this may make the condition worse. After preparation, the leg is held by the practitioner and 5 ml local anaesthetic injected at both sides over the palmar nerve at the side of the distal end of the sesamoid bones, using a 25G needle 16 mm in length; it is advisable to inject the medial nerve first. To locate the nerve in the thick-skinned horse, the clinician should feel for the beating of the palmar artery; the nerve runs just caudal to the artery. Allowing a minimum of 10 min, the block can be tested by pushing a ballpoint pen into the coronary band on the dorsal aspect of the hoof: the horse should not react. In the event of failure, the clinician should wait a further 10 min, then the block should be repeated.

Coffin joint block

Attainment of this joint block is not easy. However, it is much easier in a diseased joint as the slight joint effusion will aid placement of the 21G, 40 mm needle. For blocking a normal-sized joint, 5 ml local anaesthetic will be required; the larger foot will require up to 10 ml. *Full aseptic precautions must be taken.* With the foot on the ground and an assistant holding up the opposite leg, a skin bleb of 1 ml is placed 2 mm above the coronary band and 2 mm laterally from the midline. After 10 min a 21G needle is inserted at an angle to meet the midline at the level of the coronary band; the needle should also be angled slightly caudally. Joint fluid should be seen on the hub of the needle before either the local anaesthetic or the medication is injected.

Fetlock joint block

Once again, this joint block is not easy, but again it is easier in a diseased joint as the slight joint effusion will aid placement of the 21G, 40 mm needle. For blocking, at least 10 ml local anaesthetic will be required, more for the heavier horse. *Full aseptic precautions must be taken.* Initially, with the leg bearing weight and an assistant holding up the opposite leg, a skin bleb of 2 ml is placed laterally palmar to the cannon bone and dorsal to the lateral sesamoid bone. After 10 min the hoof is lifted by an assistant and the joint flexed. Next, a 21G, 40 mm needle is inserted directly into the leg through the collateral ligament caudal to the cannon bone and past the distal end of the lateral sesamoid. Joint fluid should be seen on the hub of the needle before either the local anaesthetic or the medication is injected. In some instances, fluid will not emerge, even though the needle is correctly placed. Negative pressure with a syringe may be required.

Carpal joint block

In a diseased joint this block is easy. Both the carpometacarpal and intercarpal joints communicate. The joint should be blocked with 10 ml local anaesthetic. *Full aseptic precautions must be taken.* Initially, with the leg bearing weight and an assistant holding up the opposite leg, a skin bleb of 2 ml is instilled at the distal end of the carpus just lateral to the midline, i.e. lateral to the main extensor tendon. After 10 min the hoof should be lifted by an assistant and the joint flexed. A 21G, 40 mm needle is then inserted directly into the leg to the lateral aspect of the main extensor tendon, angled towards the midline. Joint fluid should be seen on the hub of the needle before either the local anaesthetic or the medication is injected. As much of the synovial fluid as possible should be drawn off before medication.

Shoulder joint block

The shoulder is a very difficult joint to penetrate, and practitioners in the field are advised not to block this joint but only to medicate it after making an informed guess on the diagnosis of arthritis in the joint. It is a very deep joint, and therefore a 19G, 90 mm spinal needle will be required. *Full aseptic precautions must be taken.* The horse must be heavily sedated. A skin bleb of 3 ml local anaesthetic is placed with a 25G, 25 mm needle over the area of the groove between the two prominences of the lateral humeral tuberosity. After 10 min an assistant should hold up the opposite front leg so that the affected leg is bearing weight. The spinal needle is inserted into the notch between the cranial and caudal prominences and directed in a straight line towards the opposite elbow. Negative pressure will be required to confirm that the needle is in the shoulder joint.

Tarsometatarsal joint block

Another difficult joint to medicate, this is best done under good sedation and therefore nerve blocking of the joint is not advisable for a practitioner in the field. *Full aseptic precautions must be taken.* With an assistant holding up the opposite hind leg, a skin bleb of 3 ml local anaesthetic is injected with a 25G, 25 mm needle over the plantarolateral surface of the hock in the area of the fourth metatarsal bone. After 10 min, again with the opposite hind leg held up, a 19G, 40 mm needle is inserted just proximal to the head of the fourth metatarsal bone in a small depression between the head of the fourth metatarsal bone and the distal aspect of the fourth tarsal bone. The needle will need to be inserted to an approximate depth of half its length. If a bleb of joint fluid is not apparent, the needle should be rotated as this will often yield joint fluid. This joint is the one to be medicated for a spavin. The clinician should be aware that this joint communicates with the central tarsal joint and the tarsotibial joint in less than 50% of horses.

12.11 Exertional Rhabdomyolysis Syndrome

A multi-factoral condition, this is a very well-known clinical entity in the working horse worldwide. However, knowledge about its pathophysiology is being discovered at the time of writing this book. There appear to be two types of the acquired form, one sporadic and the other recurrent. There is also an inherited form called polysaccharide storage myopathy (PSSM); this condition can be diagnosed only by muscle biopsy.

The clinical picture is extremely variable but is always related to exercise. The exercise does not need to be violent but is usually more strenuous than the horse is accustomed to. Attacks often follow a period of rest – even as little as 1 day – which accounts for its old-fashioned name of 'Monday morning disease'. It also goes under the titles 'tying up' and azoturia. Onset is normally sudden, the horse being reluctant to move; there may be increased sweating and there is pain in the gluteal area; the heart rate will be raised, and the horse may paw the ground. It can be differentiated from colic as there are normal gut sounds and rolling is not a feature. The urine will be discoloured a red-brown colour, but this will take some hours to appear. It is extremely rare in ponies.

The acute disease is a clinical emergency, and therefore the handler should carry out immediate first aid. All exercise must stop and the tack removed. If the animal is sweating it should be dried off and rugged up if in cold conditions.

The clinician must then give i/v NSAIDs; there is anecdotal evidence that flunixine is the NSAID of choice. Ideally, a serum sample should be obtained to measure CK levels, which would be expected to be raised by several thousand. This measurement is useful, so that a follow-up sample may be taken in 2–3 weeks to guide the clinician through the course of the condition. NSAIDs are then continued by mouth, with the horse having total rest. On clinical improvement, and ideally on studying CK levels, the horse may be brought back slowly to very light exercise, which can then slowly be built up.

One of the main trigger factors is a high-starch diet, so prevention is based on lowering starch in the diet. The clinician has a dilemma, for if the horse is expected to work hard it will require energy and this energy is normally supplied as starch. Therefore, in cases of recurrent exertional rhabdomyolysis starch in the diet should be slowly replaced by vegetable oil; this can be given at up to 500 ml for a 500 kg horse.

References and Further Reading

Aßmann, A., Furst, A. and Bischofberger, A.S. (2023) Standing osteosynthesis of an accessory carpal bone fracture in a Warmblood mare with a 6-hole 3.5 talonavicular fusion plate and 3.5 mm screws. *Equine Veterinary Education* 35: 239.

Corraretti, G., Meulyser, M. and Gustafsson, K. (2023) Treatment of fistulous cranial nuchal bursitis by complete surgical resection in two horses. *Equine Veterinary Education* 35: 235.

Jimenez-Rihuete, P. and O'Meara, B. (2021) Three cases of olecranon fracture repair in the standing horse. *Equine Veterinary Education* 35: 131.

Mair, T. (2023) Advances in imaging of the equine distal limb. *Equine Veterinary Education* 35: 116.

Stashak, E.S. (1987) *Adams' Lameness in Horses*. Lea & Febiger, Philadelphia, Pennsylvania.

Termansen, H. and Meehan, L. (2021) Can sedation be used for equine lameness investigation? *Veterinary Evidence* 6(2). Available at: https://doi.org/10.18849/ve.v6i2.373 (accessed 1 September 2023).

Wyn-Jones, G. (1988) *Equine Lameness*. Blackwell Scientific Publications, Oxford, UK.

13

Wounds

Abstract
Wounds are common in working equines. The causation, management and treatment of wounds, and the full science of wound healing, are described in this chapter.

13.1 Principles of Wound Healing

Wound healing is a continuous process, but classically it has been divided into four phases: the inflammatory phase, the debridement phase, the repair phase and the maturation phase. It is prudent for clinicians to warn owners about these phases so that they will not alarmed by the progress of the healing. This is particularly important if they are dressing the wound themselves.

Inflammatory phase

There is always acute inflammation, whether the injury is surgical, physical, chemical or from infection, with an immediate vascular and cellular response. The blood clot will hopefully fill the wound in a sutured wound The smaller the clot the better, as excessive seroma formation will delay healing from pressure necrosis and bacterial growth. The inflammatory phase lasts approximately 6 h and is often called the golden period, as wounds sutured in this period tend to heal better. The clinician has a dilemma when trauma has occurred: should care be forfeited for speed? Should the wound be sutured immediately or should the animal be moved so that it can be cleaned more thoroughly?

Debridement phase

The second phase begins about 6 h after the incident and lasts up to 12 h, and is mainly a white blood cell response. During this phase it is important that good surgical debridement and haemostasis is carried out. Obviously, good drainage should be arranged, particularly if the wound is infected. Drainage is paramount to ensure good healing.

Repair phase

This next phase normally begins after 12 h and proceeds after barriers such as blood clots, necrotic tissue, debris and infection have been removed. There should be epithelialization, but this may be delayed until a granulating bed has formed.

DOI: 10.1079/9781800624283.0013

Unfortunately, with wounds on the horse's leg granulation bed formation may be too vigorous, so that epithelialization cannot occur quickly enough to cover the excessive granulation tissue, called proud flesh. This overzealous granulation formation is particularly prevalent in thoroughbred and Arab horses. Normally, granulation tissue is proceeded by fibroplasia, which appears after 3–4 days; this is early scar tissue and will continue for approximately 3 weeks. Tensile strength slowly increases as the collagen is laid down; in large wounds tensile strength is still only 80% of the original after 1 year.

Except when granulation is excessive, it is very beneficial, as it allows epithelial cells to migrate. It is very resistant to infection. Wound contraction is centred around granulation, as is collagen formation. However, it does not look very pleasant and owners should be warned. Wound contraction is what owners are looking forward to, but this may be slow or nonexistent if excess proud flesh occurs.

There is considerable debate about proud flesh formation: why is it so common on the legs of thoroughbreds and Arabs? When it occurs on large lacerations on the body it has a very similar appearance to equine sarcoid formation (see Fig. 13.1).

Maturation phase

The final phase is really the realignment of collagen along the lines of tension. Like bone formation, where there is constant new bone growth from the action of osteoblasts and constant bone lysis from osteoclasts, collagen is constantly produced and, hopefully to a lesser extent, lysed.

13.2 Factors Affecting Wound Healing

Age and physical status

It is stating the obvious, but younger animals heal more quickly than do older animals; equally, fit horses heal faster than those suffering from systemic disease.

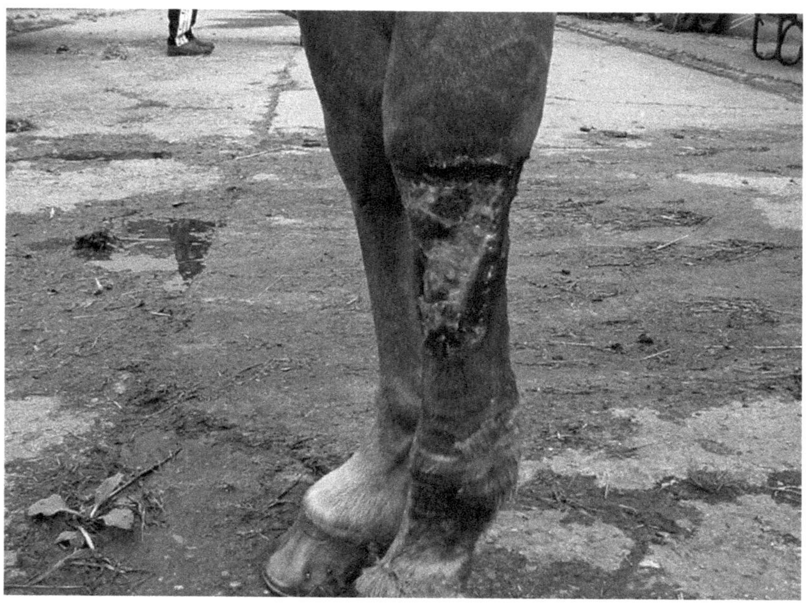

Fig. 13.1. Granulation bed.

Blood loss

There is no direct link between anaemia and delay in wound healing. However, anaemia resulting from a cause other than blood loss from the wound is certainly not beneficial and should be treated accordingly.

Uraemia

Uraemia will certainly delay wound healing, so any kidney disease should be treated and monitored.

Malnutrition and protein deficiency

Horses in this situation will certainly be slower to heal than horses receiving adequate nutrition. Fats can be synthesized by the body from carbohydrates and carbohydrates can be synthesized from protein; however, protein can be made only from ingested protein or its digestive by-products, e.g. amino acids and peptides. Therefore, a protein-rich diet should be fed to wounded horses. Certain amino acids, e.g. methionine, are particularly important for wound healing.

Trace elements

Zinc and copper are especially important for wound healing, although other minerals such as calcium, phosphorus, iron and manganese are also required.

Vitamins

Obviously, these are all important for normal body function. However, the fat-soluble vitamins A and E are very important in wound healing. Care should be taken, as excess of either of these vitamins will delay healing. Vitamin K is vital for blood clot formation, while vitamin C is essential for wound healing. Although vitamin deficiency is rare in the horse, chronically debilitated and undernourished animals will obviously benefit from vitamin supplementation.

Veterinary medicines

Certain medicines, e.g. anti-inflammatory drugs, both non-steroidal and steroidal, are known to delay healing, and so their use should be considered carefully. Certain inflammatory responses, e.g. oedema, also delay healing, so their use must be carefully monitored and controlled. A good rule is not to use either, particularly corticosteroids, unless there is a very strong indication, and then only to give them for a short period of time.

We must also consider local anaesthetics; these certainly may delay healing when they are administered into the area of the wound, but in many cases this may be unavoidable. However, nerve blocks should be used whenever possible and the amount of local anaesthetic injected kept to the minimum.

Antiseptic preparations

As these may well delay healing, obviously there must be a compromise. The skin before surgery must be made as sterile as possible, but the use of antiseptics for cleaning traumatic wounds should be limited. Foreign material must be removed or wound healing will never occur. Copious amounts of clean water are, in my opinion, much better that small amounts of antiseptic solutions. The ideal is a running hose of drinkable water.

Trauma

When considering surgical wounds, it is vital to remember that trauma will cause bruising of tissues and delay healing, and therefore should be kept to the minimum. Scalpel use is considerably preferred to scissor action and blunt dissection, from a wound-healing consideration. However, surgical technique should not be compromised.

Poor blood supply

Inevitably, this will delay healing, but in most instances the clinician cannot help the situation. Wounds around the perineum and on the head heal quickly as there is a good blood supply, but wounds on the lower limbs on the whole heal slowly on account of the relatively poor blood supply.

Movement

On the whole, movement will delay healing; therefore, stabilization should be the goal. However, certain studies have indicated that some limited movement, provided it is gentle and minimal, will encourage healing.

Infection

All infection will delay healing. Total aseptic surgery is the goal and as short a surgical time as possible is the aim. The use of antibiotics should not be a substitute for good surgical practice. Naturally, antibiotics will be required for non-surgical wounds. In elective surgery prior blood levels of systemic antibiotics are worthwhile. The role of topical antibiotics is currently under debate: rarely are they justified and they may well help in fostering antibiotic resistance.

Necrotic tissue

Another factor that will certainly delay healing, necrotic tissue should be removed by careful and systematic debridement. The resulting 'dead space' is also not conducive to healing and should be obliterated if at all possible. This may not be possible in all situations or if there is tumour growth as is shown in Fig. 13.2.

Foreign bodies

Whether these are small or large, they will delay healing indefinitely unless removed. In the case of small particles of matter, the surgeon might rely on providing good drainage, but large foreign bodies will have to be removed. Their location may not be easy to find, and so ultrasonography or radiography may be helpful. However, these modalities are in a single plane and the third dimension may be very misleading.

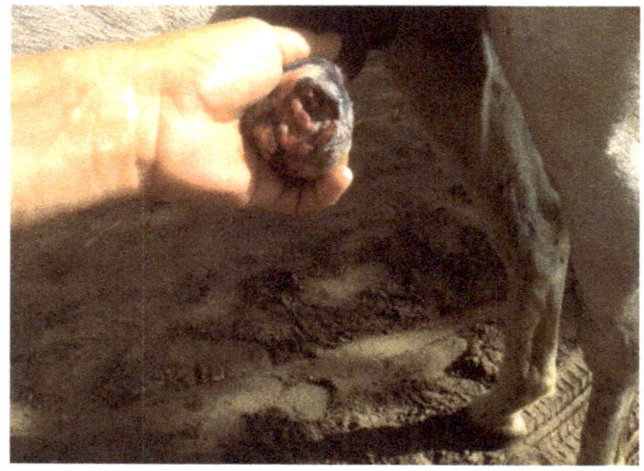

Fig. 13.2. A penis initially damaged by thorns, now showing evidence of squamous carcinomatous formation in Mozambique.

13.3 Classification of Wounds

There are many ways to classify wounds. Obviously, they can be classified by where they are on the body, e.g. a head wound. They could also be classified as to their cause, e.g. a surgical wound or a rope burn. However, the easiest way is to classify them by how they appear.

- Abrasion: often termed graze. The top layers of the skin are stripped off but the whole epidermis is not cut through.
- Bruise: caused by blunt trauma. There is usually considerable swelling.
- Haematoma: in essence, a severe bruise where the swelling is actual blood.
- Contusion: a severe bruise but there is also considerable skin damage.
- Puncture wound: a deep, penetrating wound caused by a sharp instrument; invariably infected, as there is poor drainage. This is the most common wound allowing the tetanus organism to multiply in the unvaccinated animal. *It is vital in any wound situation that the clinician establishes the*

tetanus vaccination status of the animal and takes action accordingly.

- Laceration: a large and long wound that may well involve not only the skin but also deeper structures.
- Complicated wound: may not be as extensive as a laceration but always involves deeper structures, which complicates repair and healing.
- Burn: caused by either heat or chemicals. Both the depth and extent of damage are important, and various figures are suggested: a rule of thumb is that the animal is unlikely to survive if more than 25% of its body surface is destroyed. As burns are extremely painful and invariably become infected, euthanasia must always be considered on welfare grounds. Burns should not be covered with cotton wool or gauze, as these will only make the situation worse. The first thing for the owner to do is to cool the area with cold, clean, drinkable water; then, if the burns are on the limbs these should be covered by cling film to limit infection until a veterinarian can examine them.

13.4 Advice for Owners of a Wounded Horse Awaiting Treatment

- Move the animal or make other arrangements if further damage is likely (e.g. extinguish any fire).
- Control major haemorrhage with pressure.
- If possible, move the animal to a suitable clean place for treatment.
- Clean wounds, if feasible, with running, drinkable water.
- Protect the wounds from flies.
- If the horse is required to move a considerable distance for treatment, apply oily creams to protect the wound and prevent drying.

13.5 Veterinary Approach to Wound Management

- Assuming the owner has taken the steps outlined above, the veterinary surgeon should obtain a relevant history.
- Perform a relevant clinical examination.
- Sedate the horse if required.
- Carefully examine all the wounds visually and digitally.
- Make a plan of action.

13.6 Principles of Wound Management

It should be remembered that the main goal is to return the horse to a normal functional state; it is only a secondary goal to effect a cosmetic repair. The selection of treatment will be decided upon by considering many external factors, including:

- time since the injury;
- part of the animal affected;
- depth and configuration of wounds;
- degree of contamination;
- temperament of the animal;
- nursing ability of the owner;
- physical state of the horse;
- intended use of the horse; and
- economics.

13.7 Factors to Be Considered When Deciding on a Plan of Action

- Consider the treatment of the whole horse first; this is vitally important. It is easy to get focused on repairing a wound and neglect to treat the horse for shock, debilitation, etc.
- Consider the use of parenteral antibiotics, pain relief and NSAIDs.
- Consider the deeper structures that may be damaged. If there is any possibility that a joint or a tendon sheath has been entered, lavage must be carried out, possibly several times, before wound closure.
- Consider the amount of contamination, with regard to both foreign bodies and bacteria.
- Consider how wound management is going to be accomplished – e.g. is a general anaesthetic required?
- Obviously, primary closure is the goal, but this may not be realistic. Healing by

secondary intention may be preferable to having a breakdown in primary closure.

13.8 Primary Closure

- The earlier this can be carried out the better. However, the wound needs to have a temporary covering of hydrogel cream as soon as possible.
- Clipping can then be carried out around the wound. Any hair that would then fall into the wound can be washed out with hydrogel cream.
- Hydrogel cream can be reapplied before the surrounding area is thoroughly cleaned several times with dilute chlorhexidine scrub.
- Distant local anaesthesia can be used to block relevant peripheral nerves. However, local anaesthetic should be used only if absolutely necessary, and then only after the wound has been thoroughly cleaned.
- Spray the wound with sterile water containing soluble crystalline penicillin. Do not apply penicillin or any other wound powder.
- Sutures should appose the tissues with minimal tension.
- Contrary to popular professional belief, the fewer the sutures that can carry out the purpose the better.
- Each layer should be sutured separately.
- Synthetic absorbable material should be used, as this causes the least inflammatory reaction.
- Tension suturing patterns can be used to reduce the tension on the primary suture line. These may be widely spaced vertical mattress sutures with support from small pieces of rubber tubing.
- Never hide these tension sutures under a cast, as necrosis can occur very quickly.
- Removal of sutures can be staggered.
- Drains may be used if there is dead space; they should be placed and maintained in a sterile environment. Drains should exit from a separate hole from the suture line and, ideally, be removed in 2 days, but may be left longer if drainage is profuse.

13.9 Delayed Primary Closure

- Closure is delayed until granulation tissue has started to form – normally in 5 days.
- The wound must be kept clean.
- Hopefully, the swelling will be reduced.
- Debridement is carried out before delayed primary closure.

13.10 Secondary Closure

- Useful for very contaminated wounds.
- Closure is delayed until the wound is clean, but this may be a considerable time after the initial injury.
- Excess granulation tissue must be removed.

13.11 Healing by Secondary Intention

- It is remarkable how wounds will heal eventually, with contraction and epithelialization.
- Patience must be exercised.
- The wound must be kept clean, and bandaged if possible.
- Once granulation tissue has formed the wound should be kept moist using oily creams.
- Flies must be controlled.

13.12 Selection of Suture Material

Naming individual brands would not be worthwhile, as practitioners can only use what is available. Monofilament nylon as used by fishermen is very useful for skin and tension sutures. Only absorbable suture material should be used in deeper layers.

13.13 Selection of Suture Patterns

In general, interrupted sutures should be used, as these allow for movement of the skin. Unless the subcuticular layer has been closed vertical mattress sutures should be used.

13.14 General Advice on Wounds

There is no point in suturing a contaminated wound, and sutures will delay healing further. Skin flaps can be secured in part until it is obvious whether the remaining part of the flap is devitalized. Obviously, the clinician wants to preserve as much skin as possible. However, the fundamental question has to asked: is there a good chance that my sutures will hold? If this does not seem likely, the wound is better left to heal by secondary intention.

13.15 Wounds on the Donkey's Leg

Naturally, all wounds should be thoroughly investigated to find out the extent of the damage.

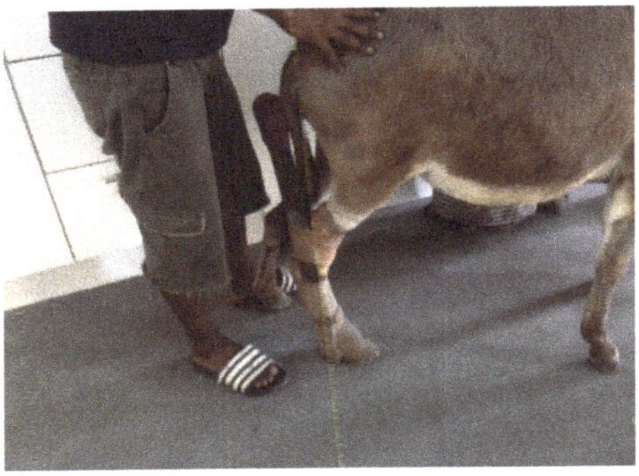

Fig. 13.3. A splint with a lack of padding.

If there is little blood or exudate, it is advisable to cover the open area with a wound gel and then clip the area; this is easier with dry hair. The whole area should then be hosed down with a garden hose; this may have to be done before clipping if the wound is very messy. The wound can then be examined carefully after drying thoroughly. Any suspected puncturing of joint capsules or tendon sheaths needs to be investigated, as in the horse; however, in this case, suturing of wounds is probably unwise and leaving full drainage is the best approach. The formation of proud flesh is a very rare occurrence in donkeys, but to be on the safe side it is advisable to bandage any wounds below the knee and hock; wounds higher up the leg can be left open; these should be liberally covered with oily creams and the area below the wound protected by petroleum jelly. Fly control is vital. After giving tetanus cover, a minimum of 5 days of antibiotics and NSAIDs should be given. It may be appropriate to start these by injection and continue with oral medication – preferably in the form of oral paste, as some donkeys are reluctant to eat medicated feed. *It is vital to remember that the donkey is very prone to hyperlipaemia*; therefore, any inappetence is dangerous.

Some wounds will be iatrogenic, as seen in Fig. 13.4. This was caused by the splint (Fig. 13.3). It was removed and then the wounds were dressed (Fig. 13.5). The animal made an excellent recovery thanks to the dedicated staff at The Gambian Horse and Donkey Sanctuary seen with the author in Fig. 13.6.

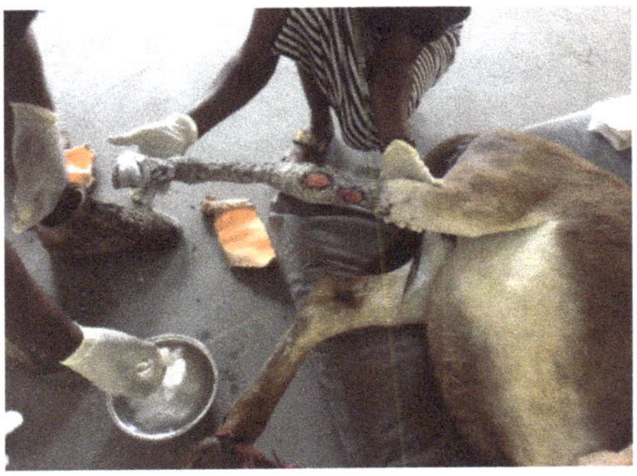

Fig. 13.4. The resulting pressure sores.

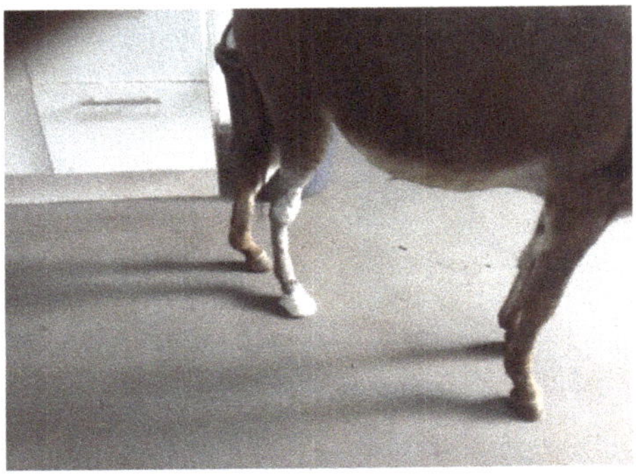

Fig. 13.5. Sores after topical treatment.

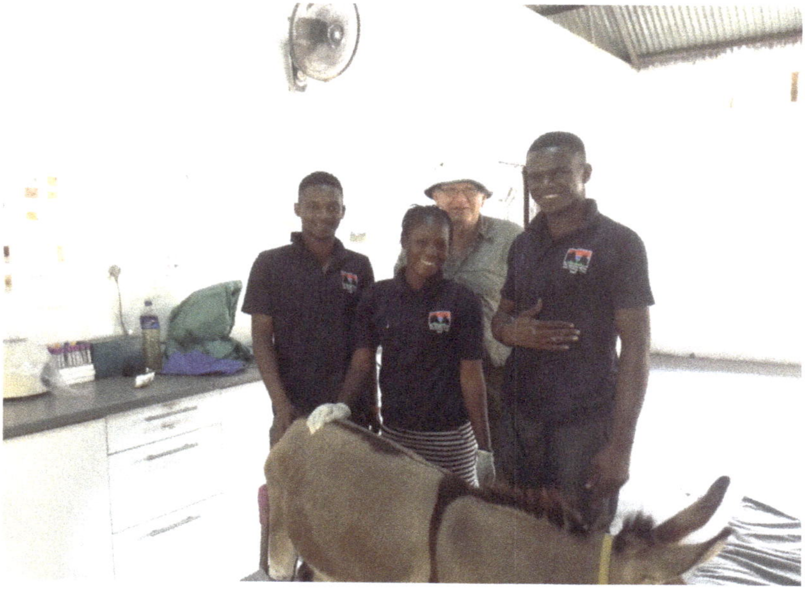

Fig. 13.6. The surgical team in The Gambia.

Further Reading

Knottenbelt, D.C. (2003) *Handbook of Equine Wound Management*. Elsevier Science, Maryland Heights, Missouri.

Stashak, E.S. (1991) *Equine Wound Management*. Lea & Febiger, Philadelphia, Pennsylvania.

14

Respiratory, Cardiac and Circulatory Conditions

Abstract

This chapter covers not only respiratory conditions, but also cardiac and circulatory disorders. Respiratory conditions are categorized as either upper or lower airway. These are then split into contagious and non-contagious conditions. Cardiac disease and circulatory disorders are described in detail as individual conditions.

14.1 Examination for Respiratory Conditions

It is very important to 'stand back' and get a general view of the horse before carrying out a full examination. The history of the case will give you some likely clues. *Don't rush in!*

You should make a mental note of the following facts from the history:

- age;
- type of horse;
- what it is used for;
- duration of clinical signs;
- coughing?
- other horses in the group affected?
- possibility of trauma?
- problems with performance? and
- normal routine changed vis-à-vis housing?

You should also look at:

- general set-up;
- actual stable (particularly size and ventilation);
- bedding; and
- long-fibre proportion of diet.

You should then look at the horse from a distance and note:

- type of respiration;
- frequency of respiration;
- any evidence of a 'heave line'; and
- presence of any discharge from the nose or eyes.

Only then should you let the owner catch the horse and put on a head collar.

After an examination of the head, paying particular attention to the nostrils and the sinuses (other than for dentistry this is the only time that you stand directly in the dangerous position directly in front of a horse), move to the left-hand side of the horse and auscultate the heart and lungs; repeat this on the right-hand side. If you suspect lower airway problems, ask the handler to cover either one nostril or the nose with a rebreathing bag (a bin liner is fine): this makes the horse breathe harder, which will render chest noises easier to hear. Then move to the rear and take the rectal temperature. Move then to the larynx: palpate it to try to perceive any asymmetry. Last squeeze the larynx to see whether that will initiate a cough reflex.

DOI: 10.1079/9781800624283.0014

14.2 Preliminary Diagnosis of Respiratory Conditions

Armed with this array of information, try to suggest to yourself whether the problem lies in the upper or lower airway; it is possible you are dealing with a combination of both. Then try to decide whether it is an infectious and/or contagious or a non-infectious disease. It is important to keep an open mind, as an infectious disease may well lead on to a non-infectious disease (e.g. an upper respiratory virus may lead to a recurrent airway obstruction (RAO, see Section 14.6)). Equally, a non-infectious disease may lead to an infectious disease (e.g. a tracheobronchial foreign body may result in pneumonia). It should be realized that many of the diagnoses described below require the use of an endoscope, either static or paced for use in a galloping horse. However, most of these conditions are those of thoroughbred racehorses and not of working horses, but they have been included for completeness.

14.3 Infectious and Contagious Upper Airway Diseases

Strangles

Caused by the bacterium *Streptococcus equi*, this highly contagious disease requires no long discussion and will readily be recognized by practitioners. Laboratory confirmation by swab is always worthwhile. The debate on the merits of antibiotic treatment, which has carried on for my whole working life of 40 years, will continue. However, in the really sick young animal the use of antibiotics is justified. There is little evidence that such treatment leads to the carrier state, with the organism lingering in the guttural pouches. NSAIDs are definitely helpful.

For decades vaccines have come and gone. The author is ever hopeful. The fusion-protein-based vaccine, Strangvac, was launched in the UK in 2022. The vaccine contains eight important and highly conserved proteins that normally help *S. equi* to attach to equine tissue, misdirect the equine immune response and cause disease.

Importantly the vaccine contains no live *S. equi* and is administered by intramuscular injection. The vaccine does not interfere with any of the available diagnostic tests for strangles. Furthermore, it does not contain the SeM protein, so avoiding the production of anti-SeM antibodies associated with cases of purpura haemorragica. There is a blood test available in the UK and some other countries, and this gives an indication of previous exposure and presence of disease, except during the 10 days when a horse is incubating the condition. The results of this test must be evaluated with care.

Difficulties in the eradication of the disease using vaccines and medical treatments make hygienic measures crucial in order to limit transmission of the pathogen during outbreaks. Practitioners will be faced with a real challenge when handling an outbreak of strangles. They will need to a basic plan on how such an outbreak is to be handled in a hygienically optimal fashion. Modern information has shown that there is a longer environmental survival time of *S. equi* than had been previously assumed. It is important to modify the surfaces for proper disinfection with appropriate disinfectants. Further efficiency can be achieved by using a colour-coding system in dividing healthy, exposed and clinically affected horses. Individual temperature monitoring twice daily is recommended for the identification of diseased horses before they pose a contagious risk. Additionally, changing clothes between visiting different stable units is likewise recommended, to minimize transmission of disease. In conclusion, veterinarians, personnel and horse owners at equestrian centres need to be aware of the importance of isolation, monitoring and dividing the site into zones according to the risk of infection. Finally, it can be concluded that, regardless of size, practical biosecurity measures can be implemented within all equine facilities.

Equine herpes virus (rhinopneumonitis)

Herpes viruses in other species give confusing clinical pictures. The equine version, with its two main distinct groups, EHV-1, which is mainly responsible for abortion and myeloencephalitis, and EHV-4, which is responsible for respiratory disease, is no exception. EHV-2 is found so commonly in healthy horses that it is hard to imagine that it is a serious pathogen; separate viruses are found in the donkeys, but these do not infect the horse. Mules are infected by both equine and asinine viruses (AHV-4). However, EHV-4 and AHV-4 produce similar disease symptoms of raised temperature and nasal discharge. There is good passive immunity to the disease.

EHV-4 should always be suspected in a case of respiratory disease. The virus can be isolated from a nasopharyngeal swab or the buffy coat of a citrate blood sample taken early in the course of the disease. Paired serum samples are also diagnostic.

Equine influenza

The veterinary profession can be congratulated on the control of this contagious disease. The problems in an unvaccinated population were well illustrated in the serious outbreaks in South Africa and Australia. Practitioners should not hesitate to send swabs for diagnosis if they suspect the disease; paired serum samples will also be diagnostic. Infected animals show a very marked pyrexia, with depression and loss of appetite. The disease is much more serious in the donkey, mainly because the loss of appetite may lead to hyperlipaemia. Both horses and donkeys show a dry cough and swelling of the submandibular lymph nodes. Usually, horses do not require antibiotic therapy as they will recover on their own, but foals and donkeys should be treated. Ciclesonide is a novel corticosteroid used in the Equihaler (a soft mist inhaler produced by Aservo). This is a prodrug that becomes activated when it reaches the airway epithelium, and so is a targeted treatment. The major advantages of this type of drug are its reduced systemic concentrations, which should reduce the chances of having undesired effects.

Vaccination is vital to maintain herd immunity and reduce the likelihood of large-scale outbreaks. Although the benefits of vaccination may be obvious to veterinarians, we must understand the perceptions of horse owners that lead to barriers to vaccination uptake if we are to educate and ignite a change in behaviour. Human motivations and views should never be underestimated as an explanation for behaviour, but we must work together to reshape the landscape and enhance protection of horses through vaccination. Protocols for vaccination at the time of publication are in a state of flux, mainly because of the shortage of vaccine from all the normal suppliers worldwide and particularly in the UK. If vaccine stocks recover, it is likely that an initial course of two injections separated by a minimum of 21 days and a maximum of 56 days will be advised and then continuous cover will be provided by 6 monthly injections. However, veterinarians are strongly advised to follow the manufacturers' instructions. Practitioners should liaise with both their national and international bodies regarding regulations for racing and all other equine sporting competitions and events.

Other upper respiratory viruses

Normally, these arrive in horse populations in waves, causing coughing and nasal discharges in groups of horses. Incubation periods of 2–10 days are seen, so gatherings of horses are often the method of spread. The infection is self-limiting. Fresh air is beneficial, and antibiotics are justified in cases showing a persistent secondary purulent bacterial nasal discharge.

14.4 Non-contagious Upper Airway Diseases

Lacerations and wounds of the nostrils

Diagnosis is straightforward, although the actual cause may not be so obvious.

Paralysis of the nostrils

Once again, diagnosis will be straightforward. The cause is likely to be damage to the facial nerve, although the actual trauma may not be apparent. The paralysis is normally permanent.

Epidermal inclusion cysts of the false nostril

Often termed atheromas, these are normally unilateral and are totally benign. They do not affect the breathing even if they grow to the size of a goose egg. Therefore, excision is purely cosmetic and is normally successful. Drainage, on the other hand, normally leads to a recurrence.

Sinusitis

There is a persistent purulent nasal discharge. If this is unilateral and malodorous it is likely to be tooth related; one of the four caudal upper cheek teeth is likely to be the cause. These should be examined very carefully with a gag, a mirror and dental picks, usually under sedation. Oblique lateral radiographs will aid diagnosis. Tooth removal is the only treatment.

If the discharge is bilateral, primary sinusitis is the likely cause. In very rare cases a fungus may be involved. Antibiotic treatment is often tried, but rarely is it effective. Surgery with copious flushing is the treatment of choice.

Ethmoid haematoma

Confusing signs accompany this haematoma: you may see a unilateral bloody nasal discharge, but often this is purulent and may well be bilateral. It is rarely true epistaxis. Confirmation of the diagnosis is normally made endoscopically and radiographically. Surgery was the previously favoured method of treatment, but nowadays laser or chemical ablation are more frequently used. Chemical ablation is achieved with 10% formaldehyde.

Guttural pouch disease

A group of syndromes that can be grouped under one heading, as they are all going to be seen as a swollen guttural pouch; whatever is causing the swelling will denominate the syndrome. Possibilities include: (i) air, as in the case of foal guttural pouch tympany; (ii) liquid pus, as in guttural pouch empyema (normally a *B*-haemolytic *Streptococcus*); and (iii) caseous, inspissated pus, as in strangles. It may also have a fungal cause, as in guttural pouch mycosis. The disease is very serious in the horse and extremely serious in the donkey.

The clinical signs are potentially very serious, as the carotid artery or several cranial nerves maybe affected. Diagnosis is achieved with the endoscope. Treatment will vary with the cause. Arterial occlusion may be required to prevent a fatal haemorrhage.

Dorsal displacement of the soft palate

A condition normally seen intermittently at exercise, high-speed treadmill endoscopy is usually required for diagnosis as the condition occurs in the tiring horse. There are several surgical options for treatment.

Pharyngeal lymphoid hyperplasia

A condition normal in the young horse, this becomes a problem only when polyps develop. Pharyngeal sprays have been advocated, but the evidence of their effectiveness is lacking. Laser treatment is a better option.

Laryngeal hemiplegia

Normally affecting the left side, the horse is heard to make a noise on inspiration. It is relatively common in the larger horse. Unless the horse is to be used for strenuous exercise, this condition is unlikely to be a problem. Unfortunately, the well-known Hobday operation does not actually cure the condition, although it does often reduce the respiratory noise. Permanent tracheotomy – 'tubing' – is no longer aesthetically acceptable. The so-called tie-back operation is the treatment of choice.

Epiglottic entrapment

A rare and normally intermittent condition, it requires high-speed treadmill endoscopy for diagnosis. The horse will normally have been presented for poor performance.

Arytenoid chondritis

Another rare condition, it involves the formation of granulation tissue on one or both arytenoids, and is a disease mainly of young thoroughbreds. Historically, treatment consisted of a prolonged course of antibiotics with some steroid, but nowadays NSAIDs are used instead with the antibiotics. Diagnosis is simple with an endoscope.

Fourth brachial arch defects

Seen as congenital defects in the thoroughbred, up to 2 in 1000 may be affected. These are normally untreatable and are diagnosed on endoscopy.

Tracheal stenosis

May be either congenital or as the result of a kick and, provided the case is not too severe, it is best left alone. Surgery in severe cases is likely to be heroic.

Abscesses

Liable to occur in structures close to the upper respiratory tract, the signs will vary with their position. Surgeons are well advised to carry out paracentesis before lancing, as abscesses may well lie adjacent to very vital structures.

Neoplasia

Tumours are extremely rare in the respiratory system. Haemorrhage from the mouth will be seen with tumours of the pharynx, the nostrils or the upper airway. Melanomas may be seen in the guttural pouch, with the appearance of a bunch of black grapes. In this latter case, euthanasia must be advised on account of the danger of rupture of the carotid artery.

Foreign bodies

Although extremely rare in the pharynx or upper airway, these may be visualized and possibly removed with an endoscope.

14.5 Infectious and Contagious Lower Airway Diseases

Pneumonia in the foal

The foal can develop pneumonia from inhalation of bacteria, e.g. in the case of a severe cleft palate. They will also develop a stress-induced streptococcal pneumonia as a result of either overcrowding or transport. However, the normal cause is *Rhodococcus equi*. This organism, which produces life-threatening effects, should always be considered. Radiography and ultrasonography will aid in diagnosis rather than resorting to a transtracheal wash. Prolonged treatment by mouth with a combination of erythromycin (25 mg/kg) and rifampicin (10 mg/kg) every 12 h is required.

Pneumonia in the adult horse

Yearlings and 2-year-olds appear to develop a type of pneumonia not seen in the older horse. The rectal temperature is raised but the animal is not severely ill; the chest is noisy. The cause is likely to be a mycoplasma, but the evidence for this is not conclusive. Treatment is by i/v oxytetracycline (6.6 mg/kg) daily for a minimum of 3 days. The concerns over the use of this antibiotic are exaggerated.

Pneumonia in the adult is very rare but it is always extremely serious, particularly if associated with pleural effusion. The clinical impression is that stallions are more susceptible. The disease seems to follow either a long journey or major trauma, e.g. a bad fall. There is thoracic pain, respiratory distress and a raised rectal temperature. Aggressive antibiotic therapy with NSAIDs is required. If ultrasonography indicates pleural effusion and a fluid line, thoracic drainage is vital. The prognosis is always grave.

Chronic fibrosing interstitial pneumonia

A condition seen only in the donkey, the cause is unknown and therefore it has been termed idiopathic pulmonary fibrosis (IPF). It is just possible that it is contagious. The signs are of very severe

RAO (see Section 14.6), with a secondary bacterial bronchitis. The recommended treatment is a prolonged course of antibiotics and clenbuterol hydrochloride, a bronchodilator and decongestant.

Tuberculosis

This is a rare disease in equids. It is normally of a chronic nature and may remain silent for long periods of time. Clinical manifestations of the disease can be non-specific and easily confused with more common diseases. Workers in Poland (Siwinska *et al.*, 2022) describe a case in a 30-year-old donkey with enlarged peripheral lymph nodes which was carefully examined without a definitive diagnosis being made. Sadly, 2.5 years later the owners noticed a deterioration in the body condition and dullness. The donkey died naturally on the farm after unsuccessful symptomatic treatment. On gross post-mortem examination, the BCS of the donkey was 1.9/5. The examination revealed enlargement and concretion of numerous nodes. Small, numerous whitish-grey, firm nodules were observed throughout the abdomen and chest cavity, as well as in the tongue. Ziehl-Neelsen smears revealed single acid-fast bacilli. PCR results indicated the *Mycobacterium bovis* ssp. *bovis*. This was confirmed by a positive GenoType CM test.

14.6 Non-contagious Lower Airway Diseases

Recurrent airway obstruction (RAO)

Common things commonly occur, and that is certainly true of RAO in recent years. Surveys indicate that over 20% of stabled horses suffer from this condition, which was rare 40 years ago. It is often called equine asthma (EA). The epidemic that results is likely to be due to poor quality hay. It is now so common that many owners are complacent; many are happy to use expensive treatments, which at best only control the symptoms rather than remove the underlying cause, which is exposure to airborne environment particles resulting in a lower respiratory inflammatory response. The clinical signs are bronchospasm, mucus hypersecretion, decreased mucocilary clearance and inflammatory cell recruitment. The predominant complaint is coughing. Horses suffering from RAO must have a completely dust-free environment. It is miraculous how they will respond to being turned outside and fed haylage and soaked hard food. The practitioner is caught in a trap: a massive amount of time can be spent explaining the problems to the owner, who then either does not believe you or does not want to believe you. You can carry out an invasive, expensive diagnostic protocol involving endoscopy with either tracheal wash or bronchoalveolar lavage (BAL) to confirm diagnosis. Inhalation therapy, if carried out correctly, is very worthwhile. However, education of owners is better therapy. Oral therapy with clenbuterol hydrochloride is very effective. If severe, the attack can be treated with corticosteroids. Caution needs to be taken as often affected horses and ponies are susceptible to laminitis. Owners are normally very against removing hay from the diet. Soaking of hay is very labour-intensive and rarely results in total avoidance of the disease. Steaming hay is arguably more effective. However, the equipment is expensive and not environmentally friendly.

Summer pasture-associated airway obstruction (SPAAO)

The time of year and the climatic conditions are the only things separating SPAAO from RAO; a similar picture is seen microscopically from a tracheal wash or BAL. The problem for the clinician is what to do: steroids certainly improve the condition, and naturally they are better given in small doses to the target organ via an inhaler rather than by i/v injection or orally. Prednisolone at up to 2 mg/kg daily by mouth is a good treatment and is very unlikely to cause laminitis, but this minimal risk should be pointed out to the owner. Dexamethasone is more effective, but unfortunately is even more likely to cause laminitis. There is a dilemma for the clinician when faced on a summer's night with a horse in acute respiratory distress: there is a particular danger in using dexamethasone with a fat horse or pony; equally, atropine will control the distress but is also hazardous as it may cause ileus. The most prudent therapy is to use a horse inhaler/spacer with a human corticosteroid inhaler; inhalation treatment can be given there and then.

These cases will recur, and if the worst comes to the worst the affected horse could be moved to another area of the country, with a different climate and therefore different plants and pollen, for the critical 6 weeks of the year. They often calm down permanently, so that there are no problems the following year.

Inflammatory airway disease (IAD)

A condition seen in the young horse showing poor performance, diagnosis is made on BAL and current treatment is likely to be corticosteroids by inhalation.

Exercise-induced pulmonary haemorrhage (EIPH)

The horse showing actual epistaxis is just the tip of the iceberg. The majority of thoroughbred racehorses have this condition, which some authorities consider follows IAD. However, it may well be a physical phenomenon of violent exercise. It is diagnosed on endoscopy. Furosemide, a loop diuretic, is the classic treatment; there is no evidence that it prevents EIPH but there is evidence that it does lessen the haemorrhage. Its use is allowed in the UK for horses in training but not when racing. Practitioners should take care that withholding times are observed.

Lungworm

With the advent of the ivermectin wormers, this parasite appears to be a thing of the past in both horses and donkeys. A raised eosinophil count would indicate an allergic condition, not parasitism. It is just conceivable that migrating parascarids in the foal might cause pneumonia.

Hydatid cysts

The intermediate stage of the tapeworm *Echinococcus granulosus* is found in dogs and cats, with the horse being a host for the adult stage. Cysts are seen more commonly in the liver. In both instances this tapeworm is likely to be asymptomatic, unless there are multiple cysts. Drainage using ultrasonography might be tried if lung function is compromised. Cysts are more frequently seen in the donkey.

Neoplasia

Tumours of the lower respiratory tract are extremely rare, and are likely to be secondary, either a malignant melanoma or secondary spread from a lymphosarcoma of the gastroenteric tract.

14.7 Cardiac Disease

Introduction

It is very important to judge the whole horse and assess whether, if at all, cardiac disease is relevant at the time of examination. Nearly all horses showing colic signs have a heart murmur. It is important not to frighten the owner. The clinician might well remark that the circulation is compromised because of dehydration and pain, but the murmur is probably the least of the horse's problems. Equally, many newborn foals will have a murmur that is unlikely to be significant in later life.

The term 'heart failure' can also be misleading to owners: its real definition is when the heart cannot circulate sufficient blood to meet the metabolic requirements of the body for nutrients. This might be seen only at altitude or during very vigorous exercise, with the horse being normal at other times. Equally, it may be manifest at rest and the horse is near to collapse. Heart failure can be categorized into four classes:

- Class 1: Clinical signs are manifest only at times of very strenuous exercise.
- Class 2: Clinical signs are seen with ordinary levels of exercise.
- Class 3: The horse is normal at rest but shows clinical signs with any exercise.
- Class 4: Clinical signs are seen at rest.

The dilemma for the practitioner is to decide whether the signs are due to primary heart disease or are secondary to some other problem. The practitioner obviously will auscultate the heart and note any abnormalities of sound and rate. Also, the practitioner should examine the peripheral circulation: the feel of the pulse as well as the rate is important. Right-sided congestive heart failure will cause peripheral oedema with swelling in the legs, prepuce and ventral abdomen. In marked disease there may be ascites and swelling of the head. It should be remembered that there are many other causes of peripheral oedema in the horse, e.g. hypoproteinaemia, vasculitis, cellulitis and even pregnancy. On the other hand, left-sided congestive heart failure will cause pulmonary oedema. This will manifest as an increased respiratory rate and even blood-tinged froth at the nostrils.

Horses may adapt to cardiac disease so that these signs will subside after a few hours, only to return when the circulatory system is again compromised.

Heart sounds

There are four heart sounds that may be heard in the normal horse. The first sound heard is at the beginning of systole and the second at the end of systole. The third may be heard as a very quiet sound immediately after the second; the fourth is heard just before the first. So the heart sounds like l–lub–da–s, with the fourth sound at the start. These heart sounds are called transient sounds, to distinguish them from murmurs. The ease of hearing them will depend on the type of animal – they are always easier to hear in the thin individual. They will sound muffled if there is pleural or pericardial effusion; abscesses or neoplasms will also make them sound dull.

Cardiac murmurs

Cardiac murmurs are defined as noises heard during the normal silent period of the heart. It is important to define the type of murmur so that the clinician can decide whether it is of clinical significance, and the timing and duration are also important. A murmur may occur in either: (i) early, middle or late systole, i.e. between heart sounds one and two; or (ii) early, middle or late diastole, i.e. following sound two. A pansystolic murmur spans the phase from the beginning of sound one to the end of sound two; a holosystolic murmur only from the end of sound one to the beginning of sound two; and a holodiastolic murmur from the end of sound two to the beginning of sound one. The intensity and the pitch of the murmur can both alter, and these are described accordingly.

Most murmurs are functional murmurs and not of clinical significance – the lower the intensity the less likely they are to be significant. Intensity is graded between 1 and 6, with the highest being 6. Where the murmur can be heard loudest is important; also, if the murmur can be heard over a wide area it is more likely to be significant.

Therefore, an intense holosystolic murmur is likely to indicate a problem with the left atrioventricular (AV) valve (also termed the bicuspid or mitral valve); this condition is likely to degenerate and so is significant. A late systolic rising murmur is likely to be diagnostic for a problem with the right AV (tricuspid) valve, and is also likely to be significant. Last a holodiastolic decreasing murmur is likely to indicate aortic regurgitation, and therefore is significant.

When considering cardiac murmurs in the working horse, the main aspect is welfare, unlike the situation with the riding horse, where the clinician has to consider the safety of the rider. Therefore, if the horse appears to cope physically with a level of work the murmur can, to some extent, be ignored. The handler should be warned that a sudden increase in the workload, either in the amount of energy required or the duration of the work, should be avoided in the horse showing a possible pathological murmur. The use of echocardiography is useful for pinpointing diagnosis. However, the equipment is expensive and not likely to be available to the practitioner in the developing world where working equids are vital.

Cardiac arrhythmias

A normal cardiac rhythm shows that the heart is functioning in a coordinated manner and therefore at maximum efficiency. This may not be so important at rest, but when exerted the horse may have to compensate for an arrhythmia by a greater increase in heart rate. If an arrhythmia is detected at rest, it is wise to examine the horse again after exercise. The clinician should spend some time on auscultation; obviously, electrocardiography is helpful but is not essential. The clinician can give useful advice to the owner from auscultation alone regarding the suitability of that horse for work, bearing in mind that welfare aspects should be paramount. The arrhythmia should be classified and related to any other cardiac or systemic disease.

Heart rate should be recorded when the horse is examined when quiet at rest; it is also suggested that the peripheral pulse be examined at the same time to establish whether there is a pulse deficit. This, however, is extremely difficult, as the horse is likely to show severe cardiac signs before such a deficit can be detected. Both the timing and frequency of the arrhythmia should be noted so that a cause can be suggested. In simple terms, the clinician needs to know whether the heart rhythm is regularly irregular or totally irregular. By far the most common arrhythmia is atrioventricular block; this is seen when the heart sounds as if it has totally missed a beat, but the main rhythm is totally regular – often called a dropped beat. In fact, some horses may drop two beats and, if the rate is really slow at, say, 20 beats/min, the clinician will wonder whether the horse is going to collapse. However, this arrhythmia is totally physiological and will be overridden as soon as the heart rate increases with exercise, or indeed excitement.

A less common arrhythmia is atrial fibrillation (AF), where the heart will sound irregularly irregular. There is normally a long period of diastole followed by several very rapid beats; this is pathological. However, it is important to judge AF in relation to the whole horse: if there is no weight loss and the horse appears to be able to work normally, then there is no reason for the horse to be rested or retired. However, if the horse becomes compromised by work, then either the workload or the time spent at work must be reduced. If this does not help then, for welfare reasons, the horse must be retired. There are treatments available, using either quinidine sulfate or electrical shock treatments given under general anaesthetic, but these are rarely successful in the long term. There may also be side-effects with these treatments, so it is better to control the amount of work for the horse rather than carry out expensive treatment.

Ventricular fibrillation (VF) is fatal. There will be no clear heart sounds and the pulse will be absent. Jumping on the horse's chest with a knee over the heart may be tried, but is unlikely to be successful.

Horses are not prone to coronary heart disease and so do not suffer from a 'heart attack', but this provides an easy explanation for an owner in the event of a sudden and unexplained death. In reality, a horse with any of the heart conditions described above is no more likely to die suddenly than any other horse. The only real cause of sudden death related solely to the heart is rupture of the major chordae tendinae of the heart valves, which cannot be predicted. The most likely cause of sudden death associated with the circulation is rupture of a major blood vessel, the most common being the pulmonary artery, the aortic root, a major pulmonary vessel, the carotid artery (normally as a result of damage in the guttural pouch from mycotic infection or a malignant melanoma), a major intestinal artery (likely to be caused by damage from migration of large strongyles) and, last, a uterine artery. These ruptures may follow an aneurysm.

14.8 Iliac Thrombosis

An extremely rare, though well-documented condition, a large blood clot – possibly of nematode origin – is released from the mitral heart valve and proceeds rapidly and unimpeded down the dorsal aorta, coming to rest at the iliac bifurcation. It is very unlikely that the owner will see the actual event. The normal history is for a horse's rear end suddenly to become very stiff, with a reluctance to move, resembling a case of rhabdomyolysis (see Section 12.11). However, there is no pain in the gluteal muscles and the horse will be more lame on one hind leg, the extremity of which will be cold. It will be extremely difficult to feel a pulse anywhere on this leg. Rectal examination will reveal the solid lump of fibrous tissue at the bifurcation, with a much weaker pulse on the affected side. Rest in these cases is contraindicated. Light work will help the horse form a collateral circulation, and it should recover. There is no evidence to suggest that treatment with either warfarin or heparin is beneficial.

14.9 Thrombophlebitis

An iatrogenic condition, normally of the jugular, this is the result of either perivascular injection of some irritant substance or an infection following the placement of an i/v catheter. If the clinician knows that an irritant substance has been injected perivascularly, then the area should be infiltrated with isotonic saline containing very dilute lignocaine; antibiotics and NSAIDs should be given. If there is any infection around a catheter it should be removed, then antibiotics given both parenterally and locally. Normally, the swelling on the neck, which may be massive, will subside, but it is likely that the jugular will remain corded and therefore useless for further i/v injections. The owner should be told, and the information logged in the horse's notes so that future clinicians do not struggle to find the jugular vein on that side of the neck. Sarcoid formation, as described in Section 20.13, may also follow i/v catheter placement.

14.10 Other Circulatory Disorders

Equine viral arteritis (EVA)

A disease caused by a togavirus and having a worldwide distribution, this condition causes a severe panvasculitis, which can be fatal. As one would expect, the main signs are oedema and petechiation, although the classical sign described is of blood-stained tears. It will also cause abortion. The actual cause of death is renal failure. Viral isolation is very difficult. It is spread from horse to horse via the respiratory tract, resulting in symptomless carriers that can be detected by serology. It is also spread venereally, as the virus is stored in the testicles. There exists, however, a good vaccine; this is not a marker vaccine and so previous blood testing is important prior to vaccination to ensure that the horse, particularly if a stallion, is not a carrier.

Purpura haemorrhagica

Although appearing very similar to EVA, this is a non-contagious, sporadic disease that normally follows another disease, e.g. strangles or equine influenza (see Section 14.3). It is nearly always fatal, even with aggressive antibiotic therapy. Large doses of dexamethasone are advised, unless the horse is considered to still be infected with a bacteria or a virus; in this case, NSAIDs are safer. The horse will have swollen, painful joints and large areas of oedema and there may be spontaneous haemorrhages.

Disseminated intravascular coagulopathy (DIC)

Inevitably fatal, this disease follows severe stress, e.g. a bad dystocia, acute diarrhoea, endotoxaemia, severe laminitis or even snake bite. There is a very marked thrombocytopenia. The signs are of either multiple haemorrhages or multiple blood clots; if either of these occur in the CNS the end is very quick. Early euthanasia is advised.

Immune-mediated thrombocytopenia

A condition of the newborn, seen when the foal inherits a platelet alloantigen from the sire that is not present on the dam's platelets. The dam produces alloantibodies against this antigen, and these are then secreted into the colostrum that the foal receives after birth. There is marked nasal bleeding and petechiae on the mucous membranes. A secondary form may be seen in the adult following endotoxaemia or some cases of lymphosarcoma. The prognosis is grave, though treatment in the form of dexamethasone can be given daily at 0.1 mg/kg, with antibiotic cover. Any surgical procedure must be avoided. Medication should be injected through a very fine needle to avoid unnecessary haemorrhage.

Equine infectious anaemia (EIA)

An untyped virus disease with a long incubation period of 14 to 42 days, this is seen in wet areas throughout the world and is usually called swamp fever; it is thought to be spread by mosquitoes or biting flies and can cause fatalities, with fever, jaundice and anaemia. Subclinical infections commonly occur. There is likely to be pyrexia (which may be recurrent). There will be lethargy and depression with inappetence and weight loss. Equally, there are horses that can survive to become carriers. It is rarely fatal in donkeys or mules, and zebra may become symptomless carriers. Spread may occur through semen and milk, and also by contaminated needles. There is neither vaccine nor specific treatment, except for supportive treatment with fluids, antibiotics and NSAIDs; steroids should not be given. A specific serological test is available, the Coggins test. The disease is notifiable in the UK. It occurred in the country in 2012, associated with an import.

Anthrax

The disease in the horse is very different from that in cattle, although it is caused by the same organism, *Bacillus anthracis*. The horse ingests the organism, which then attacks the tonsil and causes a hot and very painful neck swelling; high fever and septicaemia soon follow, and the swelling may spread to the ventral areas of the thorax and abdomen. The organism may be found in thin smears made from either blood or the serosanguinous neck fluid; smears should be fixed on the slide with heat and then stained with a solution of methylene blue (MacFadyen's stain). After 30 s the stain should be washed in running water and then dried; the classic blue rods with a purple capsule will readily be seen on examination under oil immersion. The anthrax bacillus is very sensitive to high doses of penicillin, and so most cases are worth treating.

Epizootic lymphangitis

A bacterial disease caused by *Histoplasma farciminosum* and seen in Europe around the Mediterranean, throughout Africa, the Middle East and Asia, this is often wrongly termed 'farcy' – a term that should be reserved for glanders (see below). The horse becomes covered in nodules that ulcerate, with yellow and infective pus; there follows a long incubation period with chronic weight loss. The condition does not appear to respond to antibiotics, but the majority of animals will recover; owners, however, may decide on euthanasia to prevent spread of the disease.

Glanders

Described some thousands of years ago in the Middle East, where it is still found today, this is a much-feared bacterial disease; it is also found throughout Asia and in South America. The causative agent is the bacterium *Burkholderia (Pseudomonas) mallei*. Animals develop a high fever after an incubation period of 2 weeks; nodules are formed under the skin, and also in the respiratory tract. These ulcerate, producing a thick, mucopurulent nasal discharge; normally, the animal dies rapidly, although some individuals may survive and spread the bacteria. *The disease is a zoonosis and can be fatal in man, as the organism is resistant to antibiotics*. There are enzyme-linked immunosorbent assay (ELISA) tests available, so euthanasia is advisable on confirmation of the disease; there is no vaccine available.

Acute equine respiratory syndrome

Another zoonosis, caused by a morbillivirus – the Hendra virus – this originated in fruit bats and is found in Papua New Guinea and Australia. The virus has an incubation period of 5–10 days. There is a high fever with acute respiratory signs; membranes are cyanotic and there is a frothy, blood-tinged nasal discharge. Mortality is high and euthanasia is advised. Veterinary practitioners treating the disease are most at risk. There is no treatment or vaccine.

African horse sickness (AHS)

Caused by an orbivirus, this condition requires a vector, a *Culicoides* midge, and there are several different serotypes that are *not* cross-protective. Although the disease originated in Africa, it is now seen throughout the world, except in Northern

Europe and Australasia. The disease has an incubation period of 3–14 days. The disease is extremely serious: in the naive horse nine out of ten will die, although severe suffering beforehand is the real welfare issue. The horse appears to have pleural pneumonia, but the pulmonary fluid is actually in the interlobular spaces. You will not see a fluid line on ultrasound, nor will you perceive one on percussion. The horse will be extremely ill, hanging its swollen head to the ground and with a heart rate in excess of 80 beats/min; the rectal temperature will be >40°C (104°F), and the splashing of pericardial fluid is audible on auscultation. In the rare case where recovery occurs, the horse will not be fit for work. Although treatment with antibiotics and corticosteroids is widely used, it is rarely helpful; NSAIDs may improve the demeanour of the horse. From a welfare perspective, unless there is some improvement within 48 h euthanasia is the only option.

It is a myth that the donkey does not suffer from clinical disease, but is affected in only a subclinical form: the naive donkey readily develops the disease. Mortality is less than in the horse, but is in the region of 50% and it is still a very nasty disease. However, donkeys will recover and will have developed a solid immunity to that serotype. The donkey foal will have acquired some passive immunity from its mother.

Management of AHS through controlling the vector is unlikely to be effective: vaccination is the only choice. This is complicated, however, as there are at least nine serotypes; there is some crossover of immunity but certainly not between all the nine types. Even with the correct serotype included in the vaccine, 100% immunity cannot be achieved, but vaccination certainly increases recovery rates quite markedly. In endemic areas, before the rains arrive with an increasing midge population, owners should be urged to vaccinate all equine animals. It is likely that zebra are resistant to the disease. The disease is notifiable in Great Britain and Northern Ireland. But it has never occurred on these shores.

Babesiosis

A protozoal disease spread mainly by ticks, the foal can also become infected *in utero*. The organisms involved are *Babesia equi* (the other name for this organism is *Theileria equi*) and *Babesi caballi*. These are found worldwide, but are much more common in tropical and subtropical areas, mainly on account of the distribution of the tick vector. A recent study in Scotland (Coultous *et al.*, 2023) carried out a risk assessment on Equine Piroplasmosis (EP), and concluded that EP positive animals are able to enter and are currently present in the UK, and that conditions do exist that could allow forward transmission of the disease. The study highlighted a gap in existing policy where the UK falls behind OIE guidelines and has suggested steps to address this discrepancy and improve national biosecurity. Tick species involved are the genera *Rhipicephalus*, *Dermacentor* and *Hyalomma*. *Babesia equi* is a much smaller parasite than *B. caballi* and is more pathogenic. The clinical signs are fever, jaundice, haemoglobinuria and oedema of the head. Diagnosis can be confirmed by direct thin blood smears stained with Giemsa. The best treatment is diminazene at 3.5 mg/kg, prepared in a sterile manner and injected slowly i/v. There is some danger if injection is not carried out very slowly, or if there is perivascular leakage. The other treatment available is Imidocarb, at 4 mg/kg, given on consecutive days; this causes a very marked local swelling and therefore is also hazardous. It is not notifiable in the UK. It is thought by workers in Italy, where the infection has been endemic for years (Jacopo, 2021, personal communication), that it is best not sterilize the infection but to treat the clinical signs. The protocol used is 4 mg/kg Imidocarb four times every 48 h simultaneously with buscopan and flunixin to control the colic signs induced by the Imidocarb. Dexamethasone and i/v fluids are given supportively as required.

Often anaplasmosis is detected at the same time. This can be treated with oxytetracycline given i/v at 7 mg/kg for 7 days.

Anaplasmosis

There is great confusion for the clinician dealing with this condition. It is caused by a protozoan now termed *Anaplasma phagocytophilum*, previously known as *Ehrlichia equi* and, like babesiosis, is spread by ticks. It should not be confused with Potomac horse fever (PHF), the proper name for this latter disease being equine monocytic ehrlichiosis. PHF was thought to be caused by an organism called *Ehrlichia risticii*, but this has now been renamed *Neorickettsia risticii*. The laboratory difference between the two organisms is that *N. risticii* is *not* found in the granulocytes on blood films, while *A. phagocytophilum* is.

Anaplasma phagocytophilum is found in both North America and Europe, being spread by *Ixodes pacificus* in North America and *Ixodes ricinus* in Europe. The same organism has been found in humans, so potentially it is a zoonosis, although it is spread to humans only by tick bites.

Signs in the horse vary enormously, from mild, transient fever to an acute, febrile disease with limb oedema, petechiation and jaundice. Treatment with i/v oxytetracycline at 7 mg/kg for 7 days is effective.

Neonatal haemolytic disease

The correct name for this condition is neonatal isoerythrolysis syndrome (NIS). It occurs only in foals born to mares that have had a previous foal. There is a very low incidence in the thoroughbred and an extremely low incidence in other breeds; it has not been recorded in donkeys or mules. The multiparous mare produces antibodies to a transplacental leakage in a previous pregnancy, and these antibodies appear in the colostrum. There is an incompatibility in the foal to these antibodies, with the young animal becoming progressively weaker and ceasing to suck after the first 24 h of life. A low erythrocyte count will be found, registering $<3 \times 10^{12}/l$.

The foal will be jaundiced, although this is not pathognomonic, as a foal with severe septicaemia may also be jaundiced; however, in this latter case the rectal temperature will be raised unless the foal is *in extremis*. If the foal is still sucking, the best option is to leave well alone as any stress will increase the tachycardia and tachypnoea; if the foal has stopped sucking the only other option is a transfusion, the best practice being an exchange transfusion, but this is impossible in the field. The next best practice is a transfusion of washed red blood cells, but this also is impracticable in the field. The third recommendation is to transfuse 1 litre of whole blood collected from a totally unrelated gelding.

Immune-mediated haemolytic anaemia

A similar condition to NIS but occurring in the adults, the cause is unknown. However, it normally occurs in conjunction with another disease, e.g. Lyme disease or Marie's disease. Certain drug therapies have also been blamed. Treatment is rather empirical and is centred on dexamethasone and cessation of any other medication.

Lymphangitis

A much over-diagnosed condition of an idiopathic nature, the signs are of very oedematous lower limbs. The horse appears bright and the rectal temperature is normal, unlike the main differential which is cellulitis. The horse is found to be eating normally. In heavy horses it is said to occur after a day's rest and is called 'Monday morning leg'. Normally, regular exercise will control the condition. Diuretics such as furosemide rarely help and, certainly given as multiple doses, are contraindicated.

References and Further Reading

Beech, J. (1991) *Equine Respiratory Disorders*. Lea & Febiger, Philadelphia, Pennsylvania.

Colgate, V. and Newton, R. (2023) Vaccination: Horses that will benefit and persuading owners. *Vet Times Equine* 9(1), 7 March: 10–11.

Coultous, R.M., Sutton, D.G.M. and Boden, L.A. (2023) A risk assessment of equine piroplasmosis entry, exposure and consequences in the UK. *Equine Veterinary Journal* 55: 282–294.

Grause, J.F., Ueti, M.W., Nelson, J.T., Knowles, D.P., Kappmeyer, L.S. and Bunn, T.O. (2013) The efficacy of imidocarb in eliminating *Theileria equi* from experimentally infected horses. *Veterinary Journal* 196(3): 541–546.

Holden, M.T.G., Heather, Z., Paillot, R., Steward, K.F., Webb, K. *et al.* (2009) Genomic evidence for the evolution of *Streptococcus equi*: Host restriction, increased virulence, and genetic exchange with human pathogens. *PLOS Pathogens* 5(3): e1000346.

Patteson, M.W. (1996) *Equine Cardiology*. Blackwell Science, Oxford, UK.

Robinson, C., Waller, A.S., Frykberg, L., Flock, M., Zachrisson, O. *et al.* (2020) Intramuscular vaccination with Strangvac is safe and induces protection against equine strangles caused by *Streptococcus equi*. *Vaccine* 38(31): 4861–4868.

Rush, B. and Mair, T. (2004) *Equine Respiratory Diseases*. Wiley Blackwell, Oxford, UK.

Siwinska, N., Zak, A., Slowikowska, M., Niedzwiedz, A., Ciaputa, R. *et al.* (2022) Chronic tuberculosis caused by *Mycobacterium bovis* in a domestic donkey in Central Europe. *Equine Veterinary Education* 35: 62.

Waller, A.S. (2023) Ending the nightmare of strangles. *Vet Times* 53(17), 5 May: 10–12.

15

Gastroenteric Conditions

Abstract
This chapter covers the whole intestinal tract from the gullet with choke to the anus. The teeth, pharynx and oral cavity are covered in Chapter 10 under dentistry. In equines, with their small stomach and large hindgut, problems with colic are extremely common and will receive more attention.

15.1 General

Gastrointestinal disease is very common in adult equines. Clinical signs depend on the underlying pathophysiologic processes and area of intestinal tract affected (Table 15.1).

15.2 Vesicular Stomatitis

This vesiculovirus disease with zoonotic potential is spread by insects, including biting flies and midges, black flies and sand flies. It can also be spread by direct contact through saliva or fluid from ruptured blisters and indirectly through fomites. The incubation period is 2–8 days. Blisters occur on the tongue, oral mucosa, nose, lips, coronary bands, udder or sheath. Diagnosis can be confirmed by serum with an ELISA on serum, or on whole blood, or on a swab from a lesion, or on a nasopharyngeal swab. There is no specific treatment or vaccine available. It is notifiable in the UK and has never been seen here. It is seen in North, Central and South America with a greater incidence in warmer regions.

15.3 Choke

Most cases of choke are easily diagnosed by the owner, but the clinician then has a dilemma: if the owner or the patient is very distressed then immediate attention is indicated, but if the owner is sensible and the horse relatively calm, I think it is quite reasonable for the practitioner to delay visiting the case: many cases of choke will have cleared within a few minutes. It is very important that the client knows that a horse that is choked has a blocked oesophagus and is not in an immediate life-threatening situation, unlike a human, who can become choked with a blocked trachea. A choked human needs application of the Heimlich manoeuvre immediately.

Assuming that the horse is still choked on your arrival, you will readily observe the classic action of arching of the neck and failure to swallow. Rarely is the heart rate raised above 48 beats/min, and the mucous membranes will appear normal; however, saliva and food material will be running intermittently down the nose. There will appear to be no abdominal pain and gut sounds will be normal; rectal temperature will be normal and the anal sphincter will have a normal tone.

DOI: 10.1079/9781800624283.0015

Table 15.1. Common clinicopathological abnormalities seen with chronic intestinal disease.

Clinicopathological abnormality	Common cause
Anaemia	Chronic disease
Leucopenia and increased serum amyloid A concentration	Acute inflammation
Eosinophilia	Endoparasitism or generalized intestinal inflammation
Hypoalbuminaemia	Protein-losing enteropathy
Leucocytosis, hypoglobulinaemia and hyperfibrinogenaemia	Chronic inflammation

In a study of 100 cases of choke attended in general practice between September 1997 and April 2003, 100% showed drooling and nasal return of saliva and food. Equally, 100% made repeated attempts to swallow, 92% had a palpable mass on the left lateroventral aspect of the neck, while 81% had repeated spasm of the neck muscles. Marked anxiety and distress was not a feature, with only 5% affected; 11% had a cough.

It will be rare that you will have a problem with diagnosis. However, the possible differentials are:

- colic;
- grass sickness;
- botulism;
- tetanus; and
- chronic lead poisoning.

Other causes of dysphagia are:

- dental abnormalities;
- guttural pouch disease;
- foreign bodies in the naso-/oropharynx; and
- palatal defects.

Choke is normally caused by dry concentrate feed, particularly pelleted feed, but the very worst cause is dry sugarbeet pulp.

Accepted wisdom is to attempt to pass a nasogastric tube to confirm your diagnosis. This is obviously sensible if there is any doubt in your mind but, if there is no doubt, caution should be exercised. First of all, the owner will assume that you are going to clear the obstruction, which is rarely the case; you are then faced with an even more worried owner who will want a result. Second, you will find the tube harder to pass into the rostral oesophagus in a choked case than in a normal one; this will cause you some anxiety and the owner even more anxiety.

A better approach, therefore, is to sedate choke cases with romifidine (e.g. 1 ml Sedivet/100 kg i/v) after normal clinical examination. This dose will cause the horse to lower its head, thus reducing the risk of aspiration pneumonia; a full oral examination should then be performed. It is prudent to give the horse antibiotics by injection to guard against the danger of inhalation pneumonia. Strict instructions should be given that the animal is to be stabled with a non-edible bed. All food is to be removed, as some horses will start to eat again even if the choke remains. Ask for the water to be removed. The rationale is that many horses will play in the water, so that after 4 h the owner will not be able to see whether the animal has drunk or not. It is much better to present the water to the animal on a regular basis; one can then see whether the animal has drunk and therefore swallowed. Reassure the owner that you will visit the following day, unless you receive a telephone call to say the horse has recovered: this is an advantageous psychological ploy – the owner does not get the impression that you think the horse will be clear within 24 h.

In a study of 100 horses treated in general practice without passage of a nasogastric tube (see Fig. 15.1), 71 were clear within 12 h and a further 15 within the next 12 h. The other 14 horses had to be visited after 24 h; these were not sedated again but received i/v antibiotics and NSAIDs. In temperate countries it is reasonable to wait a further 24 h, but in hot climates the horse that has been choked for 24 h will require i/v fluids at that stage. Of those 14, 9 had managed to clear the obstruction within a further 24 h, leaving 5 horses out of the original 100 still choked and obstructed after 48 h. The lesson from this study is that the majority of choke cases will clear themselves.

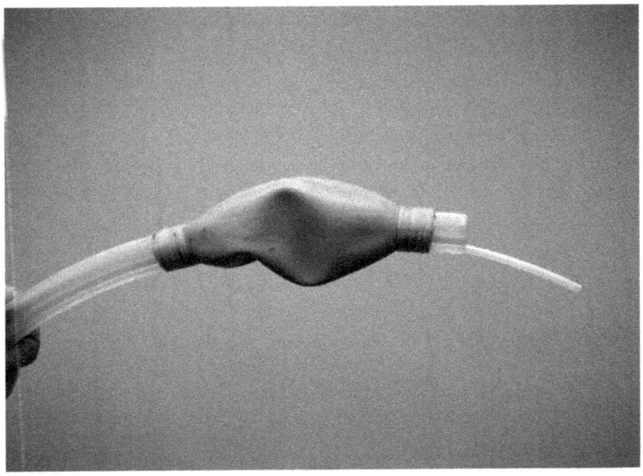

Fig. 15.1. Cuffed nasogastric tube.

The clinician has two options if the horse is still choked. First, the horse can be given a general anaesthetic following premedication, then intubated with an endotracheal tube; the cuff is next inflated and the anaesthesia maintained with gaseous agents. A nasogastric tube is passed and the blockage cleared with large volumes of water. This is a hazardous procedure, as it is possible for water to inadvertently find its way into the trachea, even with an endotracheal tube in place, and to set up pneumonia. Second, the choke can be cleared without a general anaesthetic, but with sedation and a cuffed nasogastric tube.

Clearance is relatively straight forward. There is good evidence that the use of neither oxytocin at 10 IU/100 kg i/v nor butylscopolamine and metamizole (Buscopan®) i/v helps the horse move the choke.

To summarize, the best advice on treating cases of choke in horses is:

1. Pass a nasogastric tube only if the diagnosis is in doubt.
2. Time will solve 95% of cases.
3. A cuffed nasogastric tube is extremely useful in the choked horse, but has its limitations in the small pony.
4. Intravenous fluids are useful in preventing dehydration.

15.4 Colic

The causes of colic will vary enormously, depending upon the part of the world in which you are working. Dry, sandy areas will predispose to sand colic, particularly after the annual rains have started, whereas in areas of high rainfall with lush pastures, gassy colics will predominate. There are, in reality, almost 100 different causes of equine colic. Age will have an influence: young animals are more prone to intussusception or larval cyathostomosis (see Section 15.5), while strangulating lipoma is seen in the older animal. Gender also has a marked influence: uterine torsion occurs only in the last trimester in the mare, while inguinal herniation and testicular rotation are seen only in the stallion. There have been few epidemiological studies on breed or type of horse influencing the cause of colic, although Standardbreds and Cleveland Bays appear to have a predisposition to inguinal herniation. A horse that has previously had colic is much more likely to suffer from colic a second time, though any horse that has undergone colic surgery is at a very high risk of repeated attacks of colic. Poor dentition or lack of dental care has been suggested as a predisposing cause of colic, although this has never been proved. A multi-centre study in donkeys with abdominal lesions showed that they may present with a range of signs often not including colic. Surgical findings were diverse and survival to discharge appeared to be lower than in horses.

On the other hand, the presence of tapeworms, particularly at the ileocaecal junction, has been shown to predispose to colic. Large redworms cause damage to the small intestinal arteries, leading to infarctions later. Obviously, cyathostomes that have become encysted will cause larval cyathostomosis. Administration of anthelmintics, particularly in the presence of large numbers of either roundworms or tapeworms, will trigger a colic episode. The influence of management factors, e.g. feeding and housing,

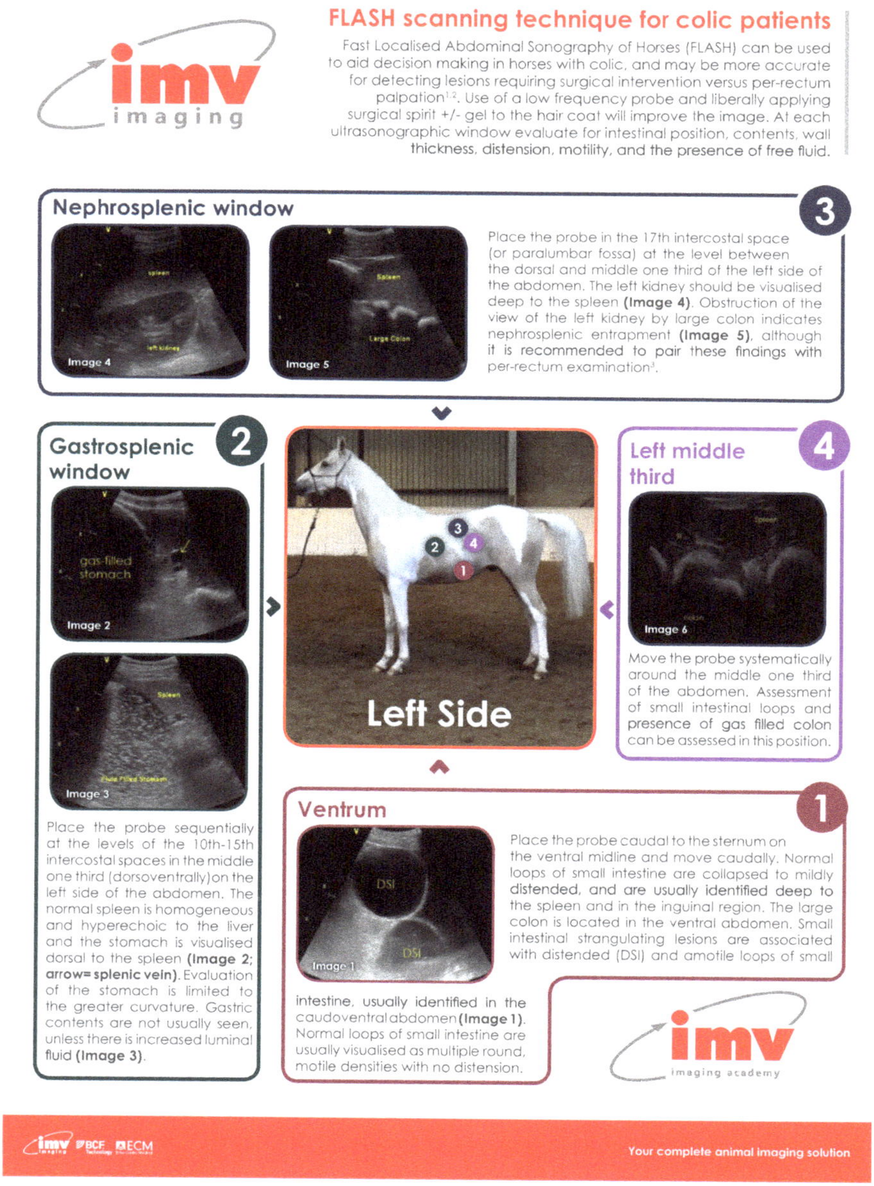

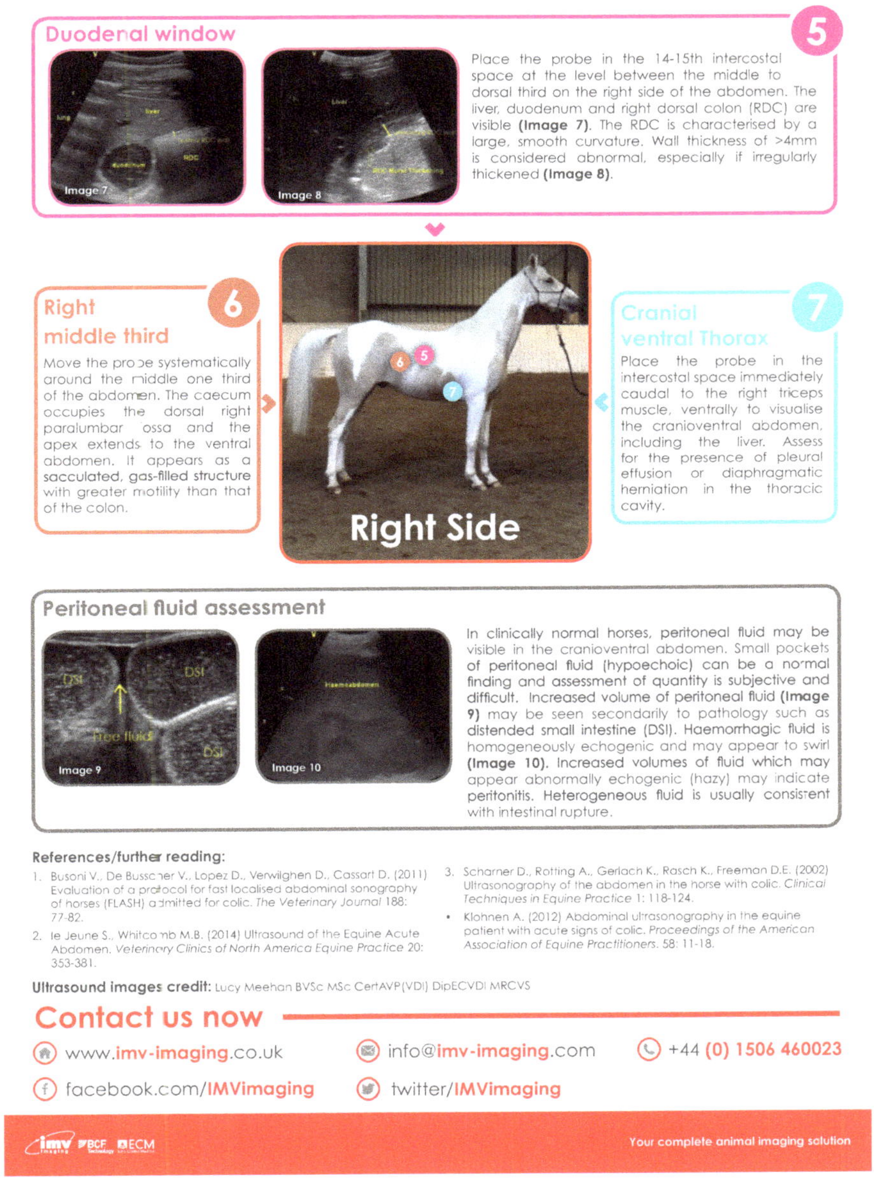

Fig. 15.2. An example of a useful technique for examining the horse's abdomen trans-abdominally in a quick but thorough manner to help with diagnosis and treatment developed by IMV (Quiney, personal communication, 2023).

is likely to influence the rate of colic attacks: the nearer a horse is kept to a natural environment the less likely it is that a colic episode is going to occur. Horses, left to fend for themselves, will feed and move for at least 18 h out of 24, and any change in this pattern will predispose to colic.

All these factors will influence the numbers of colic attacks within a population. However, the actual cause of the majority of cases is never ascertained. Even with surgical intervention the original cause is often not established, e.g. why a volvulus has occurred (see Section 15.8), why an enterolith has formed, why there is an intussusception or even why a horse has developed grass sickness (see Section 15.9).

Of all the improvements made in equine surgery and medicine, the greatest have been in the treatment of equine colic. There have been massive benefits to both the horse and its owner, and these advancements have been brought about through excellent research, evidence-based medicine (EBM) and clinical audit (CA). The veterinary schools and referral practices are to be congratulated for all their hard work.

Gone are the seemingly endless days and nights of worrying about horses with colic, although in areas of the world where there are no surgical facilities the practitioner has to do the best with the facilities available. Below is presented an approach to colic cases. With all these excellent advancements, it is still very important that we have in the forefront of our minds the welfare of the horse. The following questions need to be answered by the owner:

1. How old is the animal?
2. Has the animal had colic before and did it have surgery?
3. When did they last see it in a normal state?

The clinician needs to make an assessment as to:

1. Whether the owner is prepared for considerable expense.
2. Whether the owner is prepared to care for the animal properly.

The clinician should then perform a full examination of the horse, which will vary enormously in different scenarios. However, the following signs and symptoms should always be checked:

1. Check the general body condition and look for signs of trauma.
2. Measure heart rate and pulse; a raised pulse indicates pain, dehydration or enterotoxaemia.
3. Measure respiratory rate; a high rate also indicates pain.
4. Assess the gut sounds; intermittent bursts of sound in the right quadrant are related to the caecum, while sounds in the left quadrant tend to relate to the small intestine or left colon. Either increased or decreased sounds are abnormal; the normal response of the bowel proximal to an obstruction is hypermotility.
5. Look at the colour of the mucous membranes and gauge capillary refill time.
6. Take the rectal temperature (this is useful to assess the danger of a rectal examination. If a horse kicks when you take rectal temperature it will certainly kick when you perform a rectal examination). It will be raised in colic cases if there is anterior enteritis, colitis (*Clostridium* or *Salmonella*) or peritonitis.

It is normal to perform a rectal examination, but the clinician should be mindful of the danger to the horse and to him- or herself. The use of a spasmolytic and analgesic, e.g. butylscopolamine and metamizole, or sedation, e.g. with a combination of detomidine and butorphanol, may well be the way forward. Clinicians with large hands and forearms should not attempt to perform a rectal on a small pony or donkey. When performing a rectal examination, the serosal surfaces should be checked – these will feel tacky in cases of peritonitis or bowel rupture. The position of the bowel is then checked and any pain associated with palpation noted. The bowel is next checked for distension, i.e. gas or firm ingesta. Even at this stage the clinician should have the answers to the second group of history questions in the back of their mind. If ultrasound is available performing a FLASH scan, Figure 15.2 will be very helpful.

This information is required to decide whether at this initial visit the clinician is going to treat this as a surgical or a medical case. If it is decided that it is a surgical case, the decision has to be made whether the horse is going to be referred, surgery is going to be undertaken by the first-opinion veterinary surgeon or the owner needs guidance towards making the decision of euthanasia.

The clinician may carry out nasogastric intubation. It is useful here to apply suction to create a siphon; drawing off a large volume of fluid may be lifesaving, as gastric rupture will be prevented. A large volume gives a poor prognosis, as this indicates gastric impaction or a blockage in the anterior section of the small intestine. In either of these conditions the horse will often sit in a dog-sitting position to relieve the pressure in the anterior abdomen.

Very careful thought must be given before deciding that surgery should be undertaken:

1. There must be an upper age limit for colic surgery, which will vary depending upon whether the patient is a pony or a horse. Realistically, ponies over 25 and horses over 20 years of age are not suitable surgical cases.

2. If an animal has previously had colic surgery, this must make the prognosis more serious. Where it has had colic and recovered medically that must make the prognosis more encouraging.

3. The possible duration of the colic symptoms aid decision making: if the animal is known to have been well within the previous 2 h, a trial with analgesics is acceptable (obviously, if the signs have not indicated a surgical case). Otherwise, prompt referral is indicated if in any doubt. However, if the symptoms have been obviously long-standing and there is likelihood of severely damaged bowel, from a welfare point of view immediate euthanasia is the only option. Naturally, no practitioner should feel totally alone; if one is in doubt a second opinion from within the practice or from a neighbouring veterinarian is certainly worthwhile.

Consideration must be given to assessment of the owner:

1. If the owner is not prepared for considerable expense, then everyone has a problem. The costs of sedation for a rectal, passing a nasogastric tube, performing a peritoneal tap, scanning the abdomen, etc. are going to enlarge the bill. Multiple visits might end up being more expensive than hospitalization. One thing is certain – immediate euthanasia may be the least expensive option and, from a welfare standpoint, cannot be faulted. Surgery is not an option.

2. If the owner is not prepared or is unable to provide adequate care for the animal, medical care at home is not an option.

Last we come to the vital signs, and these are useful guidelines:

1. Heart rate is a very good predictor.
2. A rising heart rate is an adverse sign.
3. A heart rate remaining high after analgesia is also an adverse sign.
4. Signs of pain, including the respiratory rate, are helpful but should be judged with care.
5. Absence of gut sounds, particularly after analgesia, is an adverse sign.
6. The presence of gut sounds that then disappear is an adverse sign.
7. The colour of the mucous membranes is a good predictor.
8. Dehydration is a bad prognostic sign.

Regarding treatment of the surgical case, this must be aimed at keeping the animal comfortable until it reaches the referral centre. If the decision has already been made that surgery should be carried out, then any analgesic that will help control the pain is acceptable. However, if the clinician in the field wishes a further diagnostic work-up, the analgesic must be chosen with care. The analgesic must not mask the signs and deceive the referral practitioner, so flunixin is not advisable; a combination of butylscopolamine and metamizole (Buscopan®) and phenylbutazone is useful. If the transit time will not be unduly long, xylazine is acceptable.

If it is decided that the case is non-surgical, for treatment there are two important goals:

1. Controlling the pain.
2. Providing fluids.

Initial pain control is likely to be by i/v injection of NSAIDs, which can then be followed by oral administration. It should be remembered that the horse is likely to be inappetent, so the medication should be made into a paste and forcibly squirted into the mouth. In extremely severe cases fluid will have to be given as a drip, or even faster if the animal is suffering from severe dehydration. However, in most cases it can be given by nasogastric tube; the clinician will have to use judgement on volumes and frequency. If the horse is very fractious and has to be sedated, larger volumes less frequently will be better, whereas in the quiet horse frequent small volumes will be tolerated. Fluids are very important in cases of impaction. Psyllium should be given to animals with sand impaction; this medication absorbs excess fluid while promoting normal bowel movement. Successful treatment can be confirmed by collecting some faeces into a rectal sleeve and adding water; the sleeve can then be hung up. Sand should accumulate in the fingertips.

Impaction from fibrous ingesta will usually be felt per rectum in the pelvic flexure of the large colon. There is good evidence that these cases benefit from lungeing exercise. Mineral oil is often used in cases of impaction – 0.5 l/24 h for a 500 kg horse.

It should be remembered that the horse with diarrhoea will often show colicky pain.

15.5 Diarrhoea

Diarrhoea in the horse is normally classified as either acute or chronic, and these two types may be subdivided with respect to age – foal or adult.

This subdivision is confusing: When is a horse an adult? Where do yearlings fit in to this? A further subdivision is whether the cause is infectious or non-infectious, which adds further confusion since our knowledge of diarrhoea in horses is far from complete, and so an organism may well be found that causes what previously was considered to be a non-infectious diarrhoea. To try to simplify the subject, the following text will be divided into causes in alphabetical order, with a full description of possible agents and potential age groups affected.

Chronic inflammatory bowel disease and intestinal neoplasia

If this condition occurs in the small intestine, there will be chronic weight loss but no diarrhoea, making diagnosis difficult. A glucose absorption test, as described in Section 2.2, will be helpful. Alternatively, if this condition occurs in the large intestine, there will be diarrhoea as well as weight loss. The wall of the large intestine will feel thickened and the mesenteric lymph nodes will be felt to be enlarged; even the rectum may feel thickened. In these cases – and only in these cases – will a rectal biopsy be helpful with diagnosis. There is no realistic treatment, although oral prednisolone has been suggested. Euthanasia is the recommended course of action.

Clostridial diarrhoea

The pathogenesis of *Clostridia* spp. causing disease in the horse is unclear. Normal horses, particularly pregnant and lactating mares as well as foals, have *Clostridia* spp. in their large intestine, the most common being *Clostridium perfringens* and *Clostridium difficile*. Some trigger factor is required to cause the disease that is manifest as sudden death, or acute diarrhoea, often haemorrhagic. A positive diagnosis is rarely made in life, as confirmation of the bacterial toxin involved is extremely difficult. On post-mortem the necrotic enteritis is readily seen; smears will reveal large numbers of gram-positive rods, which are difficult to grow even in anaerobic conditions. Isolation of toxins requires very specialized laboratory facilities. The clinical picture will normally be mares and young foals that have received some stress factor, e.g. a long journey or sudden access to very lush grass. Treatment with NSAIDs and fluids is rarely successful.

Coronavirus

Coronaviruses are now much more commonly found in species other than the horse, and it is likely that they will also be seen in the foal. They will cause diarrhoea and may be associated with antibiotic usage, so clinicians should be careful with the use of antibiotics in the foal, particularly by the oral route. Treatment for coronavirus must be by fluids, with NSAIDs as support. An outbreak was confirmed on one farm in Switzerland (Fouche *et al.*, 2022). There were 26 horses, 7 developed clinical signs and 1 died.

Equine monocytic ehrlichiosis

The more common name for this disease is Potomac horse fever. It will cause diarrhoea and colic in all ages of horse, and will also cause abortion in the mare. The causal agent is *Neorickettsia* (formerly *Ehrlichia*) *risticii*, which is distributed throughout North America. It is likely that spread is via a vector associated with water. The organism can be isolated from the blood to confirm diagnosis. There must be a subclinical form, since high numbers of normal horses are seropositive. Treatment is supportive and symptomatic, while vaccines are of doubtful value.

Equine right dorsal colitis

Unusually, this condition is linked with NSAIDs; however, although all formulations can trigger the condition, the main cause is phenylbutazone. Classically, the condition is seen when excessive dosages have been given for an extended period, although it has also been recorded in animals receiving the recommended dosage of 4.4 mg/kg by mouth twice daily. The donkey does not seem to be affected. The presence of *Salmonella* spp. does not seem to be relevant, since these may be present in the normal horse. Diarrhoea may be profuse and even life-threatening. However, by immediately stopping the administration of the medication fatalities are normally avoided. The best treatment is psyllium mucilloid – 30 g daily for ponies and 60 g daily for horses. This treatment should be continued for a minimum of 2 weeks or longer if the diarrhoea persists, and can also be used in cases of sand colic.

Giardiasis

The pathogenesis of the protozoan *Giardia equi* is controversial, since it has been found occasionally in the faeces of normal foals and adults. However, it has also been demonstrated in very large numbers in cases of chronic diarrhoea in the adult horse. The treatment of choice is metronidazole, at 20 mg/kg by mouth 3 times daily. This often causes a depression in appetite, and it may be that this is what helps control the diarrhoea and that the protozoan is not the real problem.

Idiopathic chronic diarrhoea

As the name suggests, there is no known cause for this condition, and it is the common diagnosis when no cause for chronic diarrhoea can be found. There are welfare implications: the horse with chronic diarrhoea may develop sores on the backs of its legs and be plagued with flies. One helpful measure is to cover the upper part of the tail with cling film or polythene, so that it can easily be kept free of faeces. Codeine is a useful treatment, at the rate of 1–4 mg/kg twice daily; this is supplied normally in 60 mg tablets, which need to be crushed in the food. Hopefully, the diarrhoea can be controlled nutritionally by cutting out laxative food, but it should be stressed that water should never be withheld. It is also useful to give the horse extra electrolytes, as these will have been lost through the diarrhoea.

Intestinal tuberculosis

Both *Mycobacterium tuberculosis* and *Mycobacterium paratuberculosis* have been isolated post-mortem from horses that have clinically shown chronic diarrhoea. The lesions on post-mortem are of thickened, granulomatous areas in the colon that ulcerate; acid-fast organisms can be seen on smears made by scraping the mucosa. Because the horse is not a normal host it is not possible to grow the organisms, nor to isolate them, from faeces samples; multiple smears from the faeces, particularly if bloody, may reveal acid-fast organisms. Diagnosis is therefore extremely difficult since serology for *M. paratuberculosis* is unreliable, as is the intradermal skin test. Treatment would consist of isoniazid together with rifampicin, both at 10 mg/kg twice daily by mouth; this treatment will need to be given for a minimum of 2 months.

Larval cyathostomosis

Although this disease can occur in all age groups, it is mainly restricted to young yearlings and 2-year-olds; these animals will be found to be poorly fleshed and have been exposed to cyathostomes. Small strongyles invade the mucosa of the large intestine, this mainly occurring during the summer in temperate climates and during the rains in the tropics. The trigger factor that stimulates the mass emergence of cyathostome larvae is not fully known, but it is known that stressful conditions will bring on a life-threatening attack. Stress factors include: (i) severe weather conditions, e.g. autumn weather in temperate climates and drought in tropical situations; (ii) transporting animals; or even (iii) mixing groups. Faecal egg counts (FEC; see Section 1.8) are not useful diagnostically, as it is the non-egg-laying larvae that cause the disease, these being normally seen in large numbers on a rectal sleeve.

Diarrhoea is acute and watery; prevention is vital, for once the larvae emerge the chance of survival is slim. Treatment with dexamethasone and moxidectin (an anthelmintic) is rarely effective. Good worm control will prevent numbers of small cyathostomes building up on the pasture. Large numbers of eggs will then not be available for ingestion, and larvae will not become encysted. Horses should be wormed with moxidectin or double-strength fenbendazole (for 5 days) before the critical period, i.e. autumn in temperate climates.

Lawsonia

A rare cause of diarrhoea in the yearling, this disease is age specific and has not been isolated from the non-weaned foal. It is mainly sporadic, affecting just one or maybe a second animal in a group. The causal organism is the bacterium *Lawsonia intracellularis* and, as the name implies, it resides in the cells of the mucosa. Diagnosis is difficult, as the organism cannot be isolated in the faeces, but it can be found in histological samples of the intestine; a blood test performed by specialized laboratories is also available. The disease is of a chronic nature and is non-febrile, with a steady loss of weight, and therefore a clinical diagnosis is possible. Treatment is by a combination of erythromycin at 25 mg/kg three times daily and rifampicin at 10 mg/kg twice daily, both given orally. Tylosin injection, which is one of the treatments for the disease in pigs, should *never* be used in the horse, for given i/v it will cause death and given i/m or s/c will cause a massive necrotic reaction.

Nutritional diarrhoea

In the foal this condition is so common that it might be considered normal. It occurs when the foal first starts to eat food other than its mother's milk, which is normally 7–10 days after birth. It may also commence at the same time as the mare comes into oestrus post-foaling. It used to be thought that there were hormonal changes in the milk causing the diarrhoea, but this is not correct – diarrhoea is caused by change in diet. Antibiotics are not indicated, and most cases are self-limiting. However, a rise in temperature will indicate a more serious condition, and this is particularly likely if the foal has not received sufficient good-quality colostrum within the first 12 h of life.

Nutritional diarrhoea will also occur in the adult, when a sudden dietary change is imposed; obviously, any changes should be made slowly. Nutritional diarrhoea is particularly likely when a horse suddenly receives a large amount of lush, green grass.

Rotavirus

Rotavirus attacks the suckling foal at any age, it is highly contagious and has a 2-day incubation period. It is rarely fatal, however, if the foal can be kept hydrated. The use of antibiotics is contraindicated, as is the use of NSAIDs; the latter may cause gastric ulceration. The virus destroys the intestinal villi, and so the diarrhoea may persist but will eventually subside. Good hygiene is required to prevent spread of the disease.

Salmonellosis

Frequently a fatal disease, it is nevertheless not a simple one, being normally acute in both adult and foal. It appears to be infectious and then highly contagious, and yet some 15% of adult horses harbour the organism in their bile ducts. Some stress agent is required to trigger the disease (this is often surgery, which typically triggers an attack 2 days later), or the animal's defences are overwhelmed by the numbers of organisms in the environment. These organisms may have come from an equine carrier, be contaminants from another species, normally a rodent, or from the feed or water. The most common isolates are *Salmonella typhimurium*, *Salmonella enteritidis*, *Salmonella anatum*, *Salmonella heidelberg* and *Salmonella newport*.

The condition may present as a relatively mild illness with fever, anorexia and depression; the faeces are of a 'cow pat' consistency. Such a disease may be self-limiting, with the animal appearing to recover in a few days, without treatment, although such animals may become active carriers. The more common form, which is seen in adults as well as in foals, is acute, watery diarrhoea. There is high fever with abdominal pain, these signs possibly appearing before the onset of the watery diarrhoea. This then causes confusion with the diagnosis, since the animal appears to have colic, but the high fever and severe depression will alert the clinician. There is also a marked neutropenia. When the diarrhoea begins it often contains blood and strands of mucosa, and has a distinctively foul smell.

Treatment requires i/v fluids and electrolytes; NSAIDs are extremely useful, particularly flunixin; antibiotics need to be used with care, although they are certainly worthwhile in the early stages. The antibiotic of choice is trimethoprim-potentiated sulfonamide (TPS), which must be given i/v; oral antibiotics should be avoided.

It must always be remembered that this is a zoonosis as well as being contagious to equines.

Strongylosis

A disease of mixed aetiology, it may be caused by the small strongyles (cyathostomes) described above under larval cyathostomosis, although it may also be caused by the large strongyles. The most pathogenic is *Strongylus vulgaris*, the large redworm, whose larvae invade the wall of the small intestine and enter the arterioles. They damage these and cause emboli; historically, these emboli and the resulting infarctions were said to be a major cause of colic. With the advent of modern wormers their prevalence has diminished markedly, but they are still a threat. They will cause weight loss and diarrhoea; very little resistance to anthelmintics has been reported.

Trichomoniasis

The protozoan *Trichomonas equi* is found in normal faeces as well as in cases of equine diarrhoea. Knock's postulates, the long-established criteria for infectious disease, have not been fulfilled, and so I think this organism can be ignored as a cause of diarrhoea.

15.6 Diseases of the Rectum

Rectal prolapse

An extremely rare condition, this can occur spontaneously, in which case euthanasia is the best course of action. Any surgery may initially appear worthwhile, but recurrence is a certainty. If the condition occurs after a bad foaling, the rectum must be replaced as soon as possible; the mare should be sedated and local anaesthetic instilled around the anal ring, and a purse-string suture then put in place with uterine tape. The organ can then be replaced and the purse-string tightened: it should be tight enough to fit around no more than two fingers. This may seem tight to the surgeon but there will be a large amount of swelling, which will reduce with time and NSAIDs. The suture should be removed in 2–4 days and the horse given a very laxative diet.

Rectal tears

Rectal damage will occur when practitioners are performing rectal examinations, but provided care has been taken and a suitable amount of lubricant used, a rectal tear is *not* the fault of the clinician: there should be no blame or guilt. However, there are certain predisposing causes that should be avoided. (i) The ratio of the size of the rectum to the size of the clinician's hand and arm is important. If in any doubt do not perform a rectal examination – it should be remembered that a rectal examination is a diagnostic tool and not a treatment, and is therefore of only secondary importance to the horse. (ii) The temperament of the horse is important – the lively horse should be sedated. The use of the drug butylscopolamine, at 20 mg/kg i/v 5 min before a rectal examination is particularly effective in reducing the danger of a rectal tear.

Blood on the rectal sleeve may indicate a tear, but is not positive proof. Quite severe haemorrhage can occur when a rectal biopsy is performed, but not necessarily with dangerous consequences. If the clinician is inexperienced then no further action should be taken, but a more experienced colleague should be consulted. If such a referral is not possible then the animal should be given antibiotics and NSAIDs, then monitored. Normally, the clinician will have felt the tear; if it has penetrated the entire rectal wall, euthanasia must be the course of action. Tears such as these are graded as 4, while lesser tears may be graded as 1, 2 or 3, depending on the structures that have been torn. Most grade 1 and 2 tears will heal on their own, provided the horse is fed on a laxative diet and given antibiotics and NSAIDs. Unfortunately, a horse with a grade 3 rectal tear is likely to die, but it is reasonable to give it some time for recovery. Surgery of such a tear is likely to be heroic and unlikely to be successful.

15.7 Hepatic and Biliary Tract Diseases

Introduction

Classification of hepatic disease is very difficult, because the clinician and indeed the owner often cannot be certain when the disease started;

therefore, classification into acute and chronic disease is difficult. The liver is a marvellous organ in that it has great capacity for regeneration, and equally has a basic overcapacity, and therefore a rise in liver enzymes on a blood test needs very careful evaluation. The clinician is normally presented with one of two different clinical pictures, an acute-onset disease or a chronic disease.

Acute hepatic disease

In ponies and donkeys the most common cause of acute hepatic disease is hyperlipaemia, which is very common and extremely serious; it is discussed separately later in this section.

The main acute hepatic disease is Theiler's disease, which was originally thought to be caused by administration of tetanus antitoxin, and hence was termed serum hepatitis. This, however, is not the cause of the disease, which is as yet still unknown. It is more common during the summer and autumn in temperate countries and therefore it may be caused by a virus with a vector. The disease is manifest as acute liver failure, evidenced by jaundice and orange-coloured urine, with resulting neurological signs. Treatment, which can only be supportive, is rarely successful, and so euthanasia is advised on welfare grounds.

Chronic hepatic disease

The most common cause is pyrrolizidine alkaloid-containing plants, of which there are many, but the best known is ragwort (*Senecio jacobaea*). This yellow flower, common in temperate climates, is not palatable to the horse when mature; however, early in the spring when there is no other green herbage available, horses will ingest the young florets. They also may eat the mature plant if it has been cut and left on the pasture or made into hay or haylage. The liver will be damaged and, unless regeneration can occur, the horse will be lethargic and eventually suffer liver failure. Neurological signs will then be manifest, and after that the disease is fatal. However, if the animal can be totally removed from further access before neurological signs develop, a cure is possible with supportive treatment, i.e. no stress and a low-protein diet with extra vitamin B supplementation. As SDH and AST are both enzymes associated with acute liver disease, these will be raised initially and go undetected, but will often have returned to normal when a blood sample is taken. Raised GGT and ALP are more reliable diagnostic indicators, as these will remain high (see Table 1.2).

Hyperlipaemia

A condition of donkeys, mules and small ponies, it is not seen in young animals below 18 months of age; the incidence rises with the age of the animal. Lactation and pregnancy are predisposing causes but, regardless of the reproductive state of the mare, it is more common in the mare than in either geldings or stallions. The main predisposing factor, however, is stress, and thus the condition can be brought on by *any* other disease, particularly those that cause inappetence. It can also be brought on by any physical factor affecting the animal's ability to keep eating. The clinical signs therefore are amazingly variable, as they will depend on the underlying cause; however, cases will show a general malaise and will not want to eat.

Hyperlipaemia occurs when the body's fat reserves are rapidly mobilized to combat any energy deficit, and thus overweight animals are more at risk. It is such a common condition in the donkey that any overweight donkey which is off its food is vulnerable. Diagnosis is not hard for the experienced clinician, but even experienced clinicians may miss the early signs. Obesity leads to insulin insensitivity; stress leads to cortical release, which in turn inhibits insulin effects. Adipose tissue is mobilized and triglycerides are released from the liver – any rise >5 mmol/l should alert the clinician. Voluntary feeding with tempting, succulent foods – particularly grass – should be commenced immediately. If the disease is more advanced, fat will actually be seen in a blood sample, as a whitish grey band; laboratory confirmation is then not required.

Treatment requires a two-pronged attack: (i) the underlying cause must be promptly addressed; and (ii) adipose mobilization must be reversed. The pathogenesis indicates that both insulin and heparin would be helpful, but sadly this is not the case. Flunixin, initially at the normal dose of 1.1 mg/kg, is helpful and this must be continued every 6 h at 0.25 mg/kg. Fluids, carbohydrates and vitamins should be given by nasogastric tube if the animal will not eat, but ultimately i/v therapy may be required. However, welfare and economics must be considered, since often these cases will recur. Euthanasia is likely to be the option in such cases, or in very severe first-presentation cases. Dexamethasone *must never* be given in the hyperlipaemia case.

15.8 Diseases of the Stomach

Gastric impaction, dilation and rupture

All three of these conditions will be seen as severe colic. Differentiation will be very difficult except on post-mortem. A volvulus of the small intestine in its upper third will give similar colic signs. The signs are of a very high pulse rate and severe pain. Often the horse will sit like a dog with its back legs and rump on the ground but its front legs in extension. Unless there is a fibrous impaction in the stomach there will be a copious gastric reflux. There will be an absence of gut sounds. The mucous membranes will look toxic. Euthanasia is the only outcome. If the clinician has made an error and it is not a disease of the stomach but a volvulus of the upper small intestine, it is likely to be extremely difficult to correct surgically and so once again euthanasia is indicated. One author (Prutton, 2023) considers that some horses with gastric impaction will have more variable chronic signs over several weeks such as weight loss, lethargy, inappetence and abdominal distension. These pose a diagnostic challenge as the size of the stomach can vary enormously on gastroscopy. Starvation for 24 h prior to examination is helpful as the appearance of a large ball of food is far from normal. Treatment with cola by nasogastric tube has been suggested by German workers (Witt *et al.*, 2021).

Gastric ulceration

The clinical signs are poor performance and recurrent colic, with no other cause found. There can be a loss of appetite and a subsequent loss in condition. There may also be changes in behaviour. The rise in prominence of this condition, called equine gastric ulcer syndrome (EGUS), in recent years is due to the advent of the 2 m-length gastroscope, which represents the only way in which the condition can be positively diagnosed. It includes two distinct syndromes: equine glandular gastric disease (EGGD) and equine squamous gastric disease. Ulceration is normally seen in the horse under stress that has been fed too much corn, too little long fibre and has undergone intensive training, e.g. the young racehorse; it is unlikely to be a problem in the working horse, although I suspect that the condition is under-reported. Ulcers will heal as soon as the horse is removed from the stressful environment. It has been reported that there is evidence that phenylbutazone increased gastrointestinal dysbiosis and increased the frequency of ulceration (Whitfield-Cargile *et al.*, 2021). It is likely that other NSAIDs do the same. Diet can play a significant role in the treatment of the condition, as can increasing the amount of turn-out time. There is a specific treatment available, omeprazole, a proton pump inhibitor; oral dosage is 4 mg/kg daily for 28 days, followed by 1 mg/kg for a further 28 days. There is also an injectable form.

Neoplasia

Tumours of the stomach are extremely rare, those diagnosed being mainly the squamous cell carcinoma, although leiomyosarcomas have also been recorded. The horse will show chronic weight loss; colic is not a feature, except in the terminal stages. Diagnosis in life is possible only with a 2-m gastroscope, otherwise the clinician will see the condition only at post-mortem.

15.9 Grass Sickness

In only a few isolated areas of the world is this condition seen frequently; it was first recorded in 1907 in western Scotland, UK; however, it does occur in all northern European countries, and sporadically in the southern countries of South America. It is classified as a dysautonomia; related diseases are found in man and other animals, e.g. the brown hare, and have been recorded in all equine species. The cause is unknown, although there are various trigger factors recorded: the animal will have been out at grass, and arrival on new premises is a common trigger. Recent dry weather or anthelmintic treatment also seem to be related to this disease. It is a disease primarily of the young adult horse, although it has been recorded in horses of all ages; there is perhaps a higher incidence in the mare. Normally at onset, the animal is in above-average body condition.

The disease is divided rather arbitrarily into acute, subacute and chronic forms; there is certainly an acute form, which will appear like a colic attack, with very similar signs. However, there are some signs that will alert the clinician: the rectal temperature is often raised, and bilateral ptosis is also often seen. The horse's inability to swallow is present in these cases, but not obvious, as it is not actually eating or drinking. Squirting water or gruel into the mouth may help to demonstrate this tell-tale sign. There is often copious salivation; a nasogastric tube should be passed to eliminate the differential of oesophageal obstruction – there is normally copious gastric reflux. The pain is unresponsive to pain relief, and euthanasia is the kindest option.

In subacute and chronic cases, the disease has a much more insidious onset, when the classic tucked-up, 'greyhound-like' appearance will be seen and the inability to swallow will be obvious. The amount of pain demonstrated in these cases will be much more variable, the bouts of pain often bearing little relationship to the administration of pain relief. Animals try to get comfortable by bringing all four legs directly underneath them. All these signs will help the clinician make a diagnosis, which can be confirmed only by histology of the autonomic ganglia; the classical ganglia chosen are in the coeliacomesenteric area. Such histopathology can be performed at laparotomy or, more usually, at post-mortem.

In reality, the likelihood of any grass sickness case recovering is extremely small but, if the horse has some interest in food and is able to swallow, treatment might be considered provided that pain, which can be monitored by heart rate, can be controlled. Good nursing is a fundamental requirement. There is strong evidence that cisapride given at 0.6 mg/kg three times daily by mouth is helpful as an intestinal motility enhancer. Survivors have been recorded as returning to work.

15.10 Umbilical Hernia

The cause of umbilical hernia may be either genetic or, more commonly, acquired through failure of the umbilicus to close fully on account of umbilical infection. No action need be taken in the young foal, but the presence of hernia noted. At 4 months of age the foal is re-examined and, if the hernial ring will admit only a single finger, the hernia should be left as there is a very good chance that it will heal spontaneously. If the hernial ring will admit two fingers, the clinician can proceed in the following manner:

1. The animal is heavily sedated and cast into dorsal recumbency.
2. The hernial sac is then drawn down vertically, ensuring that all the abdominal contents have been returned to the abdomen.
3. A very tight ligature of umbilical tape or an elastrator castration ring is applied to the sac, as close to the body wall as possible.
4. Tetanus antiserum is given.
5. The area must be kept dressed with fly repellent until 1 week after the sac has sloughed off.

If the hernial ring is larger than two fingers, the following procedure is recommended:

1. Full aseptic surgery should be performed under general anaesthetic, with the foal in dorsal recumbency.
2. An elliptical skin incision is made around the hernia, removing some of the excess skin but leaving sufficient to close the wound without excessive tension.
3. Using blunt dissection, the skin is separated from the abdominal wall; if the surgeon feels that the hernia can be obliterated by closing the abdominal wall without too much tension, this should be performed by removing some of the hernial sac.
4. Multiple mattress sutures should be laid across the defect in the abdominal wall, without tying them.
5. When the surgeon is satisfied that the defect can be totally closed, the sutures can be drawn

tight, making 100% sure not only that there is no bowel trapped in the suture line but also that the abdominal wall is everted, so that the peritoneal lining is apposed to the opposite side.

6. A continuous layer of subcuticular sutures should be used to bring the skin together and thereby reduce wound tension.

7. The skin is then sutured with a line of interrupted horizontal mattress sutures, using monofilament nylon.

8. The foal must be given antibiotics, NSAIDs and tetanus antiserum.

9. The foal and its mother should be confined until the stitches are removed 10 days later.

10. It is quite reasonable for colt foals to be castrated at the same time as hernial surgery.

If the hernial ring is very large, the abdomen should not be opened. In this instance a piece of nylon surgical mesh is sutured with individual, absorbable sutures over the area of the hernia, pushing the hernial sac back into the abdomen. The wound is then closed in a similar manner. The mare and foal should both be confined for 1 month to allow the body wall to fibrose over the mesh.

References and Further Reading

Fouche, N., Remy-Wohlfender, F., Blau, D., Franzen, J., Gurter, C. *et al.* (2022) Characterization of an outbreak in Switzerland. *Schweizer Archiv für Tierheilkunde* 164: 733–739.

Haggett, E. (2021) Gastrointestinal disorders: Update on types, causes and treatments. *Vet Times* 6(3), 15 January: 6–9.

Merridale-Punter, M.S., Prutton, J.S.W., Stefanovski, D., Worsman, F.C.F., Payne, R.J. *et al.* (2023) Outcome following emergency laparotomy in 33 UK donkeys: A retrospective multicentre study. *Equine Veterinary Journal* 55: 222–229.

Prutton, J. (2023) Equine gastric disease and disorders. *Vet Times* 53(19), 15 May: 10–11.

Robinson, N.E. (1997) *Current Therapy in Equine Medicine*. W.B. Saunders, Philadelphia, Pennsylvania.

Rose, R.J. and Hodgson, D.R. (1999) *Manual of Equine Practice*. W.B. Saunders, Philadelphia, Pennsylvania.

Whitfield-Cargile, C.M., Coleman, M.C., Cohen, N.D., Chamoun-Emanuelli, A.M., Desolis, C.N. *et al.* (2021) Effects of phenyl butazone alone or in combination with a nutritional therapeutic on gastric ulcers, intestinal permeability, and faecal microbiota in horses. *Journal of Veterinary Internal Medicine* 35(2): 1121–1130.

Witt, P., Hagedoorn, S., Kranenburg, L.C. and van den Boom, R. (2021) The use of cola for the treatment of gastric impactions in equids. *Pferdheilkunde* 37(6): 588–596.

16

Neurological and Locomotory Conditions

Abstract

Neurological conditions are often linked to locomotory problems, so they are both included in this chapter. The problems appertaining to the eye are described in a separate chapter (Chapter 17), as are orthopaedic problems (Chapter 12).

16.1 Neurological Locations and Associated Signs

The brain

- Cases involving the brain will show abnormal behaviour, e.g. wandering and head-pressing.
- There may be apparent blindness.
- More advanced signs will include seizures, dementia and coma, which will lead to death.

More specific areas of the brain

- The cerebellum regulates the rate and range of motion, and correlates proprioceptive information. Signs will include the lack of both menace response and blink reflex to light. There may be head tremors, a base-wide stance and ataxia.
- The brainstem includes the cranial nerves. There may be ptosis and an altered eye position with damage to the third, fourth or sixth cranial nerves. There will be a loss of facial sensation with damage to the fifth cranial nerve. Damage to the seventh cranial nerve will show facial paralysis. There will be a head tilt and nystagmus with damage to the eighth cranial nerve. Damage to the ninth and tenth cranial nerves will be manifest as dysphagia. The brainstem includes long tracts to the spinal cord, and damage to these may be seen as weakness, ataxia and spastic limbs, all with concurrent cranial nerve deficits.

The spinal cord

- There will be a loss of coordination and weakness caudal to the lesion, and possibly sensory deficits. Focal sweating due to sympathetic fibre damage or tectosegmental spinal tract damage may also be evident.
- Tetanus is the classic upper motor neurone disease. The associated neurotoxins block

DOI: 10.1079/9781800624283.0016

inhibition of the spinal motor neurons, leading to an over-response from the lower motor neurons.

Peripheral nervous system

- There will be a regional loss of motor function.
- There will be muscle atrophy and profound weakness localized to specific areas.
- With equine motor neurone disease (see Section 16.15), there is profound and progressive diffuse muscle atrophy and weakness.
- The botulism toxin affects neuromuscular junctions, causing poor muscle tone (as evidenced by a flaccid anus), weakness, stumbling, dysphagia and eventual recumbency.

Assessment of cranial nerve function

The 12 cranial nerves and their respective functions are listed in Table 16.1.

16.2 Approach to the Equine Neurological Case

Is the horse ill and does it have neurological signs? Is there a neurological disorder? The following checklist is recommended:

- mental attitude (cerebrum);
- normal behaviour, e.g. nystagmus, eye position (cranial nerves III, VI);
- check menace tests (cranial nerves II, VII);
- pupillary light reflexes (cranial nerves II, III);
- swinging light test (cranial nerve II);

Table 16.1. The 12 cranial nerves and their respective functions.

Cranial nerve	Type	Major function	Reflex/response/assessment
I Olfactory	Sensory	Sense of smell	
II Optic	Sensory	Afferent pathway for vision and light	Menace response; pupillary light reflex; swinging light reflex
III Oculomotor	Motor	Pupillary constriction; extra-ocular muscles	Pupillary light reflex; medial movement of globe (ipsilateral response strongest)
IV Trochlear	Motor	Extra-ocular muscles (dorsal oblique)	Ventrolateral rotation of globe
V Trigeminal	Sensory	Sensory to side of head and face	Ear, eyelid and lip (facial) reflexes; pain perception (head, nasal septum)
	Motor	Motor to masticatory muscles	Chewing, jaw tone (temporalis, masseter, digastricus)
VI Abducens	Motor	Extra-ocular muscles (retractor oculi, lateral rectus)	Eyeball retraction (corneal reflex); lateral movement of globe
VII Facial	Motor	Motor to muscles of facial expression	Ear, eyelid and lip (facial) tone, reflexes and movement; facial symmetry
	Sensory	Taste	
VIII (i) Vestibular	Sensory	Afferent branch of vestibular system	Head posture; induced eyeball movement; normal vestibular nystagmus; normal gait; blindfold test
(ii) Cochlear	Sensory	Hearing	Response to noise
IX Glossopharyngeal	Motor/sensory	Sensory and motor to pharynx	Swallowing (palpation)
X Vagus	Sensory/motor	Sensory and motor to pharynx and larynx	Gag reflex (nasal tube)
XI Accessory	Motor	Trapezius muscle	Endoscopy
XII Hypoglossal	Motor	Motor to tongue	Tongue size and symmetry

- funduscopic examination;
- symmetry of the head;
- inspection of the tongue;
- nasal septum response; and
- gait at walk and trot, turning and faster gaits if not dangerous.

Is the neurological disorder primary or secondary? The following checklist is recommended:

- depression from systemic illness, e.g. endotoxaemia;
- Horner's syndrome with guttural pouch empyaema;
- patchy sweating from excitement or distress;
- abnormal limb placement due to dullness, lethargy, pyrexia from other systemic disease;
- unusual lameness, e.g. equine granulocytic ehrlichiosis;
- difficulty in rising, e.g. muscular weakness or arthritis; and
- collapse under excessive weight being carried.

Neurological examination protocol is as follows:

- perform a full clinical examination first before concentrating on the neurological signs; and
- initiate a chart to record findings and try to have a consistent order of examination.

One logical course of action is to start at the head and move caudally:

- head (brain and cranial nerves);
- neck;
- fore limbs;
- trunk;
- hind limbs;
- tail;
- anus; and
- gait and posture.

The aim of the examination is to localize the lesion(s):

- brain cortex;
- cerebellum;
- vestibulum;
- any other part of the brain stem;
- spinal cord;
- peripheral nerves;
- neuromuscular junction; and
- muscles.

Ancillary diagnostics can then be considered:

- blood tests for bacterial infections, potassium and calcium concentrations and liver disease;
- radiography for fracture lines in the head, which are often difficult to image; frontoparietal fractures are often visible externally; and
- cerebrospinal fluid (CSF) analysis, which may be unremarkable but will reveal EPM, EHV-1 (see Section 14.3) and bacterial meningitis in the foal.

Some common neurological conditions causing illness

- Liver disease (hepatoencephalopathy). This clinical syndrome occurs in severe hepatic insufficiency from a variety of causes. Toxins, e.g. ammonia, fatty acids and indoles, which would normally be detoxified by the liver increase in the peripheral blood and cross the blood–brain barrier. There is marked cranial depression. The signs seen will include head-pressing, head-hanging, yawning, ataxia, inappetence, sham drinking and even compulsive walking and aggression. Unfortunately, the prognosis at this stage is hopeless and euthanasia is advocated.
- Hyperlipaemia (see Section 15.7). This condition is restricted to donkeys, mules and small and miniature horses. The animal is usually overweight and is undergoing a period of negative energy balance. The classical triggers are pregnancy, lactation, illness, transport or some other stress. Death of a life-long companion has been reported as a trigger.
- Neonatal hypoxia.
- Cerebral trauma.
- Bacterial meningitis.
- Abscess in the CNS.
- Tetanus.
- Botulism.
- Equine grass sickness (see Section 15.9).
- Equine herpes virus 1.

Some less common neurological conditions causing illness

- Toxicity (bracken, lead, organophosphorus compounds; see Chapter 19).
- Electrolyte imbalance.
- Equine motor neurone disease (EMND).
- Equine protozoal myeloencephalitis (EPM).
- Rabies.

16.3 Liver Disease

See Section 15.7.

16.4 Hyperlipaemia

See Section 15.7.

16.5 Neonatal Hypoxia

The foal will stop sucking and will be weak and depressed; it may even start wandering and not bond with the mare. Some practitioners call these 'barker foals', as they can make a grunting noise on expiration similar to the noise made by a deer. The signs will progress: the legs will become rigid, the foal will appear blind and then will have convulsions. Respiration will be laboured although the rectal temperature is raised. The cause of this condition may not actually be a lack of oxygen at birth but the fact that, although the foal in theory has reached term, it is not yet ready for birth, i.e. it is premature. Euthanasia is the best course of action, as these foals will require 24/7 nursing for many days, and even then will not make useful working horses.

16.6 Cerebral Trauma

Diagnosis in this condition is not necessarily easy. Obviously, if a horse has been hit by a truck, there is no problem, but in other cases when the horse is violent and causing itself further damage the initial cause is not so clear. If the horse is violent the first cause of action is to sedate with an alpha-2 agonist.

16.7 Bacterial Meningitis

Any age of horse may be affected by this condition, but is very much more common in the foal following septicaemia. The foal will have a raised rectal temperature and will be slightly older than the neonatal hypoxic foal. Early treatment with antibiotics and NSAIDs is vital.

16.8 Abscess in the CNS

An abscess normally occurs as a sequel to either strangles or an ascending infection from cauda equina (see below). There will be a fever, the signs being associated with the location of the abscess. The prognosis may not be hopeless as long as there is prompt treatment with antibiotics should *Streptococcus equi* be involved.

16.9 Tetanus

Tetanus should be a disease of the past, as vaccination against the toxin-producing bacillus is readily available and inexpensive. Only two injections are required to give a minimum of 3 years' immunity with some vaccines, and the length of immunity may well be longer than that. Classically, the disease follows 10 days after a wound or castration; often, there is no visible wound and clinicians should be alert for the horse showing general stiffness, which within 24 h will turn in to classical tetanus. Spastic gait, erect ears and flared nostrils are the major signs. The horse will show the pathognomonic sign of protrusion of the third eyelid as a menace response, but 'lockjaw' 48 h later is not so often seen. The well-described 'sawhorse' stance may soon lead to recumbency, and in these circumstances euthanasia is suggested on welfare grounds. However, if the horse can be kept standing, treatment can be tried and may be successful; avoidance of any stimulation is important. Usually, the horse is able to drink small quantities of gruel. Constant use of a nasogastric tube may not be warranted, or indeed humane, and once again euthanasia may be indicated.

The horse should be given high doses of penicillin. Antitoxin in large doses is useful only very early in the course of the disease: regular injections every 6 h of acetylpromazine at 0.5 mg/kg are helpful. Clinicians should remember that if the horse has to be destroyed, extra care has to be taken. The horse will die in spasm and lunge forward; if shooting the horse, the clinician must stand to the side or risk being fallen upon. Obviously, i/v euthanasia is not so hazardous.

16.10 Botulism

A disease caused by the toxin produced by the bacillus *Clostridium botulinum*, botulism is only seen commonly in certain areas and is rare elsewhere. It may be associated with the feeding of contaminated silage; this type of botulism depends on preformed toxin. In rare cases the bacillus actually reproduces in a wound and produces the toxin in a similar manner to *Clostridium tetani*.

The disease has a slow onset, with the horse showing weakness and a tendency to lie down more frequently. There is trembling of the large muscle groups. Internally, there may be ileus so there will be colic signs. The classic sign of the flaccid rectum is not 100% reliable but is a useful diagnostic sign. Botulism is also seen in the foals, which will have difficulty sucking and show a reduced tongue reflex.

Treatment with botulinum antitoxin is vital as early as possible, otherwise treatment needs to be supportive; ileus needs to be treated. The outcome is quite good, provided large doses of the toxin have not been ingested. If silage is the cause, that batch must be destroyed.

16.11 Equine Grass Sickness

See Section 15.9.

16.12 Equine Herpes Virus 1

This is potentially a very confusing condition, as equine herpes virus 1 is normally associated with abortion. A vaccine is available, but the incidence of this myeloencephalopathy condition does not seem to bear any relationship to vaccination status, whether past, current or unvaccinated. It appears that there is a propensity of certain virus strains to attack the nervous system and cause paralysis, particularly of the hind limbs, in a sporadic manner, but in clusters on certain holdings. There may be urinary incontinence and decreased tail tone. Animals will recover in some instances, so nursing is vital. Some authorities suggest the use of dexamethasone given i/m twice daily at 0.1 mg/kg as being helpful; however, this does not seem to be a logical approach to a disease known to be caused by a virus. Diagnosis is by virus isolation from pharyngeal swabs. Isolation would be prudent.

16.13 Toxic Neurological Conditions

Bracken poisoning

Not normally eaten by the horse unless starved, this common plant causes chronic poisoning, shown as muscle weakness and other neurological signs. The specific antidote is vitamin B_1 (thiamine), which should be given i/m daily at 1 mg/10 kg.

Lead poisoning

Normally chronic in the horse, this heavy metal poisoning is usually from pasture contamination caused by mining. The main sign is stiffness, which may appear to have an acute onset following exercise, reminiscent of rhabdomyolysis (see Section 12.11). There will be raised lead levels in both blood and urine. The specific treatment is i/v calcium edentate, but this is rarely necessary in the horse if removed from the contaminated pasture and given NSAIDs.

Organophosphorus poisoning

Organophosphorus (OP) insecticides are very potent poisons, their acute toxicity being due to cholinergic overstimulation. This is shown as neurological signs: the horse is very nervous and constantly urinates; there is copious salivation and constricted pupils. Treatment is specific, with atropine sulfate at 0.2 mg/kg given slowly i/v; this may be repeated every 3 h, until signs subside.

16.14 Electrolyte Imbalance

For electrolyte imbalance to occur, the horse would normally be exhausted or have been deprived of water. There is a decrease in muscle tone and general weakness; evidence of profuse sweating and muscle fasciculation will be seen, along with a synchronous diaphragmatic flutter and ataxia. If symptoms are not too severe the horse may be given electrolytes dissolved in water by nasogastric tube; severe symptoms will warrant i/v fluids.

16.15 Equine Motor Neurone Disease (EMND)

A very rare degenerative condition of the somatic neurons, the cause is unknown. The affected horse will often show low vitamin E levels but, as it can occur at grass, such a causality is unlikely. The signs are very variable, which makes diagnosis difficult until the disease has really progressed. There is no ataxia, and the horse seems more comfortable when walking, but will also lie down more frequently. Muscle fasciculations lead to muscle atrophy; the head is held low but there is often a high tail carriage. Diagnosis is by a process of elimination. Muscle biopsy may be required to differentiate this condition from polysaccharide storage myopathy. Definitive diagnosis rests on histopathology of the cranial nerve nuclei corresponding to the degeneration of the relevant motor nerves. There is no treatment.

16.16 Equine Protozoal Myeloencephalitis (EPM)

A protozoal disease occurring throughout North and South America, it causes disease elsewhere only in exported horses from the Americas. The causal organism is *Sarcocystis neurona*; however, another protozoan, *Neospora hughesi*, has also been implicated, and its occurrence mirrors that of the main host, the Virginia opossum (*Didelphis virginiana*). It is a two-host parasite, the secondary hosts being the armadillo, the skunk and the raccoon, with the horse as the end host. It occurs in all breeds, but is rare in the pony and has not been recorded in the donkey. Mainly, it occurs in horses under the age of 5, but has been recorded in all age groups; there is no sex predilection. Diagnosis is normally on clinical grounds, although there are elaborate tests that can be performed on both blood and CSF. Blood contamination of the CSF creates false positives. The simplest test is the Western blot analysis, but this shows only exposure to the disease and therefore is not definitive.

The main initial signs are fever, inappetence and diarrhoea, which are quickly followed by neurological signs like ataxia and head-pressing. Longer-term signs are muscle wasting, occurring in muscles at random and resulting in marked asymmetry. The most common muscles affected are one of the masseters, the supraspinatus and infraspinatus on one side and one gluteal. There are two oral medicines used for treatment, both requiring to be given over a 28-day period and both 70% effective: (i) ponazuril, at 5 mg/kg daily; and (ii) nitazoxanide, initially at 25 mg/kg for 5 days followed by 50 mg/kg for 23 days. Supportive therapy with NSAIDs and vitamin E injections has also been used. Pyrimethamine at 0.1–0.2 mg/kg, together with 15 mg/kg of potentiated sulfonamide, both by mouth, was previously used; its effectiveness is less than 50%. There are no licensed vaccines available, but there may well be one soon.

16.17 Rabies

The horse is the end host for this disease and, although the presence of virus cannot be ruled out from a horse's saliva, it is very unlikely that a rabid horse will infect another horse or indeed any other type of animal. It is just conceivable that a human could be infected if cut, through performing dentistry on a rabid horse. The horse is likely to become infected from the bite of a rabid dog or wild carnivore. Signs will depend on the site in the brain that first becomes infected; if the forebrain is affected the horse will show aggressive neurological signs, but lesions in the brainstem will produce stupor and excessive salivation – this is the most common form. Last if the spinal column is affected there is progressive ascending paralysis. Death normally occurs within 5 days.

Definitive diagnosis can be made by sending fresh brain tissue to a laboratory able to accept potential rabies-infected material or by sending formalin-fixed brain tissue to other laboratories. There is no treatment, but a reliable vaccine is available that can be given from 6 months of age.

16.18 Cauda Equina Syndrome

Caused by inflammation or neuritis of the cauda equina, which in horses starts at the lumbosacral junction and includes the caudal end of the spinal cord, the sacral and coccygeal nerves, this condition is normally seen as a result of either trauma in the area or EHV-1 infection. There is a deficit of both motor and sensory function around the tail and the anus; in very serious cases there is ataxia and lack of bladder control. Horses may show signs of colic, as there will be pain from the build-up of faeces in the rectum. There is no treatment, and euthanasia is indicated in the most serious cases.

16.19 Headshaking

Horses have numerous reasons why they might shake their heads, either at rest or during exercise, but in some this behaviour becomes persistent and frequent, such that it prevents the horse from being used for its intended purpose. The horse may be wearing tack or head covering or may be just running loose. When no explanation for the headshaking can be identified, as is true of virtually all cases, it is assumed to be due to hypersensitivity of the trigeminal nerve and is described as trigeminal-mediated headshaking (TMH). Clinical signs range from virtually imperceptible to violent and incessant head movement and although they are typically associated with exercise, they can occur at rest and may be associated with self-trauma, such that the animal's welfare is compromised. Treatment maybe attempted, but medical and surgical interventions used to date have all had variable and generally disappointing results; euthanasia is an all-too-common result. Headshaking has been recognized for over a hundred years.

Signalment

- Young adults.
- More frequent in geldings.
- More common in spring and summer.
- Associated with bright sunlight.
- Associated with wind and rain.
- Triggered by flying insects.
- Triggered by loud noises.
- Triggered by contact with the nose.
- Violent head movement mainly in vertical plane.

Management options

- Environment management.
- Nose nets.
- Face masks.
- Contact lenses.
- Modified tack.

Pharmaceuticals

- Carbamazepine.
- Cyproheptadine.
- Antihistamines.
- Melatonin.
- Gabapentin.
- Glucocorticoids.
- Sodium cromoglycate eye drops.

Most surgical interventions cannot be recommended on account of their unreliability and, more importantly, because of the welfare implications.

Further Reading

Lavoie, J.-P. and Hinchcliff, K.W. (2009) *Blackwell's Five-Minute Veterinary Consult: Equine*, 2nd edn. Wiley Blackwell, Oxford, UK.

Rendle, D. (2017) Update on headshaking in equine patients. *Vet Times Clinical Equidae*, 20 November: 28–32.

17

Eye Conditions

Abstract

This chapter is devoted to the eye and surrounding tissues. The eye is given a separate chapter from the rest of the neurological system on account of its importance.

17.1 Trauma to Structures Surrounding the Eye

Trauma is probably the most common problem seen by the practitioner concerning the equine eye. The eye is very prominent and horses suffering any irritation tend to rub the area around the eye quite violently. Careful examination, normally under sedation, is vital; hopefully, the orbit itself will not be affected. The clinician should make a visual examination followed by careful palpation. This will provide almost as much information as sophisticated diagnostic techniques, e.g. radiography, ultrasound (the modality of choice), CT or MRI. Some very bad head wounds will require a general anaesthetic and repair, but these are rare. Fractures to the orbital rim or zygomatic arch may well be left to heal on their own. Skin lacerations must be repaired as soon as possible under a regional block or local infiltration: the clinician will be pleased at the fast rate of healing. Antibiotics should be given parenterally to prevent infection, and NSAIDs given cautiously to control the swelling.

When suturing the eyelids it is important to use small, single interrupted stitches using a soft suture material, to avoid irritation. If the third eyelid is torn, suturing can be attempted, but careful trimming will usually be better; rarely will the third eyelid be prolapsed, and in these cases an assistant should be shown how to keep the third eyelid in position while the clinician sutures the eyelids together. These sutures need be left *in situ* for only 48 h; the third eyelid will remain in position after this length of time. In the extremely rare event of prolapse of the orbit, the clinician will have to be mindful of welfare considerations; unless the injury is extremely fresh, replacing the orbit and suturing the eyelids is neither a humane nor viable option – the eye should be removed under general anaesthetic.

17.2 Nerve Blocks Related to the Eye

Auriculopalpebral nerve block

The palpebral branch of the auriculopalpebral branch of the facial nerve can be palpated as it transverses the zygomatic arch after emerging through the stylomastoid foramen, underneath

DOI: 10.1079/9781800624283.0017

the parotid salivary gland. The nerve innervates the powerful orbicularis oculi that closes the eye. Deposition of 1 to 2 ml of lignocaine at this site will paralyse the upper eyelid. The nerve can be blocked at other sites and the auricular branch to the pinna will be included if it is blocked more proximally.

Supraorbital nerve block

A supraorbital nerve block enables complete desensitization and akinesis of the eyelids, as well as blockade of the lacrimal nerve on the lateral aspect of the lower eyelid (ophthalmic branch of the CN V), blockade of the zygomatic nerve on the ventral aspect of the lower eyelid (maxillary branch of the CN V) and blockade of the infratrochlear nerve (maxillary branch of the CN V), which innervates the skin around the medial canthus.

Technique

The supraorbital branch of the ophthalmic branch of the CN V emerges from the supraorbital foramen that is palpable on the dorsal aspect of the orbit. Injection of 2 ml of local anaesthetic using a 23 to 25 G × 18 mm needle subcutaneously will desensitize the upper eyelid and conjunctiva.

Retrobulbar nerve blocks

Complete retrobulbar blockade results in exophthalmos, mydriasis, globe paralysis and corneal desensitization.

Technique

There are many ways to desensitize structures deep in the orbit. The author favours a lateral and medial approach involving introducing a 22G × 90 mm spinal needle subconjunctivally at the medial and lateral canthui. The needle is advanced following the contours of the orbit while flexing in a curve to enable injection of local anaesthetic deep in the orbit and close to the optic nerve cone.

Corneal desensitization

This is best achieved using ophthalmic amethocaine or tetracaine drops (Ophthaine, Minims) that are pharmacologically sparing to the cornea and have a rapid onset of action.

17.3 Removal of the Eye

This procedure can be performed in the standing horse, and with modern sedation is the method of choice. After the horse has been sedated and received pain relief, preferably in stocks, regional nerve blocks should be placed as described above. The area is prepared for surgery and the eyelids are then sutured together, and the area prepared a second time; the idea behind this is that contamination from bacteria and possible tumour cells is then contained within the orbit and will not contaminate the wound. The incision is then made very carefully through the eyelid, but not through the underlying tissue, so that the eye and the conjunctiva will be removed intact. As much of the eyelid tissue as possible is retained to allow for closure later. After the skin incision, blunt dissection is used to separate the conjunctiva from the overlying tissue; the muscles have to be cut with curved scissors. Eventually, the optic nerve is cut with curved scissors and the eye is removed intact within the conjunctiva.

The incisions made in the eyelids are then sutured together with small, simple interrupted sutures after the dead space has been filled with a sterile bandage. The end of the bandage is allowed to protrude through the suture line medially. The bandage can be removed slowly on a daily basis, or in larger quantities every 5 days until the sutures are removed after 15 days. Antibiotics and NSAIDs are given at the time of the surgery and are continued for a minimum of 10 days. Fly control is essential.

17.4 Orbital Tumours

Squamous cell carcinoma

The most common tumour affecting the eye, particularly in the tropics, it is thought to occur as a result of strong sunlight, as it is nearly always found in the conjunctiva of non-pigmented eyes. Usually, it starts in the third eyelid, where the vigilant owner will notice it before invasion of the conjunctiva. Immediate removal is required, and it is a simple procedure. The animal is sedated and local anaesthetic instilled into the eye and conjunctiva; after 5 min the third eyelid can be grasped with a pair of tissue forceps. The tumour with a good margin is then dissected free from the third eyelid with a pair of scissors; hopefully, the cartilage of the third eyelid can be left intact. Antibiotics should be instilled into the eye, and this continued for 5 days; NSAIDs should be given by mouth. Fly control is essential. If the tumour has spread to the conjunctiva, the whole eye will need to be removed.

Equine sarcoid

Strictly speaking this is not a tumour, but it behaves in a similar manner. It can occur anywhere on the body, but around the eye is a common site. Treatment at other sites is discussed in Section 20.13. There is specific treatment for the sarcoid near to the eye: it should be injected on three occasions at 3-weekly intervals with BCG vaccine (a human vaccine for tuberculosis that can be obtained from hospitals and dispensaries). It is important to use a fine 25G needle and inject the vaccine throughout the lesion, right up to the perimeter. NSAIDs may need to be given per os if the swelling is severe. Fly control is required. The success rate is variable, but normally >90%.

Melanoma

The predilection site for melanoma is at the junction between skin and mucous membrane in the grey horse, and this includes the eye. Normally seen as round nodules of about 2 mm on the rim of the eyelid, they rarely grow larger. However, as the animal ages more may appear. They are best left alone unless they enlarge quickly or begin to rub on the cornea, but can be removed surgically, taking only a small margin.

17.5 Foreign Bodies

An uncommon finding, but it is important that the clinician looks carefully at the eye (see Fig. 17.1). The surface of the eye should be searched, as well as the sclera and the conjunctiva. Local anaesthetic is instilled into the conjunctiva so that the third eyelid can be lifted for a search beneath. If found, they should be carefully removed. Antibiotics are instilled locally and NSAIDs given orally – the drug of choice is flunixin.

17.6 Conjunctivitis

This is rarely seen in just one eye: if only one eye is affected a foreign body or corneal ulcer should be suspected. Conjunctivitis may be a sign of systemic disease, so a full clinical examination should be performed. In the foal, conjunctivitis is often seen early in pneumonia; it is also seen in neonatal maladjustment syndrome. In the yearling, conjunctivitis may be a sign in mycoplasma infections; in the older animal, it is likely to be associated with upper respiratory viruses.

Parasites are an important cause of conjunctivitis: *Habronema muscae* and *Habronema majus* are stomach worms normally found in small granulomata in the stomach wall; their eggs and larvae are shed in the faeces and ingested by flies, which act as the intermediate host, then the horse ingests the flies. The granulomatous stage can occur in the conjunctiva and even on the eye. Ivermectin treatment by mouth is effective, although the small granulomata may remain for some months. *Onchocerca cervicalis* is a common microfilarial worm also seen in the horse, and its role in ocular disease is controversial. It may certainly be seen in large numbers in cases of conjunctivitis, but it can also be seen in the normal eye. Oral treatment with ivermectin is effective, although initially following treatment the conjunctivitis appears to get worse as the worms die. Resolution is eventually complete. *Thelazia lacrymalis* is a specific worm in the equine eye, the adult being easily seen in the eye. Its pathogenesis is in doubt, but it is unlikely that its presence is entirely benign. It is spread by flies and controlled by oral ivermectin.

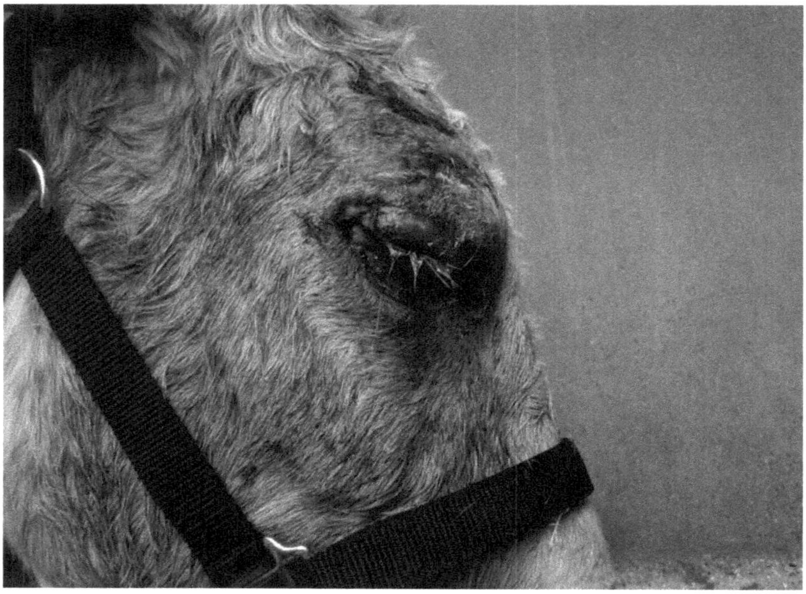

Fig. 17.1. Self-trauma following foreign body in the eye.

There are no specific bacteria associated with conjunctivitis in the horse, but if horses are kept in close contact with cattle, they may well develop bovine keratoconjunctivitis (commonly called 'pinkeye'). The aetiology of this condition is contentious: the causative agent is thought to be *Moraxella bovis* linked with a virus or a mycoplasma. Certainly, no specific pathogen has been isolated to date in the horse, but the clinical condition does exist.

Another equine condition is keratoconjunctivitis sicca (commonly called 'dry eye'); diagnosis can be confirmed via the Schirmer tear test, as described in Section 2.9. Treatment with a mixture of artificial tears and cyclosporin A, although expensive, is usually effective.

17.7 Dacryocystitis

Blockage of the nasolacrimal duct is common in the horse and is usually caused by inflammation and infection. In this instance it will respond to local instillation of antibiotics and corticosteroids. Fluorescin dye is instilled into the eye to test patency, at least 45 min being allowed for the dye to reach the nostril. If the duct does not appear to be patent, it may be cleared from the rostral opening in the nostril. A thin catheter, 16-gauge, 40–60 cm, is slowly inserted with a small amount of K-Y Jelly; when it reaches the blockage, local anaesthetic solution is syringed down the catheter under pressure and, on clearing the duct, it will be seen welling up in the eye. The blockage may have a physical cause, e.g. an injury from a kick to the face or a headcollar that has been put on a foal too long so that it has become too tight. An apical maxillary tooth root abscess might also cause a blockage, but this will show as a unilateral swelling. A young foal may show dacryocystitis through a congenital deformity, but other physical facial deformities will also be seen.

17.8 Corneal Ulceration

A very common condition seen in the equine eye, it can be both sight-threatening and cause considerable pain, so early diagnosis and treatment is vital. The clinician seeing a swollen eye should always eliminate the presence of an ulcer. It is reasonable to treat with antibiotics locally and NSAIDs orally for 24 h to see whether the condition will settle down and allow examination of the cornea. However, it should not be left any longer than this without sedation and instillation of local anaesthetic and fluorescein dye; an ulcer will take up the dye and become visible.

Ulcers can be classified as: (i) micro-erosions, when only a few epithelial cell layers have been removed (these will still take up fluorescein); (ii) superficial, when the whole epithelium has been removed; (iii) deep, when some of the stroma has been removed; (iv) descemetocele, when the entire stroma has been removed; and (v) rupture of the cornea with prolapse of the iris. The cornea will heal provided there is no infection or further trauma; the clinician must give the cornea protection. The cornea is nearly 1.5 mm thick in the centre, but less than half that at the perimeter. The rate of healing will depend on the thickness of the ulcer; micro-erosions will heal in <7 days, superficial ulcers will take 14 days or more, while deep ulcers will not be fully healed for 56 days. The latter type will show pronounced fibrovascular healing but, provided infection is prevented, healing will proceed leaving only a thin scar, visible with difficulty by the clinician and not impairing the vision of the horse.

Corticosteroids must never be put into an eye with a corneal ulcer – if applied the ulcer will not heal (Fig. 17.2). If a fungal infection occurs, again the ulcer will not heal; early fungal ulcers do not stain with fluorescein and require staining with Rose Bengal stain for visualization. To detect bacteria or fungi, the cornea has to be scraped with the handle of a sterile scalpel to yield any organisms. In both these conditions the ulcer may in fact start to melt, with disastrous consequences. If a melting ulcer is suspected, local treatment with the horse's own plasma (using EDTA as an anticoagulant) should be started as often as 6 times per day.

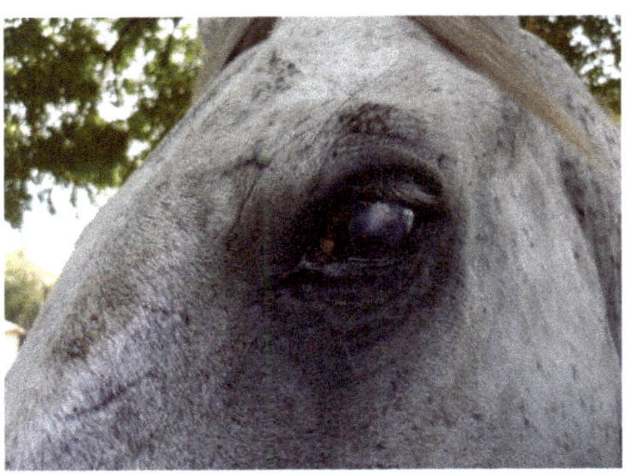

Fig. 17.2. The resultant long-term healing of a cornea with blood vessels and scarring.

Deep penetration of the stroma to Descemet's membrane with perforation of the cornea is a possible sequela to all corneal ulcers. To prevent this disaster, non-healing ulcers should be treated aggressively. If superficial, the ulcer can be scraped superficially to stimulate healing, using local anaesthetic; if this does not improve the situation, the cornea should be protected by a conjunctival flap, which is preferable to the more old-fashioned treatment of stitching the eyelids together. If the clinician is not happy to carry out the delicate surgery of a conjunctival flap, a third-eyelid flap may be used.

Medical therapy is difficult in the fractious horse or when the eye is very painful, and therefore in such cases a subpalpebral lavage system can be installed.

The antibiotics of choice initially are chloramphenicol and gentamicin. If an infection of *Pseudomonas* is suspected, amikacin and polymyxin B are indicated. In the event of a fungal infection, natamycin, miconazole or silver sulfadiazine can be used topically. In all cases, systemic NSAIDs should be given.

17.9 Iris Prolapse

Iris prolapse normally follows a sharp perforating injury to the cornea, but can also follow a melting ulcer. Aqueous humour will be lost, resulting in collapse of the anterior chamber. Unless the iris is removed and the cornea sutured, there is no possibility that the eye can be saved, and so the clinician has nothing to lose in attempting iridectomy.

17.10 Eosinophilic Keratoconjunctivitis

This is an inflammatory condition caused in all ages of horse by immune-mediated disease, in which the affected eye appears to granulate over.

Diagnosis is made by direct smears stained with Giemsa to demonstrate large numbers of eosinophils. Aggressive local treatment with antibiotics and corticosteroids must be started immediately, and this regime will need to be continued for some weeks. The horse should be given ivermectin worm treatment in case parasites are involved.

17.11 Cataract

A cataract is an opacity of the lens causing varying degrees of visual loss, the most common being the congenital cataract, which may become worse with age. Small cataracts do not cause a problem in the horse, in a similar way that small pieces of dirt on glasses do not obstruct the wearer but are very obvious to the onlooker. However, the dangerous cataracts are flocculent; the opacities in these lenses shift with movement of the head and eyes. A horse may spook at a real or imagined fear, which will cause the flocculent opacities to move and make the horse move more violently. Cataracts will prevent examination of the retina, therefore making assessment of the degree of blindness extremely difficult. A cataract should not be confused with nuclear sclerosis, which is common in the older horse and does not cause any loss of vision. Unless the lens is dislocated and is resting on the caudal border of the cornea, cataracts do not cause pain. There are sophisticated surgical techniques available to remove them, but these are outside the scope of this book.

17.12 Recurrent Uveitis

Formerly known as periodic ophthalmia, this was first recorded in the UK at the end of the First World War, in horses returning from continental Europe. It is thought to be connected with *Leptospira interrogans*. Many other bacteria, viruses, protozoa and parasites have been implicated, but no real evidence for any of these has been shown. The disease is recurrent, as the name suggests, and is manifest as an anterior uveitis; in only 20% of horses are both eyes affected.

The first signs are increased lacrimation, blepharospasm (Fig. 17.3) and photophobia; often, self-inflicted ulcers are present and treatment of those should not be neglected. NSAIDs are important, both parenterally and locally, in

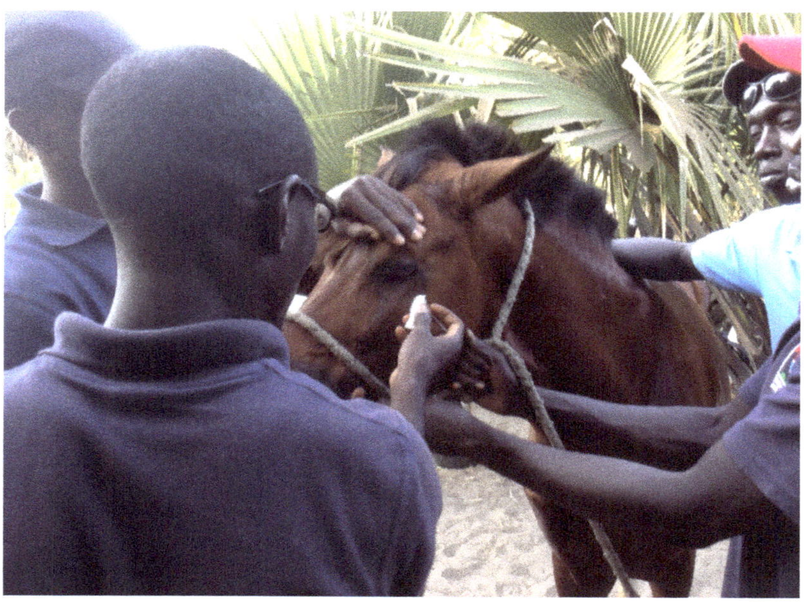

Fig. 17.3. Blepharospasm.

the treatment of uveitis. The horse should be kept in the dark or covered by a mesh fly screen – these are available with an extra covering for either the right or left eye and are suitable for the majority of cases when only one eye is affected. Some authorities recommend the use of corticosteroids, but these are risky if given locally on account of the possibility of ulcers, and problematic too if given parenterally on account of the danger of triggering laminitis.

Topical atropine is useful to dilate the pupil, and should be used intermittently as this will help drainage of the anterior chamber; it may cause impacted colic, so the horse should be monitored carefully. Cyclosporin A has been shown to be effective through suppression of the immune response. Topical antibiotics are useful; however, as treatment may be very prolonged these should be used with care as fungal overgrowth must be avoided. A very useful review article was published (Fischer *et al.*, 2023) recently suggesting equine recurrent uveitis (ERU) is the leading cause of blindness worldwide. The authors discuss treatment options, comparing non-recurrence rates, visual outcomes and associated complication rates.

17.13 Retinal Disease

The choroid and the retina become inflamed as a result of equine herpes viral infections, the lesions appearing as holes in the retina. There is no effective treatment, as topical treatments do not reach the retina. The loss of vision is related to percentage area loss in the retina.

There are various inherited conditions affecting the retina, showing initially as night blindness but sometimes progressing to total blindness.

Trauma or long-standing recurrent uveitis may result in retinal detachment. Laser surgery may be attempted but is outside the scope of this book.

Certain diseases causing an inflammatory episode, e.g. septicaemia, may result in optic nerve atrophy; the optic disc becomes pale.

Reference and Further Reading

Brooks, D.E. (2002) *Ophthalmology for the Equine Practitioner*. Teton NewMedia, Jackson, Wyoming.

Fischer, B.M., Brehm, W., Reese, S. and McMullen, R.J., Jr. (2023) Equine recurrent uveitis: A review. *Equine Veterinary Education* 35: 254–264.

Tremaine, H. (2019) Local analgesia techniques for dental and head procedures in horses. *In Practice* 41: 165–176.

18

Urinogenital Conditions

Abstract
This long chapter covers the urinogenital system in its entirety. It starts with the urinary system and then focuses on the male and female genital organs. Castration is given due importance as it is the most common surgical procedure carried out by the equine general practitioner.

18.1 The Kidney

Primary conditions

Primary kidney problems are extremely rare in the adult horse and are normally caused by an ascending infection resulting from cystitis. Both kidneys will be affected. The normal isolates are *Corynebacterium* spp. The main signs are general malaise and pyrexia; diagnosis is aided by rectal ultrasound or manual palpation. The kidneys are usually found to be painful. Urea and creatinine levels will be raised; culture of the urine is not helpful as the infection may come from lower down the urinary tract. Haematogenous infection of one kidney is possible but extremely difficult to diagnose, except on post-mortem. The recommended treatment would be a long course of potentiated sulfonamides.

The condition of idiopathic renal haematuria is extremely rare. It is more common in Arabs. Physical examination findings are unremarkable aside from pale mucous membranes. Blood clots will be seen in the bladder. Ultrasound of the kidneys may show pyelectasia and a decreased cortico-medullary ratio. There is no known treatment and euthanasia is recommended.

Secondary conditions

Also rare, these can occur with endotoxic shock or rhabdomyolysis (see Section 12.11). Heavy metal poisoning (see Chapter 19) will cause renal failure, as will overdosage of either gentamicin or phenylbutazone. Renal failure will be seen in the terminal stages of some infectious diseases, e.g. equine infectious anaemia (see Section 14.10), equine herpes virus (see Section 14.3) and bacterial septicaemia. Treatment is unlikely to be successful and is probably inhumane.

18.2 The Bladder

Primary conditions

Problems of the bladder are more common than those of the kidney; they may be related to

DOI: 10.1079/9781800624283.0018

parturition in the mare or caused by urinary stasis in the gelding through bladder stones. There will be bacteria in the urine, and also probably blood, with possible continuous dribbling of urine or total anuria in the gelding, accompanied by pain and straining; the bladder will be large when felt per rectum. A calculus may be felt in the penis, and this may either be passed following heavy sedation or removed with crocodile forceps. If the calculus is lodged at the ischial arch, it may be felt just below the rectum; a catheter can be passed until the calculus is reached. If the calculus cannot be removed, the animal should be humanely destroyed as there are welfare considerations with any type of urethrotomy. Naturally, cystitis should be treated with potentiated sulfonamides, provided there is some flow of urine. Bladder inversion may occur following foaling, but provided it is not torn it can be replaced under epidural, with a guarded prognosis. The mare should not be bred from again.

Secondary conditions

Resulting from either bladder paralysis following cauda equina syndrome (see Section 16.18) or spinal injuries, there is rarely any treatment, but supportive therapy can be attempted hoping that time will deliver some improvement.

Conditions of the foal

The most common bladder problem in the foal is rupture, which has a much higher incidence in the colt foal. The condition is thought to occur during parturition, but the signs are not normally seen until 24 h after birth, when the foal will appear weak and will stop sucking. A peritoneal tap will reveal urine in the peritoneum. Surgical repair is the only feasible treatment.

18.3 Polyuria (PU) and Polydipsia (PD)

Both of these signs can be indicators of significant disease: therefore, prompt investigation is required. Owners normally bring the problems to the practitioner on account of the extra work generated by the increased urine in the stable. The condition is rarely noticed at pasture and yet obviously it can be present. There is a wide range of the amount of water drunk by horses. The normal cut-out point is 100 ml/kg/day. Normal intake is between 25 ml/kg/day to 70 ml/kg/day. Healthy horses produce 15 ml/kg/day of urine up to 30 ml/kg/day. PU can be defined as production of more than 50 ml/kg/day.

Numerous physiologic methods of water loss exist, such as faeces (major route), via the respiratory tract and in sweat. Weather conditions, as well as altitude, need to be considered. Naturally, not only the amount but also the severity of the exercise is relevant. Horses exercising in a warm environment or encountering substantial water losses because of large bowel disease may consume water in excess of 100 l/day without a corresponding urine volume (Carlson, 1987). Increased frequency of urination can be mistaken for increased volume of urination and this ought to be considered when water intake is normal. If PD is present, it may be due to increase in thirst or due to PU. It is a chicken-and-egg situation. An understanding of normal water homeostasis facilitates a systemic approach to both PU and PD. Normal water homeostasis requires adequate pituitary release of antidiuretic hormone (ADH).

ADH is produced by the hypothalamus and stored within the pituitary. It is released primarily in response to increased plasma osmopolarity, which is detected by hypothalamic osmoreceptors. ADH acts on the distal renal tubule and collecting ducts to promote the absorption of water into the renal medullary interstitium, with the subsequent production of more concentrated urine.

Renin is released from the renal juxtaglomerular cells in response to a decreased circulating volume. This leads to angiotensin 11 production and is partially responsible for stimulation of thirst.

PU/PD can occur as the result of diseases that either increase water consumption directly or where diuresis is the driving factor. Increase in thirst is due to physiologic requirement, for example, following exercise, during hot weather or while lactating. Increased intake may also be seen following fluid loss due to haemorrhage or diarrhoea.

Horses are termed 'box wetters' when they choose to drink an excessive amount, without an increased water requirement. This is poorly understood. Owners normally accept that horses are box wetters as this is a diagnosis of a disease condition in their minds but of course, in reality, it is just a name.

Renal disease may lead to a reduction in the ability of the kidney to concentrate urine so that there is water loss and an increased requirement for water, and so can pituitary *pars intermedia* disfunction. Diabetes mellitus is extremely rare in equines and so glycosuria is likely to indicate neoplasia and is a sign of a very poor prognosis. Diabetes insipidus is also extremely rare and is normally idiopathic. Of course, it can be iatrogenic following drug use.

Owners may push for a full investigation. They need to be warned that this is likely to be expensive and not lead to a diagnosis.

18.4 Descent of the Testes

The testicles normally descend at birth, but a stallion is still said to be normal if descent has occurred before 6 months of age. After that, descent can still occur, but the animal is considered to be a rig, with the testicles in these cases being of different sizes. Castration can be carried out in the normal manner, as described in Section 18.5. If descent has not occurred before 6 months of age, the stallion should not be bred from as the characteristic of cryptorchidism is inherited. Cryptorchid males tend to be more masculine than ordinary stallions, the reason being that the abdominal testicle, although smaller and infertile, secretes more testosterone than a normal scrotal testicle.

All cryptorchids should be castrated, and it is very important that the practitioner does not just remove the single testicle, as that will cause subsequent confusion. The gelding will often display stallion-like behaviour, even showing an erection and mounting and penetrating mares; however, in this case the owner and the practitioner may have doubts regarding the previous history of castration. If there are doubts and no testicles can be felt, blood can be taken for hormonal analysis: if the horse is >3 years of age, oestrone sulfate levels can be measured in a clotted blood sample with 100% accuracy. In the horse <3 years of age and in all donkeys, two samples are required for assessment of testosterone levels. Following the first blood sampling, the animal is injected with 6000 IU human chorionic gonadotrophin (hCG) i/v; the second sampling is then performed 30–120 min later. The testosterone level from the first sample in a cryptorchid may be confusing, as this may be similar to that for a gelding, i.e. 0.3 nmol/l; however, the second sample in the gelding will show similar values to the first, but in the cryptorchid will be markedly higher, i.e. 1–12 nmol/l.

18.5 Normal Castration

Introduction

There are three general surgical options: (i) closed technique, where the testicle within its tunics is drawn down and removed only after the whole cord within the tunics has been ligatured, followed by suturing of the skin; (ii) semi-closed technique, which is similar but the skin is not sutured; and (iii) open technique, which is the most commonly carried out, where the tunics are incised and the testicle is drawn down so that the cord and blood vessels can be either crushed with an emasculator or ligatured, with the skin left open as in the semi-closed technique. Whether a general anaesthetic or local anaesthetic is used depends on the preference of the clinician.

The age at which a horse is castrated is very much dictated by fashion. There is no real reason why castration is not carried out in the foal, it being a myth that it will not grow into a strong, well-formed horse; it will certainly recover much more quickly than the older horse, although the technique is harder as it is more difficult for the clinician to grasp the testicles within the scrotum. There is little to find in the literature, except workers in France (Cognie *et al.*, 2023) confirmed in 22 Welsh ponies that early castration at 3 days did not interfere with morphological or behavioural development.

Because surgical castration is one of the most frequently performed surgery in equines it is thought to be a high cause of post-surgical complications. This is not the author's view having performed over four thousand castrations in ambulatory practice initially in Kenya, but also in Australia and the UK (Tables 18.1 and 18.2).

The place of castration

The author considers the easiest and safest place to carry out a castration with a short acting GA is in a large dry paddock. The vast majority (3909) of the cases described were castrated in paddocks. Only 67 were castrated in a knock-down box at the owner's request. Sadly, through force of circumstances 24 animals were castrated in totally unsuitable conditions (Fig. 18.1).

Weather conditions

As with any routine surgical procedure to be performed outside, I think it is best to reschedule if weather conditions are not favourable (Fig. 18.2). Postoperative haemorrhage was reported in seven cases by the owners. Six were found not to be serious.

Table 18.1. The types of equids castrated by the author.

Type	Number
Heavy horse	342
Thoroughbred racehorse	10
Standardbred (all in Western Australia)	15
Riding horse	1328
Riding pony	1808
Shetland pony	267
Mule	2
Donkey	228

Table 18.2. Ages of animals.

Age	Number
Foals	714
Yearlings	2200
Adults	1086

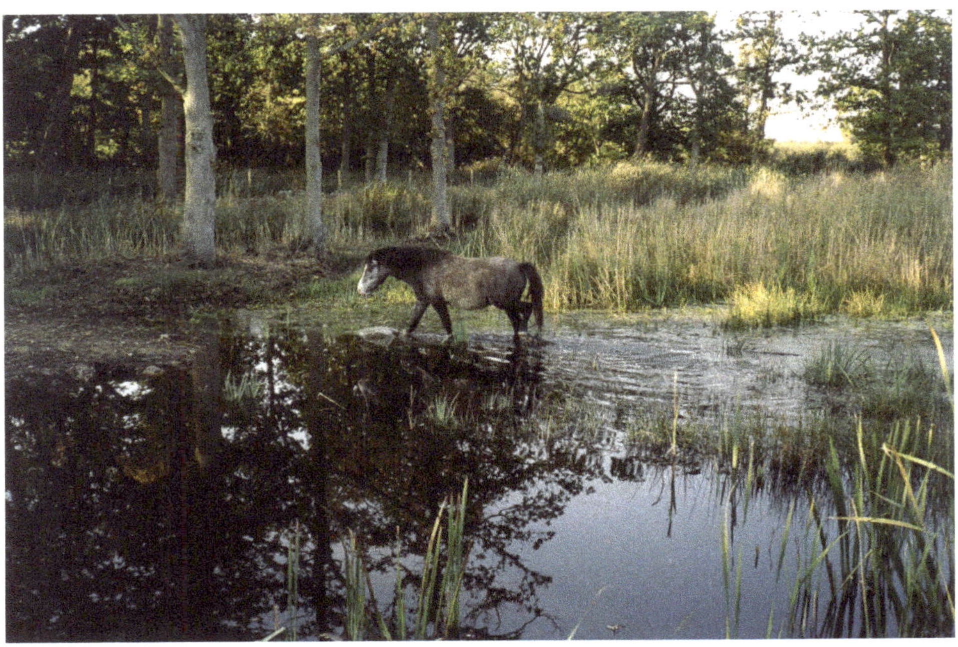

Fig. 18.1. A totally unsuitable place for a castration on the Norfolk Broads.

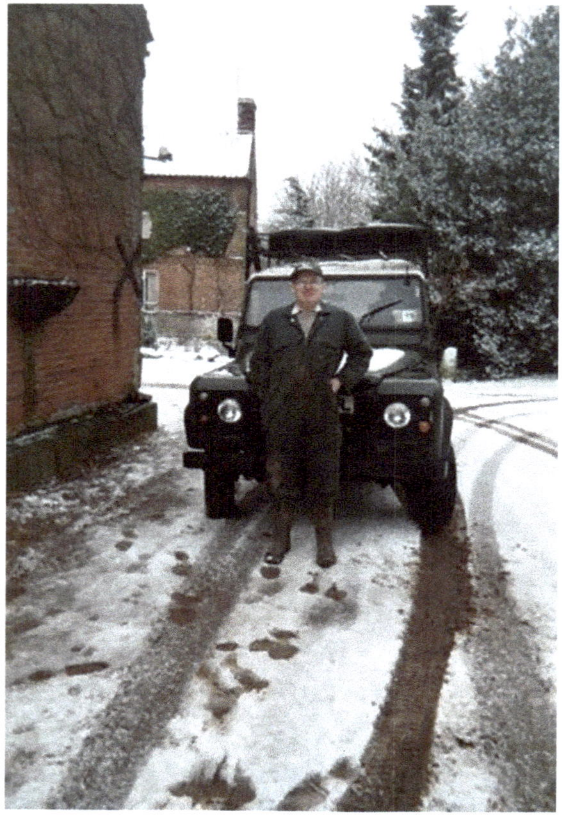

Fig. 18.2. Not ideal weather conditions for a castration.

Anaesthesia

All the castrations were carried out under a short-acting anaesthetic. The author was sure that if he had been working in a racehorse practice, he would have been forced to carry out the surgery in the standing animal because of the unproven myth that a GA adversely affects a horse's racing potential. The development of short-acting anaesthesia was relatively rapid through the early years of the author's career. The first 22 castrations in Kenya were carried out after premedication with acetylpromazine (ACP) with a bolus of thiopentone. The recoveries were often far from ideal. However, the use of courageous dedicated staff averted any catastrophes. The author was lucky that he did not see any penile prolapse in these patients, as was reported by other clinicians from the use of ACP. He did encounter a goose-egg-size swelling over one jugular because of some injection of the highly irritant thiopentone perivascularly. This resolved without treatment after three months without surgical intervention.

When the author arrived in Norfolk in 1974, the anaesthetic agent in vogue was Large Animal Immobilon. This is a mixture of an extremely powerful morphine derivative, M99 and ACP. The author used it in 72 patients. He was fortunate that only one of his patients suffered from penile prolapse, which mercifully resolved after prompt supportive treatment using a pair of tights. The main problems with LA Immobilon were on recovery. The standard protocol was to inject an appropriate dose of LA Revivon on completion of the surgery intravenously. The author experienced one case of recycling in a pony. From then on, he injected an extra half of the calculated dose of LA Revivon intramuscularly. He also experienced nine cases of recycling in donkeys and so from then on he injected an extra full dose of LA Revivon in this species.

The author was very relieved by the arrival of a protocol of intravenous premedication with romifidine, followed by intravenous ketamine. This was the author's preferred short-acting GA in 3891 castrations.

While doing three locum placements in Western Australia the author castrated 15 Standardbred yearlings. This breed is renowned for inguinal prolapse. The veterinary defence society in Australia will not cover practitioners who carry out an open method of castration. The protocol for anaesthesia was premedication with ACP and detomidine followed by a mixture of glyceryl guaiacolate (GG) and thiopentone given by flutter valve to effect.

There were no anaesthetic deaths.

Castration protocol

A total of 3905 animals were castrated using a standard open technique. The vascular and the non-vascular portions were emasculated. The instrument was held in position for one minute on the vascular part. As stated earlier, 15 animals were castrated in Australia with a semi-closed method. Each testicle enclosed in its tunics was ligatured with a transfixing ligature before being removed with the emasculators.

The 2 mules and the first 78 donkeys were castrated using a standard open technique, together with ligatures placed on the vascular and the non-vascular portions, as the author had been taught at college in 1966. He then gave a lecture in Newmarket to 58 veterinary practitioners after he had carried out 1000 castrations. During the discussion it became evident that there were some in the audience who felt that the ligatures were unnecessary. There was a show of hands: 24 practitioners did not ligature donkeys and had had no problems with haemorrhage. Since that meeting the author has castrated a further 148 donkeys without using ligatures. None of these had any postoperative haemorrhage.

Postoperative haemorrhage

The owners reported 7 cases of postoperative haemorrhage. A total of 6 were found not to be serious and received no further treatment. A single case was found to be in extremis. Euthanasia was carried out. The cause of the failure of the emasculators was never found.

Recovery from the anaesthetic

All the animals had an unassisted recovery from the GA. There were no problems.

Postoperative infection and the use of antibiotics

A total of 342 (8.5%) animals were reported by the owners to have postoperative infection, of which 338 were thought not to be serious. They were given 5 days of oral TMPS. Three animals were clinically sick with a fever. These were given 3 days of intravenous penicillin and gentamycin. A single animal was found to have an infected cord. This was removed under sedation. It was given 3 days of intravenous penicillin and gentamycin, followed by 5 days of intravenous cephalosporin. All these animals then made uneventful recoveries.

The use of antibiotics at the time of surgery is controversial. Until 1998, the author did not give any antibiotics. He was then persuaded by his younger colleagues to inject penicillin at the time of surgery. They could give no evidence of the effectiveness of this; however, they claimed that the owners expected their patients to be given antibiotic cover. They also pointed out that the author's level of postoperative sepsis was high. From his records the author could not see any advantage. The author considered that education of clients is the most important factor. Clients who did not bring their animals into a stable for at least 10 days on the author's instructions never seemed to have problems. Although the author always dressed the wounds with an oily preparation of acriflavine after surgery, he was never convinced of its effectiveness. However, possibly the oil helped to keep the wounds open to allow drainage. Certainly, the use of oxytetracycline spray is unlikely to be beneficial.

The author considers that it is vital to forewarn owners that there will be swelling after such radical surgery. There nearly always is and in the author's experience it quickly lessens with time and exercise.

The use of pain relief and anti-inflammatory drugs

The use of these drugs was not considered in 1966. However, in the intervening years they have become the norm. The author would strongly urge clinicians to support their patients with whatever they feel is the most effective protocol. The author has never used local anaesthesia. However, he thinks its use should be considered.

Tetanus

The danger of tetanus should not be forgotten and clinicians should use their own judgement. The author does not think the use of tetanus antitoxin (TAT) is required if the animal has been fully vaccinated, but is vital otherwise. It would seem prudent to start or complete tetanus vaccination at the time of surgery. The author sees no problem in giving equine influenza vaccination at the same time. However, he always tried to dissuade owners from other procedures, such as foot trimming or mane pulling, as he was concerned for the anaesthetic recovery from any unnecessary delay.

Total disasters

In the series of 4000 castrations, there was only one 2-year-old Cleveland Bay colt which was castrated in the afternoon on the paddock behind the surgery. Everything appeared to be well when the owner collected it at 17.00 for the 3-mile journey to his home. The author was called the following morning at 6.00. The patient had 3 ft of small intestine prolapsed through the left incision. It appeared to be undamaged. The author managed to anesthetize it with detomidine/ketamine and washed the bowel in sterile saline, enlarged the incision, replaced the bowel and with difficulty tried as best he could to suture the inguinal ring. He then sutured the skin. The animal recovered from the GA and there was no further prolapse. However, sadly the animal died of shock at 16.00.

Potential disaster

The author castrated a yearling pony. This animal was found the following morning with several feet of omentum protruding from the incision (Fig. 18.3). With the excellent assistance of a veterinary student, Jess Bartman, the pony was given a GA. We pulled a couple more inches of the omentum out of the wound and then removed the contaminated omentum with scissors. Jess managed to get a good mattress suture into the inguinal ring while I kept the omentum out of her way. She then sutured the skin. The colt made an uneventful recovery with antibiotics and pain relief.

Summary

Only 2 deaths were recorded after 4000 standard castrations (0.025%), 1 from haemorrhage and the other, a Cleveland Bay, from herniation. It was possible that the single animal which died of haemorrhage had a clotting disorder. However, a more likely explanation was that it was the author's error of not closing the emasculators well enough. Certainly, practitioners should beware of inguinal herniation in Cleveland Bay colts. A closed or semi-closed method would be advised.

Closed technique

The main advantage of this technique, if performed in a fully surgical manner, is that there are fewer postoperative complications: (i) there is no danger of evisceration of bowel contents through the inguinal ring and to the outside; (ii) there is no danger of haemorrhage or infection; (iii) there is less local oedema; and (iv) the horse recovers more quickly. However, it is much more time consuming, requires delicate surgery and a GA is required, which will need to be prolonged, with the resultant inherent risks of anaesthesia in the horse. It is vital that the ligature is tight enough to control the haemorrhage, and it also must not slip off or there will then be the danger

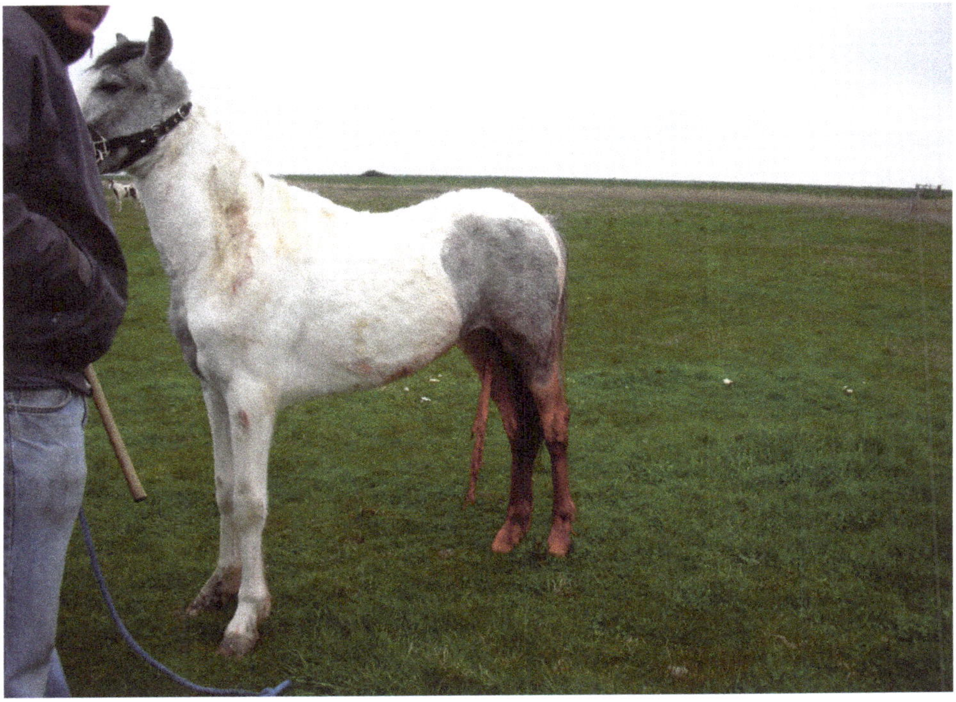

Fig. 18.3. An omental prolapse 24 hours post-castration.

of evisceration; it also needs to be strong and absorbable. There may be problems with rejection of the ligature by the body, causing an abscess or, more seriously, a granulomatous lesion called a 'champignon' (after the French for mushroom). To some extent these dangers are lessened by using a transfixing ligature and modern absorbable suture material.

Semi-closed technique

In some ways this method falls between two stools: it takes longer than the open method, so a relatively long GA is required; on the other hand, as it is not locally closed there is a risk of infection and accompanying swelling, but it does lessen the risk of evisceration. This risk is low in most horses, except in the case of Standardbreds and Cleveland Bays, where either a closed or semi-closed method should always be used; in fact, many veterinary indemnity insurance policies will not cover the clinician who fails to use a ligature in these breeds. Mules and donkeys, in particular, when castrated over the age of 2 years have very large vascular testicles relative to their size; there is a myth that these are more liable to haemorrhage and therefore should be ligatured, but this is not the case. Naturally, the clinician should make sure that emasculators are very strongly applied and kept in place for a minimum of 1 min. In one sense, the use of a ligature in a hairy donkey poses difficulties for the clinician, as it is easy to include a hair in the ligature which will then pull the ligature off. The advice therefore in this case must be to use the open technique.

Open technique

As this is a relatively simple technique surgically, it can be done standing, under local anaesthetic and sedation. However, there are welfare considerations; if the horse is very well handled and is above 15 hands then this technique may well be the method of choice. After the tail has been bandaged, the horse is sedated and a twitch is applied. The scrotum is checked to see that it contains two testicles and that there is no evidence of an inguinal hernia. The scrotum is washed thoroughly with a dilute chlorhexidine solution, and 10 ml local anaesthetic is injected into each cord. Another 10 ml of local anaesthetic is then infiltrated along the ventral aspect of the scrotum on both sides where the incisions are going to be made. The area is rewashed.

A longitudinal incision is made boldly on the ventral aspect of the scrotum the full length of the grasped testicle. The incision should cut the skin and the tunics and will often slightly score the testicle. The testicle is drawn down and a finger placed through the vascular and non-vascular portions of the testicular connections. The emasculator is first placed through the non-vascular part so that the whole of the epididymis is on the outside. *It is very important that the crushing edge of the emasculator is towards the abdomen and the cutting edge is towards the testicle.* This can be easily confirmed: if the nut of the emasculator is pointing towards the testicle, the instrument is placed correctly, i.e. 'nut to nut'. However, the clinician is well advised to check the full mechanism of the emasculator before it is sterilized. The emasculator is then closed firmly on the non-vascular part and released. The suspended testicle is next grasped and drawn down carefully so that the emasculator can be applied very firmly to the vascular part and held for a full 1 min. This procedure is then applied to the second testicle. An oily cream is applied to the two open wounds. Fly control is advised, if appropriate.

Careful instructions and warnings are given to the horse's handler; ideally, castration should be performed in temperate climates in the spring or autumn, when keeping the newly castrated colt outside is not a problem, either on account of flies or very inclement weather. However, if the colt has to be castrated in winter, it must already either be living outside, even at night, or a closed castration method must be used. In warmer climates the horse should not be allowed into any stable or shelter for 10 days, to lessen the danger of sepsis. The handler must be told that swelling of the scrotum and prepuce are inevitable. If either severe haemorrhage occurs or a piece of tissue that the horse cannot retract is seen, the handler should contact the clinician. The use of antibiotics and NSAIDs is up to the discretion of the clinician. However, all horses not fully immune to tetanus should receive tetanus antitoxin.

This technique is not so easy in ponies and donkeys, and is impossible in very small animals and foals. In these cases, a short-acting general anaesthetic should be used (see Fig. 18.4). There is no need for local anaesthesia, although some clinicians inject local anaesthetic into the cord to help with placement of the emasculator; certainly, a general anaesthetic reduces the danger of injury to the clinician and also gives more control in the event of herniation or severe haemorrhage. It should be remembered that the scrotum should be palpated before the general anaesthetic is given to ensure that the horse is not a rig and that there is no other structure in the scrotum.

18.6 Castration of the Rig

Introduction

As stated earlier, it is important that all rigs are castrated, as this is an inherited condition. It is also very important that practitioners do not remove the single testicle if a unilateral rig is presented. Planning is everything with this surgical procedure, and it is very important that the surgeon knows all the facts before the anaesthetic is administered. The horse that is presented may have no testicles in the scrotum – it may already have been castrated, and in this situation a hormone test, as already outlined above, should be carried out. If this shows the horse to be a rig, the clinician has no way of knowing for certain whether there are one or two testicles in the abdomen. Horses have been described having been born without one or both testicles, but such cases are extremely rare and will not test positive to the rig test. Some clinicians are able to palpate an abdominal testicle near to the inguinal ring per rectum.

Castration of the rig is a very difficult and highly skilled procedure. A 5 MHz linear scanner is quite useful to visualize a testicle near to the inguinal ring. Abdominal testicles, of course, can be found and removed by endoscopy. However, assuming these sophisticated aids are not available, the clinician has to rely upon

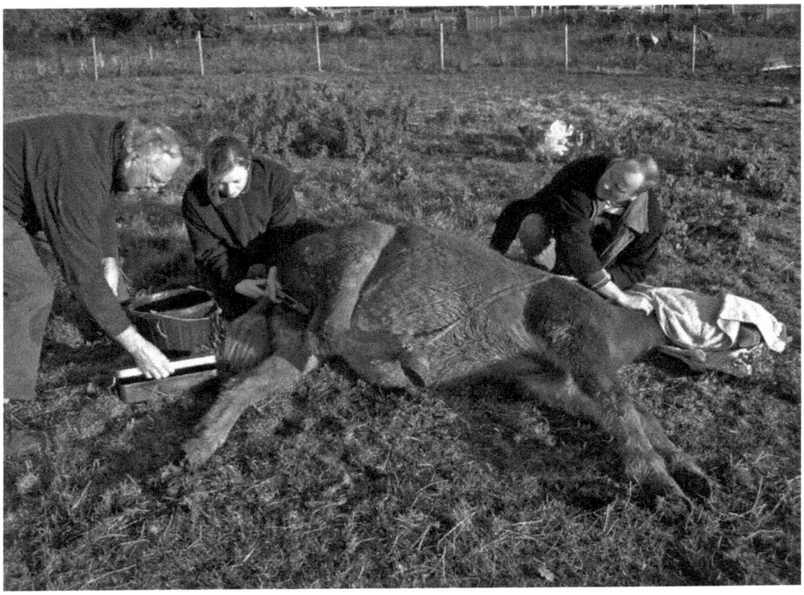

Fig. 18.4. Castration performed under general anaesthesia.

common sense. One of six different scenarios is presented to the clinician:

1. If the animal has one normal testicle in the scrotum and a second palpable in the inguinal ring, the respective sides should be noted. Although this animal is a rig, it is likely that with a good GA both testicles can be removed. The surgeon should remove the testicle in the inguinal ring first but if that cannot be removed on no account should the normal testicle be removed. There is no need to carry out a rig test.
2. If the animal has one normal testicle in the scrotum and no testicle can be felt in the inguinal ring on the other side, the animal should be examined for scars; this may require deep sedation or even a GA in the fractious animal. If there is no scar then the animal is definitely a rig, the side of the normal testicle is noted and rig surgery will need to be carried out. In my experience, if the normal testicle is on the left side the right testicle is likely to be found just inside the inguinal ring. On the other hand, if the normal testicle is on the right side the left testicle might be just inside the inguinal ring or possibly further up in the abdomen. Once again, there is no need to carry out a rig test.
3. If the animal has one normal testicle in the scrotum and no testicle can be felt in the inguinal ring on the other side, it should be examined for scars. If there is a scar, this scar must be examined carefully; if the scar is just under the skin, the animal is definitely a rig, the side of the normal testicle is noted and rig surgery will need to be carried out. There is no need to carry out a rig test. If the scar is attached to a deep structure not just beneath the skin, the animal is unlikely to be a rig because one testicle is likely to have been removed previously. The side of the normal testicle should be noted and normal surgery to remove that testicle will need to be carried out. If after a few weeks the animal stops showing stallion-like behaviour, there is no need to carry out a rig test. On other hand, if the stallion-like behaviour persists then a rig test should be carried out. If this test is positive, then the side with the earlier scar will need to be investigated.
4. If the animal has no normal testicles in the scrotum but two testicles can be felt in the inguinal rings, it is a rig. However, with a good GA it is likely that both testicles can be removed. There is no need for a rig test.
5. If the animal has no normal testicles in the scrotum and one testicle palpable in the inguinal

ring, the side of this testicle should be noted. This animal is a rig. At this stage a rig blood test would not be appropriate, as the practitioner already knows there is a testicle, albeit abnormal, present. On the other hand, appropriate surgery should be carried out. The side without the palpable testicle should be investigated for scars. If there is a scar with adhesions deeper than the skin, it is likely that the testicle on that side has been removed. The surgeon can then remove the other testicle with some confidence. If after some time stallion-like behaviour persists, a rig test should be carried out, and if this is positive then further surgery will be required to investigate the side where no previous testicle was located.

6. If there are no testicles in the scrotum and no evidence of scars, then the animal is likely to be a bilateral rig. It is prudent to carry out a rig test to make sure that the horse actually has testicles.

Inguinal approach

The horse needs to be anaesthetized, with a view to a long surgical procedure. With the back of the horse well padded, it is placed in dorsal recumbency and polythene bags placed over the hooves. The area is prepared surgically, with a ball of sterile cotton wool placed in the preputial opening. If the testicles cannot be located, a skin incision is made over the superficial inguinal ring, care being taken to avoid the large skin veins in the area. The subcuticular tissue is parted so that the superficial inguinal ring is exposed, then the inguinal canal is exposed. The vaginal tunic containing no testis will be found, this varying in size between that of a pencil and a thumb. It may be short, only just visible in the inguinal canal, or may be long enough to be attached to the scrotum. If the vaginal tunic is attached to a scrotal scar, it is likely that a scrotal testicle has previously been removed by an open surgical technique. If there has been no previous surgery the vaginal tunic will have only a tenuous fibrous attachment to the scrotum.

The vaginal tunic is next grasped by a pair of long-handled forceps. A small incision will reveal the deferent duct, which becomes the epididymal tail distally and returns up the lumen of the vaginal tunic as the epididymal body. These two structures, the epididymal tail and body, can be recognized as they consist of coiled tubes, the tail consisting of a large tube loosely coiled, with the body a fine tube tightly coiled. With a pair of long-handled forceps similar to whelping forceps but narrower, traction is applied to the body of the epididymis. The opening in the vaginal tunic may have to be enlarged, but the testicle should be able to be drawn out. The vessels are ligatured and the testicle removed. This procedure should be repeated on the opposite side.

The main problem with this method is seen when the abdominal testicle is not small and flabby like a normal abdominal testicle, but large and cystic. The inguinal ring has to be enlarged to allow exteriorization of this enlarged structure, and it is then difficult to close the inguinal ring. Many mattress sutures should be laid in place before tightening up. A substantial layer of subcuticular sutures should be put in place before the skin is closed with horizontal absorbable mattress sutures. The horse, if possible, should have an assisted recovery and be kept in a small area for 10 days to allow the wound to heal. Antibiotics and NSAIDs are given to lessen infection and swelling.

Should one testicle not be found, the inguinal ring should be closed as described above and the horse allowed to recover. A second rig test is next performed to confirm that there is still a testicle present. The horse will then have to be re-anaesthetized and a paramedian approach, as described below, performed.

Paramedian approach

Once again, the horse must be anaesthetized with a view to a long surgical procedure. The horse is prepared as described above for inguinal approach. A skin incision, just large enough to admit the surgeon's hand, is made 7 cm from midline at the level of the preputial opening; the site should be selected to avoid any major skin vessels, and the line of incision should be the same as the line of the fibres of the straight abdominal muscle. The abdominal tunic and closely adherent tendons of the external and internal oblique muscles are incised with a scalpel, but the abdominal muscle is split by blunt dissection. The transverse tendon will be seen to run at right angles to the line of skin incision; this is then punctured and opened in line with its fibres. The whole hand is then introduced and moved caudally. On most occasions the soft or flabby testicle will be felt near to the opening of the internal inguinal ring; if it is not felt, the hand has to be extended and the abdomen is swept systematically, working back from the inguinal ring to the pole of the kidney. Normally, the testicle will be found provided the surgeon is not looking for a large, hard, normal testicle – the testicle in most cases will be small and flabby; however, it may be a large, cystic structure that feels like the urinary bladder, but if the epididymis is felt the testicle can be exteriorized with confidence. The testicle is removed with emasculators in the normal way; usually, both testicles can be removed through the same incision, but if that is not possible an incision can be made in the other side.

Closure of the transverse tendon and abdominal tunic and closely adherent tendons of the external and internal oblique muscles is made with a single cruciate suture of thick Vicryl®. Great care is needed to ensure that no small intestine is trapped in this suture; however, once this is tightly tied the surgeon can relax, since small intestinal prolapse is then impossible. The outer abdominal tunic can be sutured with interrupted horizontal mattress sutures. The dead space is filled with the subcuticular sutures aligning the tissue and the skin is closed with interrupted horizontal mattress sutures of absorbable material.

18.7 The Testes

Testicular torsion

The main presenting sign here will be acute colic; the differential diagnosis is a strangulated loop of small intestine in the inguinal ring. The differentiation is not easy – the technique is very heavy sedation and pain relief, and then the scrotum – and particularly the inguinal ring – can be examined thoroughly. In either event surgery is required. It is conceivable that hemi-castration could be performed under heavy sedation and local anaesthesia, but a general anaesthetic is more prudent.

The scrotum and surrounding area are surgically prepared. A very careful incision is made over the testicle through the skin. The tunic should be incised only after careful examination; if there is no evidence of the presence of either bowel or omentum, the testicle can be removed as for an open castration. If there is bowel present it should be examined carefully for viability, and if all is well it can be returned to the abdomen; if in any doubt, a resection must be performed before returning the bowel to the abdomen. In either case the inguinal ring may have to be enlarged. Mattress sutures require to be laid before any are tightened, then the subcuticular layer is closed before suturing the skin. All layers must be sutured with absorbable material. Antibiotics and NSAIDs are necessary.

Orchitis

The cause is normally a penetrating wound, but can be blood-borne, particularly after testicular trauma as a result of a kick from a mare; trauma is also possible when a stallion jumps over a fence or stable door, but this is extremely rare. Potentially, a large number of bacteria may be involved, the most common among these being *Streptococcus zooepidemicus*, *Klebsiella pneumonia* and *Salmonella abortus equi* (see Section 18.15). Treatment with appropriate antibiotics should be carried out. Orchitis can also be caused by viral infection, the most common being equine herpes virus 1 (see Section 18.15), equine viral arteritis (see Section 18.8) and equine infectious anaemia (see Section 14.10); in these cases, the condition is normally self-limiting, but NSAIDs are helpful, particularly in lowering testicular temperature and reducing the period of infertility.

18.8 Venereal (Sexually-transmitted) Diseases

Equine viral arteritis

A disease found worldwide, the stallion is the carrier. The mare can become infected at coitus or from artificial insemination (AI); equally, the mare can become infected from aborted fetuses or horses having the respiratory form of the disease. The incubation period is 3–8 days. Normally, the signs are of a mild respiratory infection; however, if abortion occurs these may be more severe, with fever and oedema of the udder and hind legs. The disease is self-limiting, excepting that stallions remain as carriers. Diagnosis is by serology, although it is impossible on a single sample to separate an infected animal from a vaccinated one; paired samples with a rising titre are required to confirm active disease. Care should be taken when vaccinating a horse that may be exported – a blood sample showing a negative titre should first be obtained.

Coital exanthema

Often classified as a skin disease, this condition is caused by equine herpes virus 3. It is found throughout the world and is spread mainly by coitus. However, veterinary instruments have also been blamed, so the clinician should be ever mindful of disease control. The incubation period is 1 week. The vulva and the penis will develop herpes blisters, which turn into sores; these will heal in a further week but may leave permanent skin pigmentation deficits. There will be a breeding delay, but no permanent problem.

Contagious equine metritis (CEM)

A highly contagious bacterial disease caused by *Taylorella equi*, it is transmitted by both coitus and AI; teasers have also been implicated. The active disease is seen as a purulent discharge from the uterus, which is then seen at the vulva. It causes marked infertility. There is a carrier state in both the stallion (in the urethral fossa) and the mare (in the clitoris). Isolation is straightforward from these sites, provided the culture is carried out in a micro-aerophilic environment on chocolate agar plates over a 7-day period. Although most animals will eventually recover their fertility, 20% will remain as carriers. Serious hygiene precautions are required, which will be described for all venereal bacterial pathogens below under conditions associated with the mare.

Other bacterial conditions

Included here are *Pseudomonas aeruginosa*, *Klebsiella pneumonia*, *Escherichia coli* and *Streptococcus zooepidemicus*. These will all cause infertility in the mare and are likely to be spread venereally; however, only certain *K. pneumonia* strains possessing a K capsule are entirely venereal. All these organisms may be found as normal flora on the skin; it is only when they are present in large numbers that disease occurs. It is important that the stallion's penis is not washed in iodine or chlorhexidine, as those disinfectants will help promote the growth of these organisms; the penis should be washed regularly with simple, non-perfumed soap.

Dourine

The causal agent of this life-threatening protozoal disease is *Trypanosoma equiperdum*. It is found in Africa, the Middle East, Asia and Central and South America, and is a venereal disease with high mortality. It has a slow, insidious onset; initially there is a discharge from the urethra and the vulva, although often this will go unnoticed and the horse is presented to the clinician with fever and marked swelling of the prepuce, with penile paralysis or swelling of the vulva and mammary gland. The skin will be covered by raised plaques, and in the fluid from these plaques will be seen the trypanosomes on wet preparations or dry slides stained with Giemsa. The treatment is as described in Section 6.4 with diminazene aceturate; however, if the disease is well advanced, the success rate is low and euthanasia is the kindest option.

18.9 The Accessory Sex Glands

The stallion has four accessory glands: a pair of ampullae, a pair of seminal vesicles, a bilobed prostate and a pair of bulbourethral glands. Diseases of these glands are extremely rare and these are likely to go unnoticed except when semen is collected, when the semen may be blood-tinged or will culture positive for *S. zooepidemicus*, *K. pneumonia*, *P. aeruginosa* or *Staphylococcus aureus*.

18.10 The Penis and Prepuce

Infection and inflammation

Termed balanitis in the penis and balanoposthitis in the prepuce, this always occurs to some degree following castration; it is also a common sequel to a kick from a mare. Other causes include self-trauma from pruritis, insect bites or maggots, and in such cases great care should be taken to use non-irritant cleansing agents. It can also be caused by any of the venereal diseases described in the section above. Aggressive parenteral and local treatment should be started as soon as possible, i.e. antibiotics and NSAIDs.

The potentially dangerous sequel is prolapse or paralysis of the penis. If the penis cannot be returned into the prepuce, this condition is called a paraphimosis. There is also a congenital condition where the penis cannot be extruded, termed phimosis, which can be corrected by widening the preputial orifice. Antibiotics and NSAIDs are insufficient treatment for paraphimosis because the oedema of the penis will be self-perpetuating. It is vital that the penis is supported, the best support being a pair of nylon tights tied over the back and anchored by bandage to the tail head.

The penis may be affected in habronemiasis (often called 'summer sores'), initiated by the nematode *Habronema*; the horse should be treated with oral ivermectin at 0.2 mg/kg, as well as soothing, oily cream locally.

Tumours

Squamous cell carcinoma

Frequently, this will be well advanced before being noticed. If the penis alone is affected, amputation should be carried out as described below; however, if the prepuce is also involved the condition should be managed as well as possible, with euthanasia being carried out terminally.

Melanoma

Occurring only in the grey horse, often this will grow very slowly and so the horse will be able to live out a natural lifespan. However, if it ulcerates or is colonized by maggots, euthanasia is the only option since removal is very rarely successful in the long term.

Viral papilloma

Sudden onset is seen in the young horse, and equally suddenly will disappear without treatment. However, the clinician should be wary of such papillomata in horses over 6 years of age – these may well not be papillomata but equine sarcoids (see below).

Equine sarcoid

Equine sarcoids at this site are very hard to treat. Very sophisticated treatments, e.g. laser or cryosurgery, are available, but simpler treatments may be just as effective if the cases are chosen with care. If the sarcoids are multiple and very invasive, the animal should be euthanized but, if pedunculated, either a rubber elastrator ring or a very tight, non-absorbable ligature can be placed around the neck of the mass. Another course of treatment is to inject, normally under GA, a cytotoxic substance, e.g. 5-fluorouracil, into each sarcoid.

Amputation of the penis

The horse is anaesthetized and placed in dorsal recumbency; the penis is catheterized and the area surgically prepared. A tourniquet is placed well above the point of amputation. A step-like incision is made in the penis, being 5 cm longer on the dorsal aspect and with the urethra containing the catheter running along the step towards the distal end. The corpus cavernosum is closed by a very large number of single sutures of absorbable material, penetrating the urethral membrane, the tunica albuginea and the integument, but not through the corpus cavernosum. The goal by the end of the surgery is for the new urethral orifice to be on the ventral aspect of the stump of the penis, which should be totally covered by the urethral membrane. There will be some weeping haemorrhage when the tourniquet is removed; if this appears excessive, more sutures should be placed thorough the urethral membrane, the tunica albuginea and the integument. Each day the horse must receive antibiotics and NSAIDs, and the prepuce washed with warm, soapy water.

18.11 The Vulva and Vagina

The vulva

The vulva can become deformed in two ways. First, this may occur at foaling. Opinion is divided as to whether immediate repair should be carried out or the oedema be allowed to subside. On the whole minor wounds should be repaired at the time with absorbable sutures, but larger wounds – including wounds involving the rectum – should be left for several days. The clinician should weigh up all the possibilities before embarking on elaborate surgery. If another pregnancy is not of vital importance, the problem may well be left provided the mare can defecate and not have a problem with faecal contamination, with resultant myiasis.

The second problem occurs in the thin, old thoroughbred-type horse where the vulva ceases to lie in a dorsoventral plane, but the dorsal end becomes drawn in. This allows faeces and air to be drawn into the vagina, termed pneumovagina, which will decrease the fertility of the mare. The condition can be improved by performing a Caslick's operation. The mare is restrained, if possible in stocks, and if that is not possible sedation is advisable. The tail is bandaged and the rectum evacuated, and the whole of the peritoneal area is then thoroughly cleaned. Local anaesthetic is injected around the dorsal end of the vagina; the area of anaesthesia can then be enlarged by injecting more anaesthetic through the already anaesthetized area ventrally down both sides of the lips of the vulva. The area is again cleaned. A strip of tissue 1 cm wide is removed from the skin/mucosal junction, starting at the dorsal end of the vulva and reaching at least half-way down each side of the orifice. The lips are then sutured together using simple interrupted sutures, ensuring that the cut surfaces are apposed to each other; it is important to make sure there is a good seal at the dorsal end of the vulva. With a quiet mare or where stocks are available, monofilament nylon may be used instead, with the sutures being removed in 10 days; however, without the aid of stocks, it is prudent to use dissolvable sutures to save the perils of suture removal. This operation is used extensively in thoroughbred practice, but is rarely required in the working horse.

There is a further operation, called Pouret's technique, for perineal reconstruction of a more permanent nature. This requires an extremely good surgical technique, since the internal vaginal mucosa is pulled cranially to form a new vulval seal. There is a possibility of entering the rectum, so this is not an advisable procedure for novice surgeons and is beyond the scope of this book, but directions can be found in many equine stud medicine texts.

The best method for managing a horse that has had a Caslick's operation is open to debate. The most technical approach is to cut the vulva to allow penile penetration at service, and then to re-suture. Obviously, this will have to be carried out several times until the mare is known to be pregnant. In the working horse a better method is to limit the extent of the vulval suturing to allow natural service without cutting the vulva; the vulva is then left intact until parturition. The ideal is for the vulva to be cut at foaling, but some practitioners suggest that the vulva is cut before foaling is imminent to avoid the danger of tearing. This, however, is likely to be unnecessary as the so-called tear will follow the line of the incision; the tear will need to be re-sutured after foaling.

The vagina

Varicose veins

The clinical sign of intermittent bleeding from the vulva due to varicose veins is extremely rare. On examination with a vaginal speculum, the source of the haemorrhage will be seen as very small grape-like growths, which should be cauterized with a silver nitrate pencil. The problem will often recur after service.

Necrotic vaginitis

Occurring normally after a difficult foaling, the swelling of the vulva subsides but there is a continual discharge. Diagnosis is important: if the discharge comes from the cervix there is an endometritis, which may be either linked to vaginitis or occur on its own; a vaginitis may also occur on its own. The vagina will be inflamed, with lines of yellow, necrotic diphtheritic membrane. If there is no evidence of endometritis it is important *not* to irrigate the uterus, as this will spread the infection through the cervix. Once the diagnosis has been made with a speculum, the reproductive tract should be left alone to heal; repeated examinations should be avoided for the same reason.

The antibiotic of choice is crystalline penicillin, given i/v. After 3 weeks the vagina should be examined again to see whether it has healed, and the clinician should also ensure that there has been no physical damage causing urine to pool in the vagina. If urine pooling is detected, the mare should be allowed 1 year of sexual rest; if pooling is still found 1 year later, surgery should be attempted, but this is not easy. An elongation of the urethra is constructed out of the vaginal mucosa around a large Foley catheter under epidural anaesthesia. This may be successful and allow the mare to continue to breed, but the prognosis is not good.

Tumours

Squamous cell carcinoma

Tending to be strongly locally invasive, this tumour is more common in the mare with a non-pigmented vulva. Various cytotoxic human preparations have been tried, but are rarely helpful. Surgical excision is to be avoided as the carcinoma spreads rapidly. Euthanasia is the kindest option.

Melanoma

Very common in the grey horse, this rarely causes a problem. Although it will often shell out easily, it will invariably recur, so is best left alone. Euthanasia is indicated if it becomes large and ulcerates.

Benign vaginal polyp

As the name implies, this is not a dangerous tumour and, although the owner may well think that it has grown very rapidly, it will in fact have grown very slowly; it will have been hidden in the vagina and suddenly popped out. Resection is often difficult, as the neck of the tumour is situated well into the vagina, but there is unlikely to be any recurrence.

Hamartoma

Appearing as strange, benign swellings in the muscle surrounding the vagina, it is not cancerous, since the tissue cells on biopsy appear normal to the pathologist, although these can become quite large. Surgery should be avoided, as it is very difficult to separate normal tissue from the hamartoma, there being no demarcation. The surgeon is left with a large tissue deficit, which will then re-grow but will not have a good mucosal covering.

Equine sarcoid

Although very common in the groin and around the mammary gland, sarcoid is extremely rare near the vulva.

18.12 The Cervix

Prolapse

An extremely rare, once-in-a-lifetime event, this is a problem not associated with pregnancy but with chronic vaginal infection and irritation. The cervix is easy to replace, and should be retained in place using a very deep-seated Caslick's operation (see Section 18.11). The mare should be kept on daily antibiotics and NSAIDs for 14 days.

Lacerations

Associated with difficult parturition, it is amazing how these will heal in many cases. However, with some very bad lacerations, even after 12 months' rest there will be cervical incompetence, so that the clinical picture is of a permanent, low-grade endometritis. In these cases, although the mare will show normal oestrus behaviour, there will be pregnancy failure. Heroic attempts at cervical surgery are likely to be futile.

18.13 The Uterus

Endometritis

Endometritis is the main cause of early embryo loss, although transient inflammation of the uterine mucosa is a normal physiological finding following breeding in the mare. A normal mare's uterus will clear any bacteria or inflammatory cells within 12 h, and endometritis is said to have occurred if the inflammation persists for longer than this period. The main physical cause of this may be cervical incompetence, as described above; however, a much more common cause is the intrinsic inability of the mare's uterus to contract and remove the inflammatory cells and bacteria, which will be seen on endometrial impression smears stained with Giemsa, examined under oil immersion.

Transient endometritis can be treated by injecting the mare with 30–50 IU oxytocin i/m within 6 h of mating. In more serious endometritis this treatment can be linked with uterine lavage, with or without antibiotics; lavage is accomplished by running 2 litres warm isotonic saline into the uterus with a sterile 0.5 cm plastic tube, using gravity. The saline bag, when empty and still attached to the tube, is lowered below the uterus of the mare, where gravity will then drain the fluid back into the bag. If this fluid is visibly dirty, the procedure is repeated until clean saline is seen; a small volume of antibiotics is then instilled into the uterus, and 30 min later an injection of oxytocin is given to ensure that the uterus is emptied. This whole procedure can be repeated every 48 h, assuming the mare continues in oestrus and has been either served or inseminated.

Endometritis can be caused by specific bacteria transmitted sexually, as described below in Septic metritis. Naturally in these cases, service should be stopped until both the stallion and mare have been swabbed and found to be clean, on three occasions at weekly intervals.

Endometritis can also be caused by fungi or yeasts, which may be seen on endometrial swabs. This type of endometritis is rare, and it is important that treatment with antibiotics is stopped. Uterine lavage should be continued on a daily basis for a minimum of 5 days, using 2 litres warm saline with 40 ml concentrated povidone iodine added. The solution should be sucked out as described above; it will be coloured brown and have some contamination.

On rare occasions, the clinician will observe actual flocculent material coming out of the cervix from the uterus, and on rectal examination the uterus will be felt as an enlarged, doughy structure, termed pyometra. This carries a very poor prognosis for further breeding, although the mare is rarely ill. Copious uterine flushing with appropriate antibiotics can be tried but is rarely successful.

Septic metritis

Occurring after foaling and usually associated with an assisted delivery or retention of the fetal membranes, this is an extremely serious condition. The mare will have a raised temperature initially, which will drop as endotoxic shock sets in; there will be a copious vulval discharge. The most likely bacterium involved will be *E. coli*. The sequel to this condition is a life-threatening laminitis, particularly in the heavy horse, but it can occur in all equines. The mare will cease producing milk and so the foal will suffer; the foal should therefore be monitored very carefully, as its presence and attempts to suckle will be helpful in treatment of the mare. The mare should be given high levels of antibiotics, ideally penicillin and gentamicin; she should also be given NSAIDs. The uterus is lavaged with large volumes of warm isotonic saline containing antibiotics, and following each 12-hourly lavage the mare should be given an appropriate dose of oxytocin. As tetanus can also be a sequel, the mare must be given tetanus antitoxin and, if not vaccinated, should receive the first dose of tetanus vaccine. Antibiotic treatment and NSAIDs must be continued for at least 2 days after the mare appears to be normal.

18.14 Fertility Problems Associated with the Stallion

Apart from conditions of inflammation and infection of the testicles, accessory glands and penis as described above, the stallion can present problems of libido and sperm production. Libido is rarely a problem for the stallion that is too young, although the heavy-type horse rarely shows much sexual activity before puberty, which is around 18 months of age; ponies reach puberty earlier. Poor nutrition will delay the onset of puberty and may well cause a lack of libido in the mature animal; underlying disease will have a similar effect. In temperate climates the season of the year may have an effect on libido, but day length primarily affects the mare. Certain medications may affect libido, as will extreme heat or cold and sexual overwork; stallions vary enormously, but libido is definitely linked with age. Poor libido will affect the stallion's interest in the mare, and his ability to have an erection and achieve intercourse. All these factors will also affect sperm output, which is very important not only for natural service, but also for artificial insemination, although this will not be discussed here. Certain physical problems associated with the penis, for example a deviated penis from a kick or associated with skeletal conformation (e.g. arthritis of the hock), will adversely affect the stallion's ability to achieve intercourse.

18.15 Pregnancy

Pregnancy diagnosis

The normal gestation period for the horse is 335–342 days; however, there is a wide range for normal pregnancy, lengths varying from 315 to 415 days, with a mean of 340. Gestation length is more constant for the individual mare, colt foals tending to have longer gestation length. Scanning per rectum can be performed very early in the mare, even 14 days post-service; however, assuming there is no access to a scanner, an experienced clinician can have an idea of pregnancy by manual rectal examination at 17 days. The uterus at this stage feels turgid, like that of a cow in oestrus, while that of a non-pregnant uterus feels more like a thick, velvet ribbon. However, such an examination can only be an indication and should not be relied upon.

Manual examination is carried out at 42 days, when the fetus will be felt as a mass the size of a goose's egg in the gravid horn. Twin pregnancy can be diagnosed at this time, as the two fetuses can both be palpated. The clinician, however, has a dilemma, for if the pregnancy is terminated with prostaglandin injection at this time, after formation of the endometrial cups, the mare will not become pregnant again in that breeding season and will miss a whole breeding season. Twins will cause problems in that abortions are much more common in later pregnancy, and dystocia is more likely. There is also delay in uterine involution with a reduction in fertility in the following years. On balance, therefore, the clinician is advised to inform the owner of the likelihood of twins but to leave the twins *in situ*. Best practice is to use a rectal scanner early in the pregnancy, between 17 and 28 days, and to manually void the twin at this stage. Twins are rare except in the thoroughbred and some very large draught breeds; the latter, on account of their large size, are often able to carry the twins to term naturally.

Although manual rectal pregnancy diagnosis can be carried out reliably from 42 days, the clinician may find it physically a little difficult from 70 to 120 days, when the gravid uterus has dropped forward into the abdomen; later in the pregnancy the actual fetus will be felt with ease.

Blood can be taken for pregnancy diagnosis, the timing for early diagnosis being critical. Between 45 and 90 days the parameter tested is pregnant mare serum gonadotrophin (PMS; now known as equine chorionic gonadotrophin). Blood taken between 90 and 120 days cannot be tested reliably for pregnancy, but after 120 days oestrone sulfate level is a reliable parameter. In the past urine could be tested after 150 days for oestrogens, using the Cuboni test; however, this test is no more than 80% accurate and is no longer used. Oestrone sulfate can be assessed after 160 days in the faeces, but such a test is not available commercially.

Problems

Introduction

There is no reason for a mare in early pregnancy not to carry on working, but she should be confined to very light work after the start of the third trimester and work should cease over the last month. At that time the relevant vaccinations should be reviewed to ensure that the foal receives a high level of antibody in the colostrum; this is particularly important regarding tetanus.

Mares do not require very much additional feeding in the first two trimesters – they need to be 'fit, not fat'; however, nutrition needs to be increased slowly in the third trimester. Body condition should be regularly monitored.

If equine herpes virus is a problem, the mare should be vaccinated at 5, 7 and 9 months, although this vaccine is not 100% effective for the individual mare; however, its use does reduce abortion rates within a population. Should abortion from any cause occur, the mare must be treated symptomatically for metritis and/or retained fetal membranes and the aborted foal examined, all as described in the section on abortion below.

In the older mare the weight of the gravid uterus may have two detrimental effects that the clinician is powerless to help, the first being the flexor apparatus in the hind legs, which becomes stretched until the plantar aspect of the fetlock is almost touching the ground. This will improve after parturition to some degree, but the tissues will never return to normal and further pregnancies should be discouraged.

An even more serious complication is rupture of the prepubic tendon, where the abdomen will appear to drop markedly in front of the ventral pelvis. There is no treatment; however, the mare will usually be able to deliver a live foal with some assistance. The mare should not be bred from again. This condition may occur naturally in an old mare, on account of the weight of the fetus; however, it may also be caused by an excessive amount of fluid in the uterus. If the fluid is in the amnion it is called hydrops amnion; if in the allantois, hydrops allantois, or it may be a combination of both conditions. The cause is unknown but often the fetus has some defect, e.g. hydrocephalus. It is rarely noticed until the abdomen is markedly distended, with rupture of the prepubic tendon being a common sequel.

The mare becomes ill only if the uterus ruptures, and in this scenario euthanasia is the only option; the foal is usually dead, although rectal examination should be performed to check for any foal movement. If found, the mare is given a general anaesthetic using ketamine and romifidine, as described in Section 8.12 and 8.15. The foal must be removed from the abdomen as quickly as possible and resuscitated if necessary and the uterus examined in case the tear is small and can be repaired. However, the tear is normally long and extending caudally to the cervix, and is irreparable. Euthanasia should be carried out before the mare regains consciousness. In these cases the abdomen will be filled with blood.

In hydrops allantois the allantois will be opened only when the foal has been removed. The release of this large amount of fluid may well send the mare into shock, from which she is unable to recover. This is a difficult case for the clinician when diagnosed prior to such a disaster occurring: should the mare be induced early, as described above? This may be the best course of action for the mare; however, if the foal is weak and premature, its likelihood of survival is slim. Some authorities advise draining off the allantoic fluid through the cervix with a needle attached to a tube; this is not advisable, as an ascending infection from the vagina is likely, resulting in metritis and an infection in the allantois that will kill the foal. The best course of action is to continue to monitor the mare with a view to inducing the foal after 330 days of gestation, when its chances of survival are greater. If the mare can be induced into normal labour by an injection of prostaglandin, her chances of survival are good. She may develop shock at parturition, but this should not be fatal and can be treated symptomatically.

Uterine torsion

This is a very rare occurrence in the mare and is a true uterine torsion occurring at the neck of the uterus, just cranial to the cervix. The mare, which will be in the last trimester of pregnancy, will show colic signs: the heart rate will be increased, but there will be normal gut sounds. Although torsion will be felt on rectal examination, a vaginal examination must be performed, not to help with diagnosis of the torsion, as there will be no evidence of this, but to check whether the cervix is dilating, indicating that parturition is imminent. If a limb can be felt through the cervix, manual correction of the torsion can be attempted. This requires serious upper arm and body strength and a rocking motion to be successful.

Normally, the mare is not parturient. Various methods of correcting the torsion have been advised, the best being to sedate the mare and inject local anaesthetic linearly in the lower flank to anaesthetize the skin and abdominal muscles. If the torsion is in a clockwise direction the incision needs to be in the left flank; conversely, if the torsion is anticlockwise the incision will be in the right flank. With normal aseptic precautions an incision is made, *just* big enough to admit the operator's forearm but no bigger, the reason for this being that the forearm is going to act as a plug to stop any prolapse of the small intestine. The uterus is balloted (compressed) and the torsion is normally relatively easily corrected. Any colic signs shown by the mare will immediately cease, although she may still show signs of shock as blood flow returns to normal.

Suturing the peritoneum and the innermost muscle layer is extremely difficult. Interrupted horizontal mattress sutures are laid using strong absorbable suture material, but not tidied until all have been laid. An assistant suitably scrubbed can be used to help keep the small intestine back while the sutures are laid and then drawn up and tightened. It is very important that sufficient sutures are laid, as it is extremely hazardous to try to close a small hole in the peritoneum after the main closure has been accomplished, on account of the danger of involving the small intestine in the suture line. The second layer of muscle can be closed much more easily, with strong, interrupted simple absorbable sutures. A subcuticular layer of continuous sutures of absorbable material will make closing of the skin with interrupted horizontal mattress sutures of monofilament nylon easier. Although the mare will have been administered antibiotics and NSAIDs for a minimum of 5 days, she is still at high risk and should be closely monitored until term. The cause of torsion is unknown, but is thought to be violent movement of the fetus; obviously this can recur, but is unlikely.

Uterine torsion can be corrected under GA with the mare in dorsal recumbency. Repositioning of the fetus is extremely difficult in this position, unlike in the standing position, although suturing the abdomen is easier and less hazardous. On balance, considering the risk with any GA in the horse – particularly a heavily pregnant horse – the standing procedure is safer.

A third method that has been used is to roll the mare using the Schaffer 'plank in the flank' method. The advantage of this method is that the abdomen is not opened, but the first disadvantage is that once again the mare requires a GA, albeit of shorter duration. The second, and much more serious, disadvantage is that of uterine rupture resulting in fatal shock, while a third disadvantage is the possible rupture of the middle uterine artery resulting in the death of the mare.

Rupture of a major artery

Sometimes occurring in the last few days of pregnancy, this is more commonly seen at parturition or immediately afterwards. The artery usually found to be ruptured is the middle uterine, although rupture of both utero-ovarian and external iliac has also been recorded. The massive haemorrhage will occur within the abdomen and will not be obvious externally. The mucous membranes will be totally white, the mare collapsing and performing violent leg movements. Handlers are at risk and prompt euthanasia should be carried out.

In some cases, rupture of the middle uterine artery will occur into the broad ligament; in this case haemorrhage will not be extensive, as it will be contained within the broad ligament to the size of an ostrich's egg. The clinician can confirm the diagnosis per rectum, although palpation must be very gentle as further, fatal haemorrhage is possible. The mare will show colic-like pain, which can be controlled with NSAIDs. The mare should not be bred from again.

Abortion

Introduction

Embryonic loss is said to have occurred if pregnancy has terminated before 150 days; if termination occurs after this time but before 300 days it is said to be an abortion. If a foal is delivered after 300 days but fails to take a breath (this can be tested by removing a piece of lung: if it floats in water the foal has taken at least one breath), it is said to be a stillbirth. Abortion may have a specific cause, as described below, but it may be sporadic in up to 10% of pregnancies, when the cause is never discovered. The most common cause, of course, is twinning; the second most common cause is the mare suffering a systemic illness resulting in raised temperature. Physical trauma to the mare is a possible cause, particularly during a violent colic, although such a cause is rare. Placental abnormalities or insufficiency may well be the cause of an abortion, but this may never be discovered. Abortion may have a fetal cause, e.g. strangulation by the umbilical cord or a genetic abnormality. Numerous plants have also blamed for abortion, but evidence is normally limited, as is evidence of an inorganic poison, e.g. organophosphate compounds. Clinicians should be wary of administering any medicine during pregnancy – all data sheets should be read beforehand; if there is no specific guidance, the owner should be advised of any perceived risks. Malnutrition is rarely a cause of abortion, although deficiencies of iodine or selenium have been incriminated.

Equine herpes virus

This ubiquitous virus is the most common infectious cause of equine abortion; normally, type 1 causes abortion although occasionally type 4 has been implicated. However, this type more typically causes respiratory signs. Equine herpes virus type 1 will also cause neurological disease, characterized by hind limb ataxia. Equine herpes virus is spread via either the respiratory route or contact with aborted fetuses or membranes. It normally takes over 1 month for the mare to abort, which is normally after 5 months of pregnancy. The fetus is usually expelled within intact fetal membranes. A full post-mortem should be carried out on the fetus with collection of samples of liver, spleen, kidney and fetal membrane to make an accurate diagnosis. Vaccination of all pregnant mares must be carried out without delay; the standard vaccination regime is to vaccinate the mare in the 5th, 7th and 9th months of pregnancy. Any mare further in foal than 5 months should be vaccinated to a tighter schedule, with agreement from the owner.

Equine viral arteritis

Transmission of this contagious viral disease is from either the stallion venereally or AI. Although there is said to be no carrier state in the mare, she may become infected from the aborted fetus or membranes; respiratory transmission is also possible. Illness is seen in varying degrees prior to abortion, the main sign being conjunctivitis with swelling, termed chemosis; the mare may also develop swelling of the limbs. The incubation period is short, between 3 and 8 days. Diagnosis is best achieved using serology, since virus isolation is difficult. Control is accomplished by vaccination of both mare and stallion; care needs to be taken to blood-test stallions before vaccination, as it is impossible to differentiate a raised titre through vaccination from that post-infection, i.e. a previously vaccinated stallion from a possible shedding stallion.

Bacterial placentitis

The most common organisms involved are *Streptococcus* spp., although there are five others that may be involved: *E. coli*, *Pseudomonas* spp., *Klebsiella* spp., *Staphylococcus* spp. and *Corynebacterium pseudotuberculosis*. The last mentioned can infect the mare only by haematogenous spread; the others may not only be spread haematogenously but also via ascending infection through the cervix. Diagnosis is by bacteriology of the aborted fetus. Control is accomplished by strict hygiene control at the stud.

Salmonella abortus equi

The mare will become ill with this infection before aborting, after a short incubation period of 4–7 days. The mare becomes infected by eating infected grass. Diagnosis is by bacteriology on samples from the fetus and aborted membranes. Control is by vaccination and strict hygiene.

Leptospirosis

There are several species of this bacterium that will cause abortion in the mare, which becomes infected from eating food or grass contaminated by vermin or other wildlife; the mare will become ill 2–4 weeks before abortion occurs, and treatment at this stage with i/v oxytetracycline for 5 days may prevent abortion. The disease may be suspected if there is pyrexia, but jaundice is pathognomic. Diagnosis is via paired serological samples, since isolation of the organism is, under normal circumstances, impossible either from the dam or the fetus. Species involved are *Leptospira pomona*, *Leptospira bratislava*, *Leptospira grippotyphosa* and *Leptospira icterohaemorrhagiae*. Control is carried out by avoiding contamination of food and water; vermin control should be strict. There are no vaccines licensed for use in the horse, and the use of cattle vaccines is not to be encouraged as these can cause an anaphylactic reaction; in addition, the normal cattle vaccine is preventative for *Leptospira hardjo*, which is not an equine pathogen.

Fungal placentitis

This condition is caused by an ascending infection of *Aspergillus* spp., and is very rare. Initial diagnosis is on the thick, leathery texture of the fetal membranes; the fungus may be grown from uterine culture following abortion. Antibiotics should be avoided, and the uterus copiously irrigated with povidone iodine solution.

18.16 Parturition

Signs of parturition

Increase in size of the abdomen is an unreliable sign of pregnancy, and the practitioner should not advise on pregnancy without a rectal examination; equally, the size of the fetus is not a reliable means of judging the duration of pregnancy, but fetal movement provides good confirmation that the fetus is alive. The lack of oestrous behaviour is not a good indicator of pregnancy, and display of oestrous behaviour – and indeed allowing the stallion to mount – is not a 100% guide to non-pregnancy.

Prediction of foaling dates is very difficult in the mare, although the last known service date is helpful, as is the gestation length of previous pregnancies. Pelvic relaxation may give some indication; however, the wax-like excretion seen on the ends of the teats is the best guide that foaling is imminent, i.e. within the following 24 h. It is well known that most foalings will occur at night, but it should also be remembered that the mare has some mechanism for delaying foaling, i.e. if the weather is very bad or there is no available site that is undisturbed.

Multiparous mares will often produce milk for a few days prior to foaling, and then will wax up 24 h before the actual event. This is not outside normal expectations, but if the loss is really copious it is important that the colostrum is stored to give to the foal within the first 6 h of life. On the whole the owner need not be too concerned, as these mares will normally have an excess of colostrum.

Normal parturition

It is very important for practitioners to train owners new to foaling mares; many surveys have revealed that up to half of requests to practitioners to attend to a foaling mare are false alarms. The practitioner has a dilemma, since a foaling is one of the few true equine emergencies. Many requests will be followed up with alacrity only to find that the mare has already foaled; such journeys are not wasted, for the practitioner can check the mare's udder and perineal area; the fetal membranes can be laid out and examined to make sure they all have been expelled; last a foal check can be performed as described in Section 18.19 below.

The ideal place for a normal parturition will vary enormously throughout the world; in colder climates foaling under cover will be practised. The area should be large enough, at least 4.5 m^2; the floor must be soft and well bedded down and the walls free from any sharp projections. It is wise to have the area well lit at night, so that the mare can be checked regularly without disturbing her by turning on any light; ideally there would be a small peephole or CCTV camera, for observation of the mare without her being aware of any intrusion. On the other hand, in less inclement weather, foaling outside at pasture or on the range may be quite acceptable, although supervision will necessarily be greatly reduced; however, environmental contamination will be minimal. Obviously, hazards such as ditches, rivers and large predators should be avoided.

Classically, labour is divided into three stages:

1. The stage of early uterine contractions leading to relaxation of the cervix. This is painful for the mare; she will often stop eating and show colic signs such as sweating and pawing the ground. She may even roll and repeatedly get up and down; repeated urination and defecation occur and there may be some milk let-down. The whole stage may last as long as 6 h, although the norm is <1 h. This stage ends when the cervix is wide open and cannot be detected on vaginal examination.

2. The stage of expulsion of the foal, where normally, but not always, the mare lies in lateral recumbency. The fetal membranes are ruptured, releasing the allantoic and amniotic fluids; if amnion, a white membrane covering the foal's nose, is present it should be pulled away. There are active abdominal contractions and the fetus is expelled with some considerable force, this stage normally lasting 20 min. Multiparous mares may complete stage 2 in 10 min, while the maiden mare may take up to 60 min. If the foal is covered in dark yellow fluid, the meconium, this is an indication that there has been a delay in delivery; special attention should be paid in such a case as it will need extra colostrum, having suffered hypoxia during delivery.

3. The stage of expulsion of the fetal membranes, when it is normal for the mare to show some colic signs at this time as the uterus contracts; the owner should be told about this eventuality. Extremely rare is the occurrence of either of the life-threatening problems of caecal rupture or large bowel torsion, which owners may have heard about. The owner must be briefed that these are extremely rare and, if present, would be discovered by the veterinarian on arrival. There is nothing they, or indeed the veterinarian, can do and so the owner should calmly lead the mare round if she is likely to go down and injure herself. The fetal membranes will be passed normally within 3 h, but if they are annoying the mare they should be tied up in a ball. The involution of the uterus in the normal mare is extremely rapid – it will have reduced to only 150% of its non-pregnant size within 12 h.

Problems

Premature placental separation

Often called a 'red bag delivery', the placenta separates prematurely and is pushed out through the vulva before the foal has broken out of its membranes. This is a genuine emergency, as the oxygen supply to the foal will immediately begin to be compromised. However, before cutting through the 'red bag', the clinician should make sure that this is in fact the separating fetal membranes, by feeling the foot or head actually contained within.

There is another condition occurring at parturition that may cause confusion – inversion of the mare's bladder. The foal will be lying ventral to this organ, and thus the clinician will be looking at the inner lining of the mare's bladder, which will appear very similar to the fetal membranes. However, it will not contain the fetus and in fact can quite easily be re-inverted and repositioned to allow normal foaling; no suturing is required. The condition will be unlikely to recur except at foaling, when strict monitoring will need to be carried out; it is better if the mare is not bred from again. Once again, I should emphasize that *one must not incise the bladder by mistake*.

Assuming that there is a true 'red bag' presentation, the foal should be drawn out by traction as quickly as possible, and resuscitated if necessary.

Fetal malpresentations

If only one foot and the head are seen from the vulva, or just the head or feet alone, an examination must be carried out immediately; this is even more urgent if there is evidence of a limb perforating the dorsal vagina and rectum. The clinician should carry out a full vaginal examination before applying any traction; relative fetal oversize does not occur in the mare, and therefore any delay might be a malpresentation.

'DOG-SITTING' PRESENTATION. Delay is particularly to be avoided with the rare 'dog-sitting' position, when the fetus will appear to have a normal presentation but foaling will cease, although the mare will continue to have abdominal contractions. Careful examination of the ventral aspect of the foal's thorax will reveal the two hind feet. Obviously, these could conceivably be the feet of a twin, but a 'dog-sitting' malpresentation is much more likely; if the feet belong to a twin, the fetus presenting first would be expelled without difficulty.

As soon as a 'dog-sitting' malpresentation has been confirmed, the clinician should grasp the cannons of the foal and try to repel it. In attempting to stop abdominal contractions, an assistant can grasp the mare's tongue, which prevents the mare closing her airway and thus building up pressure for these contractions. This can also be accomplished by passing a nasogastric tube into the trachea, although this is generally not recommended as the mare will cough violently, which is to be avoided. At the same time as repelling the foal, the clinician should work the two front legs vigorously; if there is still life in the foal it will kick out with its hind legs and can then be easily expelled. Even when the foal is dead, if the mare can be induced to stand up the foal's hind legs will drop with gravity, allowing delivery. If this cannot be accomplished, the clinician should reach under the thorax of the foal and slip two small, looped ropes over the two hind pasterns; traction can then be applied to these limbs to bring them into an extension position, i.e. the stifle, hock and fetlock will be in extension but not the hip. The foal can normally be drawn out, with considerable traction, in this position. If this fails, the clinician has two other options: the mare can be given a short-acting GA using romifidine and ketamine. The hind legs of the mare can then be hoisted and, with the aid of gravity and the relaxation of the mare, the clinician may be able to repel the hind limbs of the foal and accomplish delivery.

If this fails, the final alternative is fetotomy. To be used only in the event of a dead foal, a noose of embryotomy wire is placed around the body of the foal and threaded into the two tubes of the embryotome. Tension is maintained on the two ends of the wire as the embryotome is inserted under the thorax of the foal as far as possible into the groin; some traction is applied to the foal to achieve this and is maintained, as is the pressure on the embryotome while the wire is sawing to cut off the trunk of the foal as caudally as possible. When this has been accomplished it should be possible to put traction on the hind legs of the foal and reverse it, so that it is expelled in a posterior presentation.

With all such radical obstetrical procedures, the mare will require aggressive therapy, including antibiotics – both systemically and locally into the uterus – NSAIDs and uterine flushing with warm isotonic saline; the last mentioned will be required not only to clear the debris from the womb but also the fetal membranes, which will rarely be expelled naturally.

'Dog-sitting' foals are much rarer than other malpresentations, which are described below. However, such a malpresentation has been described first to emphasize the fact that the clinician *must examine* the foal carefully. Severe traction should *never* be applied to the mare via calving aids

ANTERIOR PRESENTATION. Ninety-eight per cent of normal deliveries are anterior presentations, with only 2% posterior. However, in dystocia cases the level of posterior presentations rises to 15%, as does that for transverse presentations. Anterior presentations in dystocia will have many manifestations:

- One foreleg is flexed at the carpus. This should be relatively easily corrected, by placing a thin rope on the pastern of the flexed leg, then pushing on the knee and pulling on the rope at the same time.
- One foreleg is aligned totally caudal from the shoulder. Sometimes it is possible to reach the carpus and draw that up to the flexed position and then correct, as outlined above. If this is not possible, in most cases the foal can be delivered with traction on the single leg and the head, provided the affected leg is kept straight along the foal's body.
- The two conditions described above may be found bilaterally; normally, flexion at the carpus of each leg can be corrected separately. It is very unlikely that a foal could be drawn with both legs backwards from the shoulders, and in this instance fetotomy will be required. The head and as much of the neck as possible should be removed with the embryotome, via a single cut, which will allow the practitioner more room to reposition the legs. Care must be taken drawing out the foal – if there are any sharp edges on the cut surfaces of the vertebrae these must not lacerate the walls of the vagina. Obviously, if the foal is alive another course of action needs to be undertaken. The mare is administered a short-acting anaesthetic, e.g. romifidine and ketamine. The mare's hind legs are lifted with shackles around the cannon bones so that the posterior half of the mare is off the ground, after which gravity and the relaxation of the mare will allow repositioning of the front legs and normal delivery. If the clinician runs out of time and only one leg has been repositioned, hopefully the foal will be able to be delivered with that one leg and the head, while leaving the other leg placed straight back down the body from the shoulder.
- There may be one or both legs in the nape position, i.e. the legs covering the crest of the neck. These must be repositioned, as there is a grave danger of one of the legs penetrating both the dorsal wall of the vagina and the rectum.
- The neck may be deviated in three different ways: (i) the head is deviated laterally and caudally; (ii) the neck is retroflexed ventrally; or (iii) the foal is upside down dorsopubically. In all three positions it is very unlikely that the clinician will be able to correct the situation. Therefore, if the foal is dead fetotomy should be carried out, cutting the neck as caudally as possible with a single cut of the embryotome. If the foal is alive, the mare is given an anaesthetic and

repositioning attempted, and if this cannot be accomplished a caesarean section is the next logical step.

POSTERIOR PRESENTATION. Posterior presentations in dystocia will also present several manifestations:

- If both legs are straight and presented with the hocks pointing towards the dorsum of the mare, the foal will just need some traction at the head, which normally stimulates the vagina in an anterior presentation with non-widened birth canal. Care should be taken to make sure that the tail of the foal is not sticking up vertically, which would impede progress.
- If one leg is flexed at the hock, this can normally be corrected by putting a thin rope around the pastern and then giving gentle traction while pushing the hock back into the mare at the same time. It is probably advisable for an assistant to provide the traction so that the clinician can push on the hock with one hand and cup the foot with the other, to make sure that the foot does not damage the floor of the vagina.
- One leg may be presented but the other back leg is totally flexed at the hip and in a cranial position; this will be very difficult to reposition without a GA. This presentation is termed a semi-breech.
- Both hind legs may be flexed at the hocks – this is extremely difficult to correct. If the foal is alive delivery should be attempted under a GA, with the hindquarters of the mare raised. If the foal is dead its hind legs should be sectioned just distal to the hocks; the foal can then be delivered, with little traction.
- Both hind legs may be flexed at the hips, with just the tail presented – this is the full breech position. If the foal is alive, correction should be attempted under a GA then raising the hindquarters of the mare and, if this is not successful, a caesarean section is the only way forward. If the foal is dead, an attempt should be made to draw one hock up into the pelvis of the mare; this leg is then sectioned as far proximally up the leg as possible, which hopefully will give more room in the pelvis to either draw the other leg into extension or pull the hock into the pelvis so that it can be sectioned just distal to the hock. The foal can then be delivered by traction on this one leg.

TRANSVERSE PRESENTATION. Dystocia is again a feature of this type of presentation. Although described in the old textbooks, this malpresentation is extremely rare but is nonetheless of great concern to the clinician. It is difficult to differentiate this condition from twins being presented concurrently, but careful palpation of the body of the foal will usually help in differentiation. Once again, a GA and raising of the hindquarters will help to reposition the foal. If all four limbs and the head are presented and appear to be equal, repulsion of the head and traction on the two hind legs will be the best option. However, if the forelegs and the head appear to be more engaged in the pelvis, the head – with a rope over the poll and inside the mouth, coupled with a rope over each front fetlock – should be used for traction.

Delivery of twins will require similar careful examination, regarding whether the twin in anterior presentation or that in posterior presentation should be delivered first.

FETAL ABNORMALITIES. The clinician will need to use all of his/her acquired knowledge to effect the best outcome in a dystocia case; help from another colleague should be sought if possible, although this may be difficult as most foalings occur at night. It is beyond the scope of this book to describe all the possible scenarios when the deformed foal is presented, but the most common are described:

- Schistosomus reflexus. The main concern of this presentation is that the clinician must make a very careful palpation of the foal and the vagina of the mare: it is vital that the intestines that will be palpated are known to be those of the foal and not those of the mare, which could be prolapsed through a tear in the uterus, cervix or vagina. In this latter instance the mare should immediately be destroyed. If the foal is discovered to be a case of schistosomus reflexus, fetotomy should be attempted. Normally, a single cut around the reflected trunk of the foal will allow delivery.
- Hydrocephalus. If the cranium is massively large and either the fetus cannot pass

through the pelvis or the mare will be damaged by its delivery, it just justifiable to crush the foal's head to allow delivery.
- Foals with very bent legs, fused joints or extremely contracted tendons may also cause problems.

Whatever the deformity, the clinician must use judgement if the foal is alive. It is unwise to compromise the health of the mare to deliver a live foal that has no chance of developing into a normal horse; such a foal should be euthanized with triple-strength barbiturate prior to fetotomy.

Problems with the mare

In the normal course of events, any problem with the mare should be discovered before service so that a pregnancy is not started. The mare that has been in a traumatic accident, e.g. being run over by a cart or motor vehicle or having fallen off a cliff, should be very carefully examined both externally and per rectum. If any obstruction is felt per rectum, such a mare should not be served. In the unfortunate event of a mare reaching term with such an obstruction, either the mare should be destroyed or, if the foal is alive, she could be given a short-acting GA to allow an abdominal delivery before she is euthanized. Caesarean section is unlikely to be an economical or humane option.

Induction of parturition

Induction of abortion

Embryos can be dislodged before 35 days following service by a single injection of prostaglandin: either 10 mg dinoprost tromethamine or 500 μg cloprostenol is suitable. Induction between 35 and 100 days following service is much harder: similar doses of prostaglandin are suitable but need to be repeated daily for 4 days. Later induction, up to 180 days, can be accomplished with a similar regime, although aborting such a size of fetus will be much more hazardous. Termination after 180 days should not be attempted until 330 days have been reached.

True induction of parturition

After 330 days a single dose of prostaglandin will induce parturition. Such a parturition should be fully monitored. Neither oxytocin nor corticosteroids should be used to induce parturition.

Epidural anaesthetic

Some authors advise its use for repositioning the foal but, on account of the time delay if the foal is alive, it should not be considered. However, if the foal is dead an epidural can be very useful. The area of the first intercoccygeal space should be clipped and surgically prepared, then 2 ml 2% lignocaine infiltrated as a skin bleb over the site with a small, 0.5 cm needle. Next, 2% lignocaine at 1 ml/100 kg is instilled with a 7.5 cm, 18G needle into the epidural space, the needle being directed vertically in a ventral direction.

Caesarean section

The difficulty in performing a caesarean section in the field is the provision of an adequate duration of GA without gaseous anaesthesia; possible solutions are given in Chapter 8. The need for a caesarean is limited, as other methods are normally available; however, if a caesarean is decided upon it should be performed in the following manner.

The mare is first placed in dorsal recumbency, then antibiotics and NSAIDs given i/v; the abdomen is then prepared for surgery in a fully aseptic manner. An incision is made in midline from the umbilicus to the cranial border of the mammary gland. The uterus is exteriorized and an incision made over one of the limbs of the foal, ideally the hind leg. The incision length is equivalent to the distance from the foot to the point of the hock, and is made on the greater curvature of the uterus, avoiding any major blood vessels; it is very important that the uterus is not torn. The foal must be lifted out carefully, trying if possible to prevent any fluids from spilling into the abdomen; this will require the surgeon and two assistants, who should all be scrubbed up and one of whom can then be in charge of resuscitating the foal. Time should be allowed for the placenta to contract, in order to allow the blood to return to the foal before the umbilicus is clamped close to the body and the cord cut 5 cm away. If possible, provided there is not a large amount of haemorrhage, the placenta is also removed; if this is not possible it should be removed from an area of at least 10 cm from the wound edges.

A continuous blanket suture is made around the uterine incision to prevent any haemorrhage from the cut edges. The uterus is next closed with a continuous layer of Lembert sutures; only a single row is required, provided sutures are placed close together. If the surgeon is in any doubt about closure, a second layer should be used. If the placenta is still in the uterus it is vital than none of the sutures includes it. As much blood and other debris as possible is removed from the abdomen and the uterus washed with warm isotonic saline. Next, oxytocin is injected i/v at this stage, before the linea alba is closed with a continuous layer of the strongest absorbable suture material available, doubled to give extra strength. A continuous subcuticular layer of sutures of absorbable material is then sewn, before the skin is closed with closely placed sutures of monofilament nylon. The placenta, if still in place, should be left until at least 6 h after recovery of the mare; removal can be attempted with either more oxytocin or uterine washes.

Once again, it must be stressed that, although a caesarean may be initially successful in the field, there are likely to be unacceptable risks associated with postoperative infection, particularly if the foal is dead; in this case fetotomy should be attempted, or euthanasia. Welfare must always be at the forefront of the practitioner's mind.

18.17 Postpartum Complications

Prolapse of the uterus

In this extremely rare event, ideally the mare will remain standing. She should not be sedated unless she is very fractious; an epidural is beneficial but not vital, so the clinician must use their judgement. The uterus must be supported by two helpers using a strong, clean sheet, and all debris carefully removed. The uterus is checked for tears, and if any are seen they must be repaired with Lembert sutures using absorbable material (i.e. the peritoneal surfaces of the uterus are apposed). Using a large amount of lubricant, the uterus is then reintroduced back into its correct position – this will not be difficult. Once back inside the abdomen, the clinician checks that total re-inversion has been accomplished and, provided this has been done successfully, there is no need for a vulval suture. Oxytocin will be given i/m, together with parenteral antibiotics and NSAIDs, which are to be continued for 5 days. At the same time the uterus needs to be irrigated with 2 l warm isotonic saline, as well as with antibiotics.

If the mare is recumbent, the uterus must be supported by two helpers while she is encouraged to stand; if she will not rise, an attempt is then made with a large amount of lubricant to replace the uterus, which will not be easy. Should this fail, the mare can be given a short-acting GA using romifidine and ketamine; she is next lifted with shackles around her hind cannons so that her pelvis is off the ground, when the uterus will easily be replaced from that position. A word of caution: this anaesthetic is short-acting, so any suturing and cleaning of the uterus must be carried out before anaesthesia; also, the shackles and winch have to be ready for immediate action.

Retained fetal membranes

Opinions are very diverse on this controversial subject, due to variation in veterinarians' perspectives. Ponies very rarely present a problem and, if they do have retained fetal membranes, the sequelae are rarely serious; the donkey is the same. However, at the other end of the spectrum, heavy horses often retain their fetal membranes, with removal in draught breeds being difficult; the sequelae to retained fetal membranes in draught breeds are life threatening. Standard-size horses, e.g. thoroughbreds and Arabs, fall between these opposing scenarios. Clinicians need to be cautious, but it is the owner that is likely to be unnecessarily apprehensive. A good compromise is to attend any mare which has foaled more than 6 h previously and failed to pass its fetal membranes; this duration may be shortened for draught breeds but lengthened for ponies and donkeys.

First, the mare's general health should be checked. Assuming there is no systemic illness, she is injected with oxytocin i/m, a reasonable dose being 10 IU/100 kg, although some authorities advise diluting this in 50 ml saline and giving it i/v; this may work better, although the mare may show more severe colic signs. Either way, in most cases apart from in draught breeds, the fetal membranes will be expelled within 30–60 min; if after this time they are still present, a small amount of traction should be applied, but not from within the vaginal canal.

If, after the foregoing, the membranes are still *in situ*, the clinician has two options: the current method is to flush the uterus with large amounts of warm saline (3 l for a pony or donkey, 5 l for a horse and 7 l for a draught horse) and then repeat the oxytocin injection. This process may be repeated until successful. The more old-fashioned method is to manually remove the membranes, which is particularly useful in draught breeds. The perineal area and the veterinarian's arms are thoroughly cleaned with warm chlorhexidine solution, and then one arm introduced into the vagina as far as the bifurcation of the horns of the uterus, while the other maintains tension on the fetal membranes by continually twisting them in one direction. The reason for reaching the bifurcation is to help inexperienced clinicians, as they may have a problem differentiating the membranes from the wall of the uterus; at the bifurcation the difference will be very apparent. The membranes are next continuously parted from the uterine wall by the straight fingers of the hand held together, in a similar manner to parting a Velcro® fastening. All the time the membranes are being twisted and kept in tension, but at no time are they being torn. Eventually, the membranes will be removed in their entirety, after which they are checked after being spread out on the ground. The uterus is then flushed with warm saline and antibiotics and the mare given further oxytocin.

In all methods the mare must be treated aggressively with parenteral antibiotics and NSAIDs. The tetanus status of the mare requires checking and correction accordingly.

Mastitis in the mare

Mastitis can occur in the mare during lactation and at weaning, and even in the non-pregnant mare. It is particularly serious in the draught mare, as these may develop a fatal toxic laminitis. Many different organisms may cause mastitis – *E. coli*, *Pseudomonas* spp., *Corynebacterium* spp., *Staphylococcus* spp. and *Streptococcus* spp.; the strangles bacillus, *Streptococcus equi*, will also cause mastitis. The mare will be ill with a fever and often reluctant to walk. The udder is inflamed and therefore will be hot, painful and enlarged, with accompanying oedema of the adjacent belly. The mare has four mammary glands with only two teats, each teat having two orifices; all four glands may be involved or fewer, in which latter case there will be asymmetry.

Treatment is by antibiotics and NSAIDs; culture is useful since, although the results will cause delay, treatment may be altered when the organism and sensitivity are both known. Clinicians should start with penicillin and gentamicin. Old textbooks suggest stripping the udder and instilling antibiotics into the mammary gland; this may not be appropriate, as it will be acutely painful to the mare and further contamination of an already inflamed udder may occur. The acute mastitis will subside rapidly, often leaving chronic scar tissue. If only one side is affected it is reasonable to allow further pregnancies, but if both sides are affected the mare should not be served again. In rare instances the gland will become gangrenous, with part of the udder sloughing and fly strike becoming a real danger; if the area of sloughing is large, it will never heal and the mare must be destroyed.

Clinicians may be confused with differential diagnosis, if a full history is not known, between chronic mastitis and neoplasia. The latter condition is extremely rare in the mare, although melanomas will occur in grey horses; these are normally well defined and encapsulated. Adenocarcinomas are extremely rare, but are very serious aggressive tumours that will spread to the inguinal lymph nodes very rapidly. Mastectomy is possible in the mare but is to be avoided, as the results are not good; euthanasia is the better course of action. Equine sarcoids will commonly occur in the inguinal region and be present on the mammary gland; they should be treated as described in Section 20.13.

Hypocalcaemia in the mare

A rare condition in the mare, it does not occur at the time of parturition but at peak lactation, i.e. at approximately 4 weeks post-foaling. The pathognomic sign is a synchronous diaphragmatic flutter, commonly called 'the thumps'. The mare will refuse food, gut sounds will be absent and rectal temperature will be subnormal. Treatment is by 400 ml warm 20% calcium borogluconate i/v; this should be given slowly; as it is irritant if given perivascularly, catheter placement is advisable. The response to treatment will be immediate, with the abolition of the synchronous diaphragmatic flutter and the return of appetite and gut sounds. Normally, further treatment is unnecessary.

Oestrus suppression

The requirement to suppress oestrus is extremely rare in working equines. Most methods have distinct disadvantages and are not recommended by most veterinarians as the practice is rarely indicated medically or surgically. An oral synthetic progestin altrengest called Regumate Equine is the only licensed treatment in the UK. It poses risks to pregnant women.

18.18 The Newborn Foal

Immediate postoperative care

Naturally, any foal born by caesarean section is going to be at higher risk, as are any foals born to mares that have required a GA to assist delivery. The cord must be clamped close to the body before cutting some 5 cm away – the cord must not be broken by tension. After ensuring that the foal is breathing, the umbilicus is dressed with chlorhexidine; foals should be held upside down if there are respiratory problems, to allow fluid to drain. Vigorous rubbing of the chest is helpful, as are flexing movements of the legs. Constantly rolling the foal from side to side is useful, to allow the lower lung to inflate. Ideally, the foal and mare are allowed to bond; however, if the mare is weak following anaesthesia, the foal requires thorough drying and being kept warm with hot-water bottles. Hot-air blowers should not be used to dry the foal, as these will cause the core temperature of the foal to drop by latent heat. Colostrum by stomach tube is next given, but the clinician should use judgement regarding the administration of antibiotics; if there is a definite risk of infection, they are to be given daily for a minimum of 5 days, but if there is no specific risk it is better not to administer them. The tetanus status of the foal must be ascertained, and tetanus antiserum administered if the foal does not receive colostrum with the appropriate antibodies.

Assessment of colostrum quality

Ideally, colostrum quality should be checked before the foal has sucked. Only a teaspoonful is required. It should be gently heated in a candle flame for a few seconds. This will cause good quality colostrum to clot.

More scientifically, colostrum should have a specific gravity of >1.060 and contain a minimum of 300 g/l of IgG. There are colostrometers available.

Examination of the foal

It should be remembered that there is no trans-placental immune globulin transfer, so the foal is immunologically naive at birth. It is vital that it receives colostrum within the first 6 hours of birth, ideally much earlier. It will take 2 weeks to produce an effective active humoral response. The foal should be examined comprehensively from both sides before individual parts are examined in detail and any asymmetry noted, particularly of the head and limbs. Starting at the head, the following checklist is recommended:

- The incisor teeth are examined for alignment.
- The mouth will be opened to check for any defects in the hard palate that would cause ingested milk to run down the nose. These must be given time, for if small they may heal; otherwise, euthanasia is required as large defects are inoperable.
- The eyes are checked both for problems of the eyelids and cataracts.
- The mucous membranes are checked for colour: very pale membranes indicate umbilical haemorrhage, while jaundiced membranes indicate neonatal haemolytic disease, as described in Section 14.10.

- The heart is auscultated.
- The limbs are carefully examined for deformities.
- The umbilicus should be checked for infection and herniation.
- The scrotum is checked for the presence of both testicles and for herniation.
- The inguinal area should be checked in filly foals for herniation.
- The tail is checked for damage.
- The anus is inspected for atresia ani.
- Ask the owner whether the meconium has been passed. It is also helpful if the owner has seen the foal urinate. Obviously, it is vital that the owner has seen that the foal is sucking regularly.

Neonatal maladjustment syndrome in the foal (NMS)

This is one of the most common diseases affecting the foal in the neonatal period. The disease has been given many names over the years, such as dummy foals, perinatal asphyxia syndrome (PAS), barker foals and wanderer foals. Historically, NMS has been attributed to hypoxic-ischaemic injury at around the time of foaling. Most commonly this occurs during the foaling process, when problems such as foetal malpresentation and premature placental separation cause delayed delivery and a reduction in blood supply to the foal. This is undoubtedly the underlying cause for some foals with the condition and is often easy to diagnose based on a history of a difficult delivery or prolonged dystocia.

However, the condition also occurs in foals that have had a seemingly normal delivery. In these foals it has been suggested that abnormal compression of the umbilical cord, or some other factor not visible externally, exists. In foals that have experienced a significant hypoxic episode, a complex cascade of events is initiated, including cellular energy failure, acidosis, glutamate release, intracellular calcium accumulation, generation of free radicals and, ultimately, cell death via necrosis or apoptosis.

A second round of cellular injury occurs after the primary event as a result of calcium influx, excitatory neurotoxins, inflammatory mediators and oxygen-free cells. The organs most commonly affected by hypoxia include the brain, kidneys and intestinal tract.

Most foals with NMS make a rapid and complete recovery within 2–5 days of supportive care. This suggests the condition in these foals is caused by a different aetiology. One author (Haggett, 2018) suggests that the condition should be split into two syndromes – PAS for foals that have experienced a hypoxic event, and NMS for foals that have no history or suspicion of birth hypoxia.

Recent evidence suggests that NMS occurs when foals fail to complete the normal birth transition process and don't fully adapt to extrauterine life. In some foals, this transition process starts normally and then falters. In a normal foal the hypothalamic–pituitary–adrenal (HPA) axis produces a large number of progestogen-based steroids that reach high concentrations shortly before foaling. It is proposed that high levels of these steroids at the time of foaling help suppress activity during parturition to prevent injury to the mare and foal. In foals with NMS, something goes wrong with this process.

NMS affects foals between 1 and 3 days of age. The most common signs are neurologic. These range from a foal that appears slightly slow to one experiencing uncontrollable seizures. Common signs include the loss of the suck reflex and poor teat searching. The diagnosis relies mainly on clinical signs.

The majority of foals with NMS will survive if given early and appropriate supportive care. Once foals have been allowed to develop secondary complications, such as sepsis, the survival rate decreases; thus, early supportive care is the key to successful treatment. Foals that have experienced a significant hypoxic injury are much more difficult to treat and can require the highest level of intensive care. Many foals can be managed on the farm.

The main aims of treatment are to maintain hydration, provide nutrition, prevent sepsis, encourage maternal bonding and control seizures or other neurologic signs. Many foals will benefit from maintenance i/v by fluid therapy with 5% dextrose (usually 3–6 ml/kg/hr). A small indwelling nasogastric tube can often be used to allow small, frequent feeding.

Enteral nutrition should be monitored very closely as not all foals will tolerate large volumes of milk. A good initial target is 10% of body weight.

Diazepam at 0.1–0.2 mg/kg i/v is the drug of choice to control seizures. It accumulates in the tissues and so Midazolam by continuous rate infusion 0.02 mg/kg/hr should be used if longer-term treatment is required. Good hygiene is required, with the foal in a warm environment in a small but separate box, close to the mare.

A technique called the Madigan Squeeze, or more properly squeeze-induced somnolence or the foal squeeze, has been developed over the last few years to recreate the physical pressure of the birth process. The idea behind this technique is the physical pressure of foaling is an important trigger in reducing progestogen concentrations. In some foals this leads to a dramatic and rapid improvement in their clinical signs. Basically, the foal is wrapped up like a parcel using a soft cotton rope. Further instructions can be found at https://bit.ly/2QK6uT7 (accessed 4 September 2023).

References and Further Reading

Aleman, M., Weich, K.M. and Madigan, J.E. (2017). Survey of veterinarians using a novel physical compression squeeze procedure in the management of neonatal maladjustment syndrome in foals. *Animals* 7: 69.

Carlson, G.P. (1987). Fluid and electrolyte dynamics in the horse. In: *Proceedings of the Annual Veterinary Medical Forum*, vol. 5. American College of Internal Medicine, San Diego, pp. 7–29.

Cognie, J., Freret, S., Lansade, L., Parias, C., Barriere, P. *et al.* (2023) Early castration in foals: Consequences on physical and behavioural developments. *Equine Veterinary Journal* 55: 214–221.

Crabtree, J. (2012a) Peripartum problems in mares, 1. Prepartum problems. *In Practice* 34(7): 400–410.

Crabtree, J. (2012b) Peripartum problems in mares, 2. Post-partum problems. *In Practice* 34(8): 462–471.

Duncanson, G.R. (2021) Thoughts on equine castration over a period of half a century. *Vet Times*, November: 8–9.

Duncanson, G.R. (2022) Foaling mares in the sticks, no big deal. *Vet Times* 52(14), 4 May: 14–15.

Haggett, E. (2018) Neonatal maladjustment syndrome in foals. *Vet Times* 48(39), 1 October.

Knottenbelt, D.C. and Malalana, F. (2015) *Equine Formulary*, 2nd edn. Elsevier Saunders, Maryland Heights, Missouri.

Knottenbelt, D.C., Pascoe, R.R., Lopate, C. and LeBlanc, M.M. (2003) *Equine Stud Farm Medicine and Surgery*. Elsevier Science, Philadelphia, Pennsylvania.

Rossdale, P.D., Mair, T.S. and Green, R.E. (eds) (2002) *Equine Veterinary Education Manual No. 5. Reproduction, Foaling, Part 1: Maternal Aspects*. Equine Veterinary Journal, Ely, UK.

Rossdale, P.D., Mair, T.S. and Green, R.E. (eds) (2003) *Equine Veterinary Education Manual No. 6. Reproduction, Foaling, Part 2: Fetal & Neonatal Aspects*. Equine Veterinary Journal, Ely, UK.

Samper, J.C., Pycock, J.F. and McKinnon, A.O. (2007) *Current Therapy in Equine Reproduction*. Saunders Elsevier, Philadelphia, Pennsylvania.

Sprayson, T. and Thiemann, A. (2007) Castration of donkeys. *In Practice* 29: 526–531.

19

Poisons

Abstract

This chapter describes the whole range of poisons which affect equines. New poisonous plants keep being found. Specific and supportive treatments are given.

19.1 Acorns

A horse is required to eat quite large quantities of acorns for poisoning to occur; this can occur on poor pasture in early autumn after a high wind. Certain animals develop a craving for green acorns, the main sign being colic. An impaction will be felt on rectal examination and the faeces will be very dry. The colic should be controlled with NSAIDs and liquid paraffin, and isotonic saline given by mouth.

19.2 Algae

Caused by high concentrations of blue-green algae in the drinking water, the acute form will kill a horse within 1 h. The presenting sign is cyanosis, but in the more chronic case there will be photosensitization and raised liver enzymes. Diagnosis is made by laboratory identification of algae. The treatment is supportive, including the obvious removal of the animal from contaminated water and providing clean water.

19.3 Amitraz

An acaricide commonly used for dipping and spraying cattle, it is toxic to horses. It normally causes an impaction, which can be felt on rectal examination, with resulting colic. Treatment is the same as for any other colic caused by an impaction (see Section 15.4).

19.4 Arsenic

Poisoning from arsenic can arise through either an inorganic or an organic source. The source for inorganic poisoning is either rat bait or acaricide, the principal sign being severe dysentery. Diagnosis can be confirmed by analysis of the ingesta, liver or kidney. There is a specific treatment other than obvious supportive therapy, i.e. sodium thiosulfate at the rate of 3 mg/kg daily. However, the mode of administration is contentious: in other species it can be given i/m, but this causes massive swelling in the horse, which may even be life threatening; very slow i/v injection is the method of choice in the equine, as oral

DOI: 10.1079/9781800624283.0019

administration is not effective. The organic source is pig growth promoters; organic poisoning has a slower onset compared with acute inorganic poisoning and shows neurological signs. There is no specific treatment.

19.5 Avocado

Horses may become addicted to this fruit, which will then cause diarrhoea. Another feature that will be observed is oedema of the lips and tongue. Treatment is symptomatic only.

19.6 Bracken

Not normally eaten by the horse unless starving, this common plant causes chronic poisoning, evident as muscle weakness and other neurological signs. The specific antidote is vitamin B_1 (thiamine), which is given i/m daily at 1 mg/10 kg.

19.7 Cantharidin

Blister beetles (*Epicauta* spp.) swarm on to lucerne during harvesting; these secrete the terpenoid cantharidin, which is very toxic to the horse. Cantharidin causes acute colic with diarrhoea, with shreds of mucosa being seen in the faeces; it also causes haematuria. The horse will die unless stabilized through an isotonic saline drip.

19.8 Carbamates

Carbamates are commonly in use as both herbicides and insecticides and can cause poisoning in horses. The signs and treatment are as for organophosphorus poisoning, described in Section 19.31.

19.9 Castor Bean

Although sometimes included in horse feed, this will cause diarrhoea in the horse so its inclusion in the diet should be avoided.

19.10 Chlorinated Hydrocarbons

These insecticides and acaricides are very potent poisons in the horse; they cause nervous signs from overstimulation of the CNS. There are no specific antidotes and supportive treatment is rarely effective.

19.11 Copper

Copper poisoning in the horse is extremely rare, but may be seen when fed copper-supplemented pig feed. The main sign is jaundice, and if this is evident the outcome is fatal. There is no antidote.

19.12 Cyanide

Although this poison could potentially be ingested by the horse when used in the inorganic form as a rodenticide, this is not the normal type of poisoning seen. Many plants such as linseed, flax, wild black cherry, sorghum and Sudan grass contain cyanogenetic glycosides, which can be released by damage to the plants through herbicides or wilting. The main signs are bright red mucous membranes and severe asphyxia convulsions, followed by death; the blood will appear bright red on post-mortem. Tests for hydrocyanic acid can be performed on the stomach contents to confirm the diagnosis. Treatment is specific: 660 mg/kg sodium thiosulfate should be given per os hourly until the horse improves.

19.13 Deadly Nightshade

The Latin name for this plant, which is found in hedgerows in the UK, is *Belladonna atropina*. The signs of poisoning are that of atropine overdose, i.e. enlarged pupils and ileus. The specific antidote is neostigmine at 0.01 mg/kg given s/c; ileus should be treated with flunixin i/v and isotonic saline by stomach tube.

19.14 Ergot

A toxin occurring in a parasitic plant fungus that grows on various grain crops worldwide;

however, the main sign of gangrene of the extremities is seen only in cold climates; abortion will also occur. There is no specific treatment; nevertheless, the condition is usually noticed early enough for the diet to be corrected and the horse to recover.

19.15 Fluoride

Factory contamination of pasture with this element can cause chronic poisoning in the horse. There is marked excessive wearing of the teeth, together with some enlargement of the long bones and the mandible. There are increased levels of fluorine in the urine and plasma. Obviously, the horse should be removed from the contaminated pasture; feeding of calcium carbonate (chalk) will reduce fluoride levels in the gut contents.

19.16 Foxglove

Digitalis purpurea is the Latin name for this common flower. The signs of poisoning are those of digitalis overdose, i.e. bradycardia, cyanosis and collapse. In the event of collapse, a 500 kg horse should be given lidocaine i/v at the rate of 30 μg/min as a one-off injection; following ingestion of only a limited amount of foxglove causing bradycardia, give a 500 kg horse 25 g potassium by stomach tube.

19.17 Hemlock

Found in ditches, this plant is rarely eaten by the horse except after ditch clearance; it contains a very potent alkaloid. Ingestion causes severe nervous signs, staggering and dilated pupils, with death occurring from respiratory depression. There is no specific antidote. However, like all alkaloids, some authors report successful treatment with tannic acid or acetic acid.

19.18 *Kalmia*

An ornamental flowering shrub found in gardens in the UK, ingestion causes acute gastritis and colic. The pain may be controlled with morphine and an alpha-2 agonist. Atropine will aid recovery by reducing the massive amount of saliva produced.

19.19 *Lantana*

Another flowering shrub, found in the wild as well as in gardens. Ingestion causes chronic liver damage, with resulting jaundice and photosensitization. Treatment is with vitamin B and keeping the animal out of direct sunlight.

19.20 Laurel

Only when cut will laurel be eaten by the horse, and quite large amounts need to be ingested before the severe symptoms similar to those of cyanide poisoning (Section 19.12) are seen.

19.21 Lead

Mining contamination of pasture is the reason for this heavy metal poisoning, normally seen in the chronic form in the horse. The main sign is stiffness, which may appear to have an acute onset following exercise, reminiscent of rhabdomyolysis (see Section 12.11). Raised lead levels will be found in both blood and urine. The specific treatment is calcium edentate given i/v; however, this is rarely necessary if the horse is removed from the contaminated pasture and given NSAIDs.

19.22 Linseed

Often included as an oil in animal feed, ingestion causes diarrhoea in the horse and its use should be avoided. There is no specific antidote.

19.23 Lupin

Plants commonly found in hedgerows and gardens, they also are grown commercially as nitrogen-fixing plants, to improve soil fertility; the seeds contain a poisonous alkaloid. The main sign is inappetence, and so the poisoning is self-limiting provided the animal is kept quiet.

19.24 Mare's Tail

Hippuris vulgaris is the Latin name of this very common weed, which is very toxic if ingested; however, it is not palatable and is eaten only by the starving horse. Signs of poisoning include ataxia and convulsions. The specific antidote is thiamine (vitamin B_1), although care should be taken with i/v administration, as deaths have been reported. Provided that the vitamin is not in combination with other B vitamins (which are very irritant), it can be given i/m at the rate of 100 mg daily for a 500 kg horse.

19.25 Mercury

Mercury is used in seed dressings, and the horse may eat the seed as food. Red Blister ointment contains mercury and can be licked by the animal, so should not be used. The main sign is diarrhoea, which should be treated symptomatically

19.26 Metaldehyde

A lethal poison found in slug and snail baits, it is often spread on the ground surrounding crops, and the horse is liable to be poisoned by spillage of this palatable substance. The presenting signs are neurological: convulsions can occur and, although these can be controlled by anaesthetizing the animal, they normally recur on recovery from the GA. There is no antidote.

19.27 Monensin

Occurring only if cattle feed containing monensin (used as a growth promoter) is fed to horses, it is extremely toxic and will cause total collapse and death from cardiac failure. Treatment is unrealistic, but oral vitamin E has been recommended.

19.28 Mycotoxins

Poisoning results from the ingestion of food contaminated with toxins produced by fungi; they may be found in a variety of foodstuffs, although the horse is rarely affected. The main toxin is ergot, described in Section 19.14; another is found in perennial ryegrass (Section 19.36); a third is found in sweet clover (Section 19.40).

19.29 Nitrate

Although this fertilizer rarely causes poisoning, it is advisable not to put horses onto treated pasture until rain has fallen following spreading of the fertilizer. It has a bitter taste, and horses will not willingly eat it. The signs are those of vasodilation, similar to shock, i.e. a weak, rapid pulse and low rectal temperature; there may be haemoglobinuria and petechial haemorrhages, and the blood is said to appear chocolate brown. Treatment is specific: slow i/v injection of 1% methylene blue at the rate of 5 mg/kg.

19.30 Oleander

A very toxic garden plant, it will be eaten by the horse only as cut prunings. It causes sudden death; there is no treatment.

19.31 Organophosphorus Compounds

These insecticides are very potent poisons, their acute toxicity being due to cholinergic overstimulation. This is evident as neurological signs – the horse is very nervous and constantly urinates; there is copious salivation and constricted pupils. Treatment is specific, with atropine sulfate at 0.2 mg/kg given slowly i/v; this may be repeated at 3 h intervals until signs subside.

19.32 Paraquat

A common weedkiller that is very toxic to the horse; there is no antidote. Death is relatively rapid, within 6–8 h, and is the result of massive pulmonary oedema.

19.33 Propylene Glycol

Used as antifreeze for motor vehicles as well as being given to cattle with ketosis, this oily chemical is toxic to the horse and causes diarrhoea. If the horse appears to be staggering, it should be dripped with isotonic saline with added sodium bicarbonate.

19.34 Ragwort

Found throughout Europe, this plant is not eaten by the horse except when in cut form; however, in equines it is a very common toxin, causing chronic liver damage. Diagnosis is made by finding elevated liver enzymes in the blood. The animal should be denied access to any more ragwort and placed on a low-protein diet; vitamin B injections may help. Prevention is vital: ragwort should be dug up from the pasture; the toxin can be adsorbed through the skin, so rubber gloves should be worn when pulling up the plant.

19.35 Rhododendron

Horses rarely eat this poisonous plant. Signs will be those of colic with excessive salivation. Treatment is with morphine at 10 mg/100 kg given i/v at the same time as sedation with an alpha-2 agonist. Atropine can also be given at 0.2 mg/kg, slowly i/v. The prognosis is good.

19.36 Ryegrass

Caused by an endophytic fungus, poisoning triggers neurological signs, mainly stiffness. Exercise will make the condition much worse, so the horse should be walked off the offending pasture. Improvement will be quite rapid, i.e. within 3–4 days, without any treatment required.

19.37 St John's Wort

Rarely causing poisoning in the horse, ingestion of this marshland plant damages the liver. The first sign will be photosensitization, so the animal should be kept out of the sun and removed from the marshy area. Vitamin B injections may be helpful, and the horse should be put on a low-protein diet.

19.38 Selenium

In the horse selenium poisoning normally takes the chronic form as a result of eating herbage containing very high levels of the chemical. The first signs are loss of mane and tail hair, with cracking of the feet. Animals will totally recover when removed from the selenium-rich diet.

19.39 Sodium Chlorate

An old-fashioned weedkiller, this rarely causes poisoning as it has a bitter taste that the horse does not like. It has been reported to cause severe depression. There is no specific treatment, so supportive therapy is recommended.

19.40 Sweet Clover

Resulting in poisoning only when the plant has been spoiled or made into hay, haylage or silage, fungal spores convert the natural, harmless coumarins within to dicoumarol, which interferes with the clotting mechanism. Haemorrhages are seen on the mucous membranes, though haematoma is rare in the horse. Normally, treatment is not required in horses, although a dose of 1.1–3.3 mg/kg of vitamin K1 given i/m has been suggested.

19.41 Sycamore

This toxicity is an important cause of death in horses in the UK. It normally occurs in the spring at pasture when the seedlings are abundant. However, the toxin, Hypoglycin A has been found in sycamore seedlings despite mowing, herbicidal spraying or storage in hay or silage (Gonzalez-Medina *et al.*, 2019). Toxicity can occur in a single animal in a group. It is not known whether it is because a single animal is attracted to the seedlings or whether certain individuals are more sensitive. The clinical signs are an acute myopathy which is called atypical as violent exercise is not required to trigger the muscular damage. The horses soon become recumbent. There is no specific treatment and, as yet, supportive treatments have not been successful if the animal has become recumbent. Euthanasia is required immediately to alleviate further suffering. Naturally, all other equines should be removed from the pasture.

19.42 Warfarin

A common ingredient of rat poison, the horse needs to eat very large amounts before the classic sign of haemorrhage in the mucous membranes is seen. Treatment is the same as for sweet clover poisoning (Section 19.40).

19.43 Yew

As this is an extremely poisonous plant, the horse needs consume very little of the foliage or berries before death ensues. However, the horse will not eat from the live tree – the danger lies in clippings from yew hedges. Poisoning is normally peracute, with the horse found either dead or totally collapsed. There is no realistic treatment.

References and Further Reading

Forsyth, A.A. (1954) *British Poisonous Plants*. Her Majesty's Stationery Office, London.

Gonzalez-Medina, S., Montesso, F., Chang, Y.-M., Hyde, C. and Piercy, R.J. (2019) Atypical myopathy-associated hypoglycin A toxin remains in sycamore seedlings despite mowing, herbicidal spraying or storage in hay and silage *Equine Veterinary Journal* 51(5): 701–704.

20

Skin Conditions

Abstract
The whole manifestation of equine skin disease is discussed, including diagnosis, long-term treatment and client-management problems. The mantra of 'pruritus think parasites' is stressed.

20.1 Introduction

The diagnosis of skin disease in the horse often presents a real challenge to the practitioner. One problem is that the condition is often of long standing, allowing ample opportunity for self-inflicted injury and secondary infection. In addition, the owner has probably applied all manner of potions. However, every skin disease should be taken seriously; the lesion may look trivial, but it is important to the owner and it may be a disaster waiting to happen. A good history is vital:

- How old is the horse?
- How long has the horse had the condition?
- Has the condition changed?
- Are other horses affected?
- What treatment has already been used?
- Is the animal itchy? (Curnow, 2020)

There is rarely a quick fix with skin conditions, particularly if they are of long standing. Always have a treatment plan and do not be afraid to take samples and photographs to obtain further advice. It is always best to obtain this advice from specialists who you know or who have been recommended to you, as there is likely to be follow-up dialogue. Client management is vital, because treatment options may be prolonged and compliance is very important. Investigation of equine dermatological disease can present challenges, but relevant diagnostic techniques are relatively inexpensive and should be considered early in the disease course prior to potential inappropriate, expensive treatment.

20.2 Aids to Diagnosis

One of the most useful aids is to brush the feathers into a Petri dish and examine the brushings under the low-power microscope. Parasites, particularly *Chorioptes equi*, are easily observed. Skin scraping needs to be deep to detect some mites, e.g. *Sarcoptes scabiei* var. *equi*, *Psoroptes ovis* var. *equi* and *Demodex equi*. Gram staining is useful to visualize bacteria, particularly from an impression smear. The clinician has to be careful to differentiate between primary and secondary bacteria, as well as contaminants; that is why bacterial culture is rarely worthwhile. It might be considered that a biopsy, which is easily taken with either a 4 mm or 6 mm punch, is the ultimate

2nd Edition (G.R. Duncanson)
DOI: 10.1079/9781800624283.0020

diagnostic tool; however, the actual sample needs taking with care to sample some normal skin as well as diseased tissue. Also, the pathologist needs to have a full history and photographs to really help the practitioner. A needle aspirate is safer for diagnosis of nodules, as punch biopsies may aggravate equine sarcoids. If pruritus is a prominent sign, the practitioner should consider parasites in the first instance. Parasites can act either as irritants in their own right or as allergens, setting up sensitivity reactions.

20.3 Mange Mites

Chorioptes equi

Termed leg mange as the mite is not found above the carpus or tarsus, this is the most common type of mange in the horse. Some parasitologists consider it to be the same species as *Chorioptes bovis* and *Chorioptes caprae*, though clinicians should be aware that there may be cross-over with the host species. Pruritus can be so intense that the horse is continuously stamping its feet, although intensity is not controlled by the number of mites. Often a horse, with millions of mites brushed off into a Petri dish, will show little irritation and yet its neighbour having only a few mites will be very itchy. Leg mange will often start off an attack of pastern dermatitis, which will then develop a bacterial infection. Leg mange can be controlled with regular 10-day i/m injections of doramectin at a dose rate of 1 ml of 1% solution/33 kg. It may also be treated topically with benzyl benzoate applied all over all four legs, to include the carpus and the tarsus, every 10 days after they have been clipped to the knees and to the hocks. In some cases this will be extremely painful. Pain relief and sedation will be required. The legs should be washed in a good equine shampoo before. If benzyl benzoate has not been a successful treatment then Lime Plus Dip, a sulfurous washing concentrate diluted with two parts water, can be used. Gloves should be worn by the person washing the legs. It should be repeated monthly. A more modern topical treatment would be a 0.25% solution of fipronil applied over the same area twice, at 10-day intervals. A further treatment suggested is daily washing of the legs with a diluted solution of 5% cypermethrin, which should be carried out for a minimum of 10 days. It is very important to remember to treat all the animals in the group. French workers (Kondratjeva *et al.*, 2023) carried out a meta-analysis on various treatments and they agreed that several treatments were partially effective, but that further comparisons are required.

Sarcoptes scabiei var. *equi*

The most severe mange infection in the horse is caused by this mite; however, it is extremely rare. It occurs all over the body and causes very severe irritation. The mites are often hard to see unless a deep skin scrape is taken. There are invariably secondary bacteria involved and, although their treatment with a prolonged course of a suitable antibiotic is important, the condition will never be cured until every mange mite is dead. The affected horse should receive regular doramectin i/m injections every 10 days at the dose rate of 1 ml of 1% solution/33 kg. In long-standing cases where there is chronic thickening of the skin, this treatment should be supplemented by painting on a 1:1 mixture of 0.5% eprinomectin and dimethyl sulfoxide (DMSO) at 10-day intervals to the severely thickened areas of skin.

Psoroptes ovis var. *equi*

A very rare mite and not as irritant as either *Chorioptes* or *Sarcoptes*, it can be found all over the body, but it favours sheltered parts, e.g. under the tail or forelock or even behind the fetlock. The mite is a surface dweller, so doramectin injections are not effective. Topical applications to affected parts every 10 days of either benzyl benzoate or fipronil are effective, as is daily cypermethrin. Various old-fashioned – but extremely toxic and environmentally unfriendly – chemicals, such as lime sulfur, toxaphene and lindane, were formerly effective in the treatment of all the mange mites discussed above; however, these have all been banned in most countries. The most effective replacement wash available contains selenium sulfide.

Demodex equi

Although these mites live in the hair follicles and sebaceous glands, they can be found in horses not showing any sign of skin disease. However, they very occasionally appear in very large numbers with an accompanying staphylococcal infection, the treatment of which has to be addressed with both parenteral and topical antibiotics. The mite can be eliminated with formamidine washes, the only one readily available being amitraz; *however, great care must be taken if using this medication* (see Section 19.3).

Ear mites

It should be stressed that the horse is *not affected by ear mites.*

20.4 Lice

There are two types of lice seen on horses, both capable of causing intense irritation. The constant rubbing will show as hair loss and eventually infection of the skin with secondary bacteria (see Fig. 20.1). Certain individuals seem to be more susceptible, particularly if affected with another disease or malnutrition. Both species, *Damalinia equi* (the biting louse) and *Haematopinus asini* (the sucking louse), are readily controlled by topical insecticides, e.g. 5% cypermethrin. This needs to be repeated at 10-day intervals, as the eggs are not killed by the chemical. Injectable doramectin is effective only against the sucking louse. Pour-on ivermectin preparations, available for cattle, should not be used in the horse as they will damage the skin and cause permanent hair loss; oral ivermectin preparations are not effective against lice.

20.5 Ticks

Throughout the world there are many species of tick capable of infesting the horse. They can be divided into two types: the Argasidae (soft ticks) and Ixodidae (hard ticks). All have four developmental stages: egg, larva, nymph and adult. Not only are the ticks species specific, but so too are

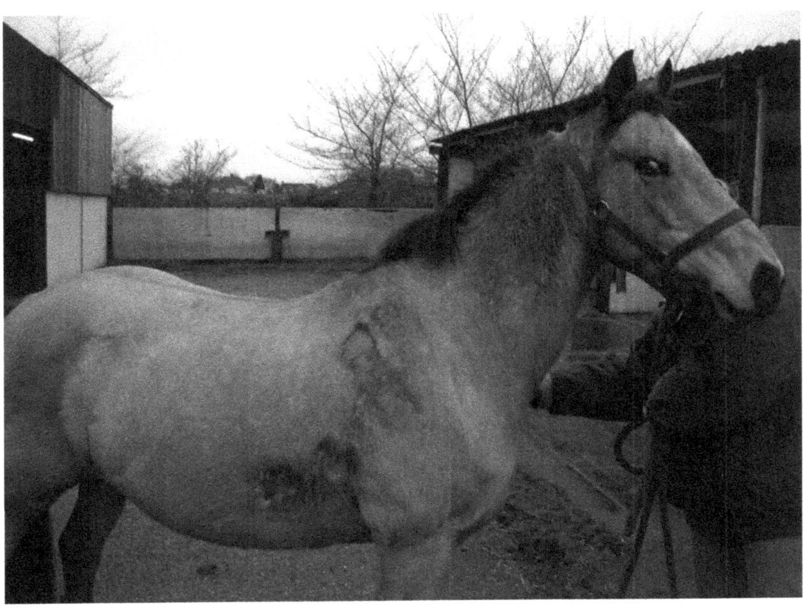

Fig. 20.1. Self-trauma resulting from louse infestation.

the different developmental stages; on the other hand, some tick species may prefer certain hosts but are very adaptable and colonize many mammalian hosts. Soft ticks very rarely infest horses, unless they are kept in close proximity to pigs in the tropics; however, hard ticks are a very serious problem in the horse, causing debilitation from blood loss, irritation with accompanying skin disease and spreading of numerous diseases. There are over 650 species of hard tick living off many different hosts that are not always mammalian. Most species have a three-host life cycle, some only a two-host and a very few have a single host. Obviously, the last of these are easier to control, except that resistance to an acaricide can build up more rapidly. Different species prefer different sites on the body, and these may vary between the immature and adult forms.

The following tick genera may be found on the horse:

- *Amblyomma maculatum* is a particular problem in horses in tropical and semi-tropical areas of North and South America; *Amblyomma hebraeum*, *Amblyomma variegatum* and *Amblyomma lepidum* are all parasitic in sub-Saharan Africa.
- *Boophilus kohlsi* is parasitic for horses in the Middle East.
- *Dermacentor nitens* is found in horses' ears in tropical areas of the Americas; *Dermacentor marginatus*, *Dermacentor reticulatus* and *Dermacentor silvarum* are found on horses in both Europe and Asia.
- *Hyalomma anatolicum* causes severe problems for horses in Asia; *Hyalomma scupense* is seen in Eastern Europe and Russia.
- *Ixodes ricinus* is found on horses in the UK, continental Europe, North Africa, and North and South America.
- *Margaropus winthemi* lives on zebra and horses in southern Africa.
- *Rhipicephalus sanguineus* and *Rhipicephalus appendiculatus* are both rarely found on the horse, the former worldwide and the latter in Africa.

Ticks can be controlled on equines with organophosphates and chlorinated hydrocarbons; however, in many countries their use has been banned. Natural pyrethrins and the synthetic pyrethroids are safer and fairly effective if applied twice weekly, or more often in very rainy weather.

20.6 Other Skin Parasites

Trombiculid mites

Although free-living, these will infest the horse's legs and cause severe irritation. As the name suggests, *Trombicula autumnalis* is seen in the autumn (fall) in the UK; it can, in fact, cause problems from June onwards, but it is killed by the first frosts. It is the six-legged larva that causes the irritation, biting firmly into the skin, so a very deep skin scraping is required for diagnosis. *Trombicula alfreddugesi* is seen in the Americas and Africa, though normally associated with poultry.

Dermanyssus gallinae

The poultry mite will also cause intense irritation on the horse. It lives in the wooden parts of the stable or hen house and feeds mainly at night, but some authorities have found it feeding during daylight hours.

20.7 Flying Insects

All the insects listed below may cause varying degrees of pruritus (see Fig. 20.2).

Stable fly

Little bigger than *Musca domestica*, the housefly, the most notable stable fly is *Stomoxys calcitrans*. It is difficult to control, as it only feeds once or twice daily. The numbers can be radically reduced by removing the dung pile from the proximity of the stable. They will cause an urticarial reaction in certain individuals (see Section 20.8).

Horsefly

Although bigger and are more aggressive than the stable fly, both *Chrysops* spp. (deer flies) and

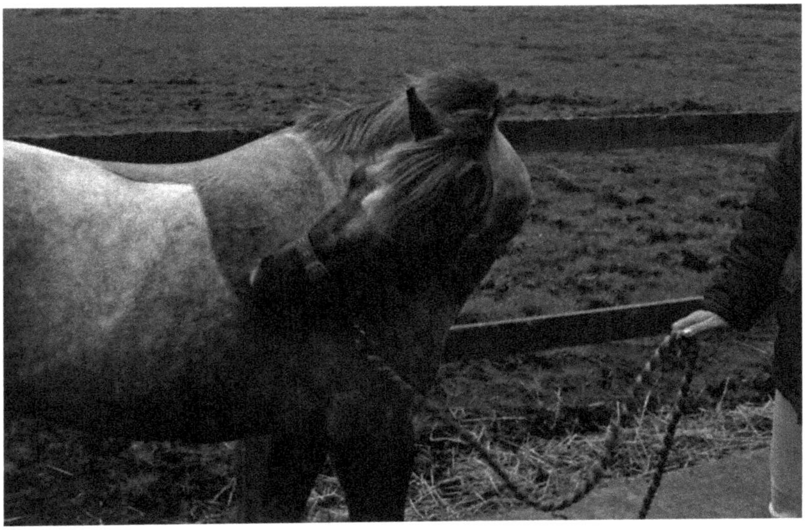

Fig. 20.2. Insect worry: acute pruritus resulting from flying insects.

Tabanus spp. cause large weals on the horse, potentially leading to more permanent lumps, particularly in the saddle area, called eosinophilic granulomata (see Section 20.8).

Blackfly

These flies will cause intense irritation to the horse but do not cause any other reactions; they are found worldwide. The most notable is *Simulium colombaschense*, which is found in the Danube valley in Europe. Survival of larvae requires fast-flowing water.

Tsetse fly

Mercifully, these flies are restricted to tropical Africa. As they spread trypanosomiasis (see Section 6.4), which is a fatal disease of equines, any localized damage is the least of the horse owner's worries. The bite is very painful, sometimes leading horses to stampede.

Bot fly

Although not actually causing any skin lesions, *Gasterophilus intestinalis* will lay a large number of eggs on the horse's skin. The horse then ingests these, which hatch into larvae in the stomach; after feeding in the stomach, larvae pass through the intestine and pupate on the soil, after which the adult then emerges and the life cycle is complete. There are two other species, the nose bot (*Gasterophilus haemorrhoidalis*) and the throat bot (*Gasterophilus nasalis*), the larvae of which bore into the tongue and buccal mucosa and will be seen when carrying out dental procedures. The best method of control is to kill the larvae in the stomach with oral ivermectin. It should be noted that, although moxidectin is claimed to kill bot fly larvae, the kill rate is not high and many survive. Regular grooming of horses helps remove bot fly eggs and thus prevent infection. In temperate climates frost will kill the adult flies, so the species has to survive as larvae in the stomach; therefore, if oral ivermectin is given after the first frost in winter the larvae will be killed and there will be no flies the following summer. Obviously, this does not occur in the tropics or subtropics.

Sandfly

As the name implies, these flies need damp sand in which to pupate. They cause constant worry to the horse, particularly around wounds; their saliva appears to delay wound healing, and so it is vital they are controlled. They are rarely recorded in temperate climates but are common in specific areas in the tropics and subtropics. Wounds should be covered or smeared with an oily cream containing acriflavin and benzyl hexachloride (BHC).

Horn fly

Attacking mainly horned ruminants, these flies are found throughout the world; however, they will also attack horses when kept in close proximity to cattle. *Haematobia irritans* seems to be the most damaging. Normal pyrethrin fly repellents are very effective for the horse; it should be noted that 'spot-on' treatments used in cattle are not suitable for horses, as the skin will be damaged.

Warble fly

Basically bovine parasites, these flies have been eliminated from the UK. They lay their eggs on the legs of cattle, the eggs hatch and the larvae then bore through the skin and travel for 9 months through the tissues to reach the deep layers of the skin on the back. The larvae emerge and pupate on the ground, the adults emerge and the life cycle is complete. Elimination in the UK has been achieved by strict treatment of all cattle with an appropriate insecticide in the spring before larval emergence. If the eggs are laid on a horse, the larvae may travel through the tissues to the back but, as the horse is not the natural host, they will form a calcified nodule and the life cycle is broken. There are two species parasitic for domestic animals, *Hypoderma bovis* and *Hypoderma lineatum*, both occurring in North America, Europe, North Africa and Asia.

Screw-worm

There is considerable confusion in the terminology of this worm in various parts of the world. They are known in North and South America as the larvae of a particular blowfly, *Cochliomyia hominivorax*, which is an obligate myiasis-causing parasite. This has been eliminated in the USA by rigid control methods using now-banned insecticides. There is a similar parasite, *Chrysomya bezziana*, found in Africa and Asia. Treatment is described under cutaneous myiasis, below.

Cutaneous myiasis

Occurring mainly in wool sheep, animals are attacked by blowfly larvae. In the sheep, *Lucilia sericata* is the most important blowfly in Europe and Australasia, the larva being termed the primary striker; there are also secondary strikers, e.g. *Phormia terra-novae* and *Calliphora erythrocephala*. There are no primary strikers in the horse. Larvae of all these species and the species of screw-worm described above require a wound before they will attack a horse or donkey, particularly if wounds remain untreated; except in the very debilitated animal, clean wounds are not attacked. However, larvae will be seen in hooves that have not been picked out, in wet conditions; they will not penetrate intact hoof. Treatment should be carried out urgently on all wounds to prevent cutaneous myiasis or, as it is commonly called 'fly strike'. In the animal with myiasis the surrounding hair is clipped away – this is particularly important in the donkey – and the wound washed vigorously with clean water; the use of a hose is particularly recommended. Any maggots remaining are removed, using forceps if necessary. The wound should be treated in the normal manner. If organophosphorus wound powder is available, this is to be dusted on; however, in countries where such powder has been banned the wound and surrounding area should be dressed with ointment containing benzene hexachloride (BHC) and acriflavin; this is marketed as 'summer fly cream'.

Mosquito

There are more than 300 species of mosquito found worldwide, the best-known being *Anopheles* sp., which spreads malaria in humans. Mosquitoes in large numbers will disturb horses. They transmit equine encephalomyelitis and West Nile fever. Diethyltoluidine is the only effective repellent, and that is effective for only 6 h under dry conditions.

Culicoides

There are over 80 species of these so-called gnats or midges worldwide. Their saliva causes a very bad hypersensitivity reaction in certain individuals, there being a genetic predisposition. The disease syndrome is called 'sweet itch' in the UK, 'Queensland itch' in Australia and many other names elsewhere. A better name is insect bite hypersensitivity (IBH), or recurrent seasonal dermatitis. In the UK, midges bite only during the warmer months of the year, but in hotter climates they bite all year round. The expected sites for the midges to bite are the mane and tail, but if these parts are denied to the insects some species will bite elsewhere, so that the horse may itch on its belly or head. Often, the animal will have been itching for some time, so the entire mane and tail hair will have been rubbed off; the skin may also be broken and a secondary infection established. It is vital to stop insects from actually biting the animal.

Culicoides *sensitivity*

A sensitivity reaction to *Culicoides* is particularly strong in certain individuals and appears to be inherited. It certainly is a welfare problem if it is not controlled. Treatment options are many and, on the whole, ineffective, and can be divided into treatments that prevent the insects biting the horse, treatments that desensitize the horse and treatments that lessen the reaction of the horse. The ultimate treatment is complete separation of insects from the horse, which is, in the main, impossible; the best option is the 'Boette' rug, an extremely fine-meshed rug that covers the horse totally excepting holes for its legs, anus and mouth. In most cases this is effective; other 'fly rugs' are useless. The midges tend to bite at dawn and dusk, so housing the horse at these times is largely ineffectual as the midges will fly inside unless there is very small-gauge netting over all the windows and doors, which makes the building unbearably hot. *Culicoides* are not good fliers, so wind is a deterrent. High-speed fans are useful, while fly repellents are generally ineffective, the only effective example being N,N-diethyl-meta-toluamide (DEET). Unfortunately, this is really only effective for 6 h under dry conditions, even less in rainy conditions, and so is therefore impracticable. Thick, oily preparations like benzyl benzoate can be helpful if smeared copiously over the bitten areas, but these are extremely messy and their application has to be frequent.

Desensitization of the horse requires expensive laboratory preparation after a blood sample has been submitted. A desensitizing injectable preparation is prepared, which then has to be injected into the horse, initially very frequently but eventually at longer intervals. This laboratory preparation is expensive and results are very variable. There are various products available containing certain fatty acids and amino acids which, it is claimed, help lessen the reaction if given before and throughout the likely period of exposure.

Last I will discuss medications that actually treat the reaction seen in the horse. As the condition is so pruritic, there is a large amount of self-mutilation, which in itself will cause more histamine release and secondary infection. Infection can be controlled by antibiotics, but the irritation is much harder to control; the drug of choice is dexamethasone, but long-term use will be extremely hazardous on account of the danger of laminitis. Prednisolone is safer but, on the whole, is much less effective; oral administration at a dose of 1 mg/kg has been recommended. NSAIDs are much safer, but also less effective. Antihistamines are largely ineffective, even at high doses given three times a day.

20.8 Urticarial Reaction

A very common reaction in the horse, owners often associate it with a high-protein diet or food allergy. Food allergies will occur in horses but are extremely rare, and are described in Section 9.9. Normally, urticarial reaction results from the bite of a fly to which the horse is hypersensitive (see Table 20.1). Raised urticarial plaques will occur all over the body or just in specific areas, the most common sites being the neck and body. These plaques may well become infected and will leak yellow serum, but are not normally pruritic. The standard treatment in the early stages is by dexamethasone, but the clinician may be reluctant to use this medication if there is any possibility of laminitis developing. The safest course of action is treatment with NSAIDs and antibiotics if the area becomes infected. Rugs should be avoided, but hosing with clean, cold water is useful. Antihistamines,

Table 20.1. Main differentials to be considered with cases of pruritus and/or urticaria.

PRURITUS	URTICARIA
Parasites in general	*Drug reactions in general*
Chorioptic mange Pediculosis Trombiculosis Poultry mite infestation Oxyuris Stronyloidosis	Topicals Antibiotics NSAIDs Narcotics Vaccines Antisera
Hypersensitivity disorders	*Hypersensitivities*
Culicoides hypersensitivity Other insect-bite sensitivities Atopic dermatitis Forage mite infestations Adverse food reactions	Insects Atopy Contact reactions Drugs Adverse food reactions
Contact dermatitis/hypersensitivity	*Associated with infections and infestations; bacterial, fungal, viral, protozoal, parasitic, including endoparasites, straw and forage mites*
Malassezia dermatitis Pemphigus foliaceous	Arthropod stings and bites Vasculitis Dermatographism Exercise/heat/cold-induced

e.g. hydroxyzine (see Section 6.9) can be tried as treatment but, like dexamethasone, this drug should *not* be used in the pregnant mare.

20.9 Eosinophilic Granulomata

Normally seen in the saddle area, these raised areas (singular, granuloma) approximately 1 cm in diameter are not painful and rarely become infected; they are caused by an overreaction to the bite of either a fly or tick. In many cases after some months they will regress spontaneously. Dexamethasone can be injected into the actual lesion and will speed remission, while steroid creams are of doubtful value. Surgical removal is an option but is not really necessary.

20.10 Viral Skin Conditions

Horse pox

Occurring in Europe (but not in the UK), the Middle East, North Africa and Asia, this is an unclassified pox virus; conditions include equine molluscum contagiosum and viral papular dermatitis. It is very rare and some experts question whether a real horse virus exists or whether horses are infected with the cow pox virus. Pox virus disease shows initially as vesicles on the mucosa and papules on the skin, these latter developing into pustules normally occurring on the mouth, nose and face, but have also been recorded on the vulva and prepuce. The disease is not venereal. Diagnosis is based on the history and clinical features, backed up by the histology of biopsies. Eventually the lesions will regress, leaving scabby areas that are then seen as areas of alopecia. There is no treatment. Autogenous vaccines have been tried, though unsuccessfully. Affected horses must be isolated and measures taken to disinfect the premises to prevent virus spread.

Coital exanthema

A venereal disease caused by equine herpes virus 3, described in Section 18.8.

Viral papilloma

A very common disease of young horses caused by a species-specific papovavirus, it presents as multiple warts mainly on the face and occurs extremely suddenly; it may even be seen on the newborn foal. It is sometimes seen on the testicles when a young horse is castrated. There is no treatment, and the warts will suddenly regress. Clinicians should be aware that if the warts suddenly occur in horses over the age of 6 they may well not regress, but such cases are extremely rare.

20.11 Bacterial Skin Conditions

Dermatophilus

Caused by *Dermatophilus congolensis*, a gram-positive organism showing branching mycelia or rows of coccoid bodies, this is a common, superficial infectious disease seen worldwide. It is sometimes called 'rain scald' or, if on the legs, 'mud rash'; as the names imply, moisture and the organisms are required in combination for signs to appear. The moisture may be sweat in hot weather; it can occur in winter when the coat is long, or in summer when there is little hair cover. The hair bunches up to form a very small tuft which, when plucked, leaves a small, triangular lesion that is often purulent. It is a self-limiting disease, although the course of the healing is aided by antibiotics and oily creams, with the affected area kept dry. The condition can be spread by rugs and clippers.

Staphylococcus

Both *Staphylococcus aureus* and *Staphylococcus intermedius* cause dermatitis in the horse. The bacteria gain entry from wounds or from micro-abrasions. They can be seen as gram-positive cocci, their spread being by saddles, blankets, girths, bridles and other tack. The disease is also common on the legs, particularly the white areas, and can be spread by continuous movement through deep mud. The notable feature of the condition is pain; lesions, particularly on the legs, will cause even the quiet horse to react violently. Cleaning the areas is important and is best carried out with running water; the area is then dried with paper towels and antibiotic ointment applied. Parenteral antibiotics and NSAIDs are also helpful.

The condition can take on a chronic nature, forming granulomatous lesions, called botryomycosis. These lesions will contain bacteria and really should be termed pyogranulomata. Unfortunately, they will not regress with antibiotic treatment as the bacteria are walled off within the lesion; the only effective treatment is radical excision.

Streptococcus

Streptococcal organisms cause systemic disease in the horse, e.g. *Streptococcus equi*, which causes 'strangles' (see Section 14.3). However, *Streptococcus zooepidemicus* and *Streptococcus equisimilis* will cause skin disease, which may take the form of an infected wound, particularly a puncture wound or a serious cellulitis. In very serious cases there may be ulcerative lymphangitis. Aggressive treatment is required, with high doses of antibiotics and NSAIDs.

20.12 Fungal Skin Conditions

If you see many horses affected with a skin condition in one group it is likely that the cause is a fungus and is called 'ringworm'. This is a real misnomer, as it has nothing to do with a worm and, in the majority of cases, the skin lesion is not ring-shaped, although it can be and in humans it is often seen as a ring-shaped lesion.

The main organism affecting horses worldwide is *Trichophyton equinum*; however, alternatively they may be infected with *Microsporum equinum*, which is the most common pathogen in the UK. Neither of these infections cause pruritus, except in the foal; on the other hand, if a horse becomes infected with a non-equine fungus, e.g. *Trichophyton verrucosum* from cattle or *Microsporum canis* from dogs, it will usually be pruritic and become secondarily infected. Luckily, the equine-specific fungal infections, *T. equinum* and *M. equinum*, are not very contagious to humans, although precautions should be observed; in addition, those infections appear to be self-limiting, so treatment for the in-contact human is rarely necessary. Although griseofulvin at 10 mg/kg daily by mouth for 14 days is said to treat the horse (provided it is not intended for human consumption), it gives rather disappointing results except for horses infected with *T. verrucosum*, when it is very effective. For treatment of either *T. equinum* or *M. equinum* infections, use topical applications of either miconazole or natamycin. The disinfectant Vircon®, used as a wash, seems to be helpful not only in reducing the level of fungal infection on the horse but also for cleaning tack, headcollars, brushes and rugs; it is rather expensive for stable cleaning, but very effective. All wooden surfaces should have creosote applied; this environmental clean-up is well worthwhile.

Equine ringworm, which is a very overdiagnosed disease, is in fact difficult to recognize. The Wood's lamp is of no use for *T. equinum*, as this fungus does not cause fluorescence, although fluorescence may be seen with *M. equinum*. Microscopic examination is difficult, but culture on dermatophyte test media is very useful; these plates, which have an added dye, should be examined daily to ensure that growth and any change in dye colour are not missed.

Environmental fungi can also cause lesions, known as cutaneous pythiosis, caused by *Pythium insidiosum*. This fungus requires rotting vegetation in a warm, marshy environment; it then appears as an opportunist pathogen on the equine skin, usually on the lower limbs, but can also affect the back, probably if the horse rolls. It may be seen on impression smears stained with Giemsa. Infection is restricted to tropical and subtropical areas.

20.13 Equine Sarcoid

The equine sarcoid is by far the most common nodule affecting the horse's skin; it also affects the skin of ponies, donkeys, mules and zebra – over 80% of the very rare Cape Zebra found in South Africa are affected, which leads to a supposition that there is an inherited susceptibility. Strictly speaking, an equine sarcoid is not a tumour but an aggressive fibroblastic nodule, but it is easier for the layperson to understand the condition if clinicians describe it as 'skin cancer'. Owners are also heartened if told that sarcoids will never metastasize to internal organs.

The cause is still unknown, although there is certainly a link with a bovine papilloma virus; it is extremely likely that they are spread by flies. The incidence varies worldwide; 9% of horses in the UK have sarcoids. They can occur anywhere on the body, the most common sites being the groin, the neck and around the ears; they are rare on the lower limbs but are very difficult to remove from these sites (see Figs 20.3 and 20.4).

Sarcoids are very variable in appearance; six types have been described:

- The so-called occult sarcoid may be little more than an area of alopecia around one

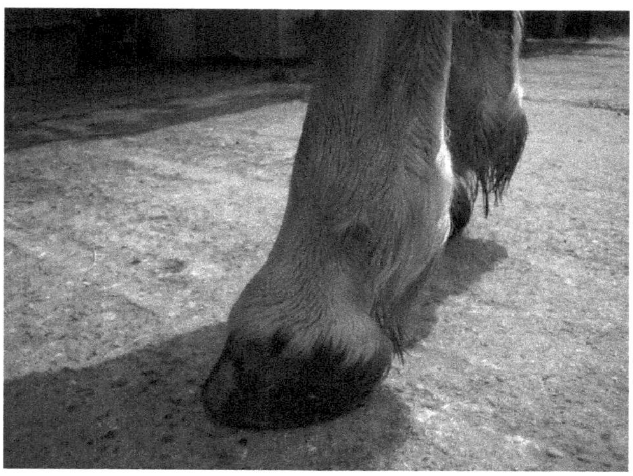

Fig. 20.3. Small equine sarcoid on the leg.

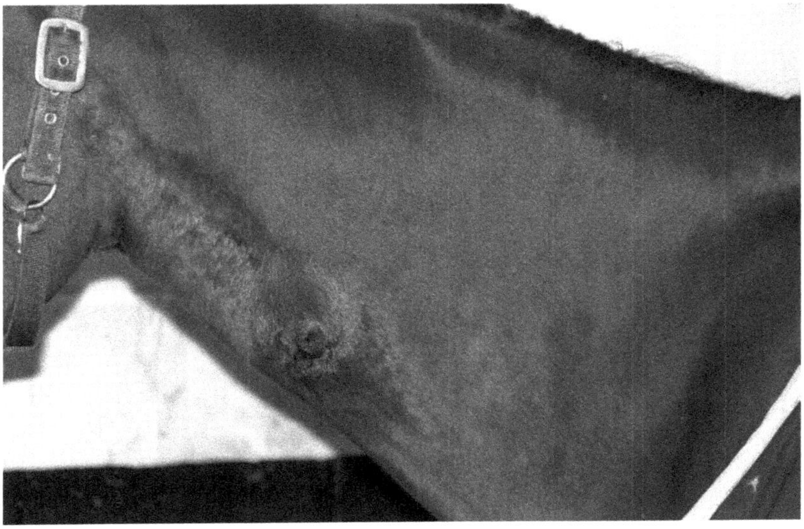

Fig. 20.4. Sarcoid in the jugular area following catheter placement.

eye. However, there will be no spontaneous resolution and these can proliferate, especially if interfered with.

- The most common type is the verrucosa sarcoid, often called wart. These are belittled by owners who are selling horses. They are *not* warts and should *not* be dismissed as unimportant. Verrucosa sarcoids may be either flat or pedunculated and are normally slow-growing unless abraded by tack. The pedunculated type can be removed slowly with a tight ligature or rubber elastrator ring, but they will never be totally removed by this method.
- The fibroblastic sarcoid is more aggressive and may involve subdermal layers. It may enlarge rapidly and then ulcerate, and is often associated with wound scars. They can occur at the commissures of the lips, presumably from harsh use of the bit. Surgical excision should not be attempted, as this invariably leads to enlargement.
- The nodular type of sarcoid lies entirely below the skin and may remain there for many years, before suddenly enlarging and bursting through the skin. It will shell out but will rapidly recur
- Occurring in loose areas of skin in the axilla or groin, the nodular sarcoid can be mixed with the fibroblastic type and so form a fifth type.
- The most serious type of sarcoid is the malevolent type, which spreads along the lymphatics and may suddenly appear at distant sites.

From the above descriptions it is hoped that clinicians can diagnose equine sarcoids on clinical appearance. Biopsy is not recommended as this tends to aggravate the sarcoid.

There are many treatments available (Table 20.2). Surgical excision should be avoided, except to debulk for cryo- or laser surgery. The best treatment available for practitioners in the field is topical or intra-lesional treatment. There are many patent creams, e.g. AW3-LUDES, produced by Liverpool Veterinary School, UK, that are very effective. These need to be applied with rubber gloves very carefully, with four applications every 48 h, or injected with a large-bore needle; a good method is to push the needle fully into the lesion and then inject as the needle is slowly withdrawn. Great care should be taken by the operator to avoid the pressure blowing the needle off the syringe. For delicate areas, e.g. around the eye, BCG vaccine can be injected with a fine needle into the lesion three times at 3-weekly intervals. Other substances, such as cisplatin, mitomycin C, arsenic paste or antimony paste,

Table 20.2. Reported success rates from different therapies for sarcoids. Used with permission from Mair (2021).

Treatment modality	Reported success rates (excluding periocular cases)	Reported success rates for periocular sarcoids
Sharp surgery	30–50%	18%
Laser surgery	62–83%	–
Cryotherapy	66%	9%
Electrochemotherapy	86–94%	–
Intralesional BCG and immunocidin	58–59%	69%
Topical chemotherapy	53–72%	35–66%
Intralesional cisplatin	96%	33%
Intralesional mitomycin C	–	100% (only reported in one abstract)
Radiotherapy	100%	75–100%

have also been used to good effect (see also Section 18.10). Radiotherapy has also been used, but is not recommended except in very specialized hands.

20.14 Neoplastic Skin Conditions

Introduction

Skin tumours are the most common neoplasms seen in the horse. It should be remembered that they can become secondarily infected with bacteria and not only will they attract flies, but they may be invaded by maggots. Removal of the neoplasm will depend on the diagnosis and the position and should not be undertaken lightly.

Melanoma

A relatively common neoplasm in grey horses, it may also be seen in the donkey. They are a condition of the older animal, being extremely rare in horses <6 years of age. They are normally found at the skin/mucosal junction, the most common position is around the anus, but they may also be seen around the vulva, the tail and around the prepuce, but rarely on the penis, and sometimes around the eyes and on the lips. They are very rarely malignant internally, but may be found in the intestine or the lungs, liver or bone marrow; one type is seen extremely rarely in bay horses, where it is invariably malignant. Additionally, they may also be found in the salivary glands; the horse so affected does not appear to suffer, even when the glands become quite enlarged, unless they obstruct the airway, in which case euthanasia is indicated. Spread to the guttural pouch is also a possibility and is life threatening, as this may erode into the carotid artery; this outcome can be averted, as in guttural pouch mycosis (see Section 14.4), by tying off the internal carotid artery. Opinions differ as to whether melanomata (plural of melanoma) should be surgically removed, as in many instances they will shell out quite easily; however, the act of surgery or even biopsy may stimulate rapid growth, so if they are not causing any problems they are perhaps best left well alone. Cryotherapy can be used.

Squamous cell carcinoma

The most common position for this tumour is in the third eyelid, as described in Section 17.3. However, they will also occur around the vagina (see Section 18.11), anus and prepuce (see Section 18.10), although extremely rarely near the mouth. As this is a very malignant tumour, prompt and complete surgical excision is advisable (see Figs 20.5 and 20.6).

Mast cell tumour

Unlike in humans, dogs and cats, in equines this tumour rarely metastasizes, and therefore the

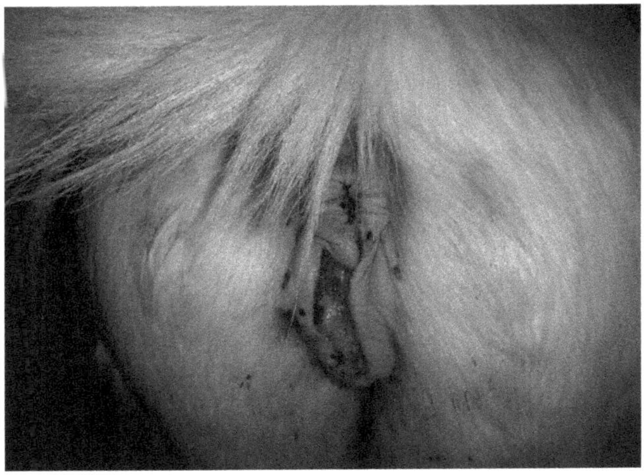

Fig. 20.5. Squamous cell carcinoma of the vulva.

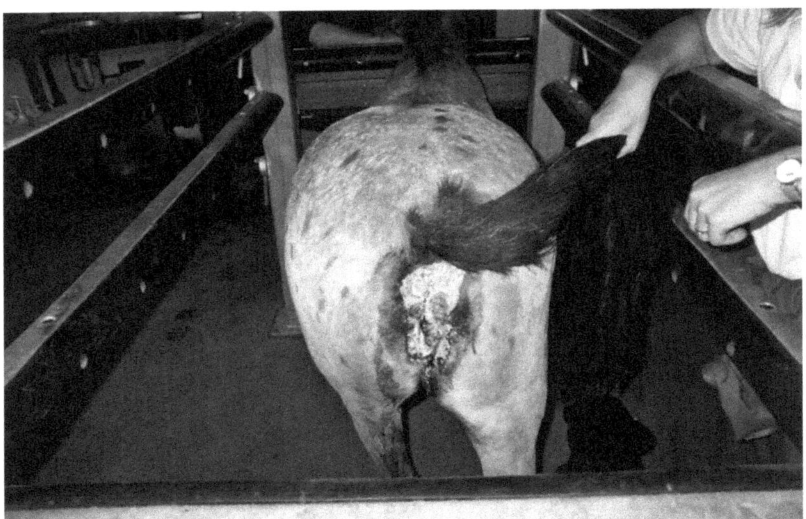

Fig. 20.6. Advanced squamous cell carcinoma of the vulva.

affected horse is an ideal candidate for surgical excision, with a recurrence rate of <12%.

Cutaneous lymphosarcoma

Lymphosarcoma in organs other than the skin invariably grows and invades rapidly, so if metastasis has occurred early euthanasia is advisable. However, when found in the skin – commonly in the perineum, axilla and subcutaneously on the shoulder, they may not progress rapidly. Diagnosis can be confirmed in many cases by spread to the adjoining lymph glands; systemic signs, indicating internal metastases, will hopefully be slow in onset.

20.15 Non-neoplastic Nodules

Axillary nodular necrosis

This is a condition similar to eosinophilic granulomata (described in Section 20.9), but differing in the fact that nodules do not contain any collagen degeneration. Although normally self-limiting, the horse may be irritated since the nodules may be abraded by the tack. If persistent, nodules can be injected with dexamethasone.

Unilateral papular dermatosis

As the name suggests, this condition occurs on one side of the body only, as firm, well-circumscribed nodules up to 1.5 cm in diameter. There are rarely problems and spontaneous regression will follow.

Amyloidosis

The cause of this extremely rare condition is unknown. Amyloid protein is deposited in plaques on the head, neck and trunk; there is no treatment and diagnosis can be confirmed only on biopsy. The condition will not regress, but often will progress over a period of years. If amyloid spreads to the respiratory system progression is more rapid, and euthanasia is indicated.

20.16 Cushing's Disease

Correctly termed pituitary adenoma, this condition is actually very common in the older horse, and particularly in ponies. It is a welfare problem as it leads to laminitis (see Section 11.5), which is extremely painful and often incurable. Interference with the endocrine system is the principal pathology, the adrenals being affected; these produce an excess of corticosteroids, hence the laminitis. Other endocrine effects may or may not be observed: there is polyuria and polydipsia, and a urine dipstick will show glycosuria. There will be an abnormal and very thick, hairy coat, which will not be shed; if the horse is clipped, which is helpful in warmer climates, the coat will grow back again quickly even if the weather is hot or the horse rugged. The heavy coat will help mask the excessive sweating and weight loss; perversely, weight loss does actually help ameliorate laminitic signs. The horse will be more susceptible to infections, e.g. dental pulpitis, oral ulcers, hoof damage. Mares may have abnormal oestrous cycles and show milk when not pregnant; ponies will show markedly bulging supraorbital fat pads. Diagnosis can be made on clinical grounds though confirmation is difficult, but it appears that the dexamethasone suppression test, as described in Section 2.8, is the most reliable method.

Treatment is not easy. The laminitis must be controlled, as described in Sections 11.5 and 11.6. Treatment with the human medication pergolide (a dopamine receptor agonist used in the control of Parkinson's disease) is the best option. This is supplied as 1 mg tablets; a daily dose of 1 mg can be started in the horse, but may have to be doubled. Clinicians need to be careful when treating ponies, as the drug may cause inappetence; this might be considered a good side-effect in the pony suffering from laminitis, but it is dangerous as the animal might develop hyperlipaemia (see Sections and 15.7), with fatal results. The dose rate should immediately be reduced to 25% of the initial dose, the pony monitored carefully and the dose increased *very slowly*. Of the neurological signs associated with side-effects of pergolide, the most prominent will be circling; once again, the dose must be dramatically reduced. Having said all that, with careful monitoring, feeding and clipping, ponies with Cushing's disease can be kept alive for many years, provided laminitis is controlled.

20.17 Autoimmune Skin Conditions

There are a large number of these conditions in the horse, but they are all very rare. Extremely difficult to diagnose on account of the inevitable secondary bacterial infection – and probably also parasitic presence – it is very difficult to differentiate among them; even skilled pathologists will have problems. Photographs, multiple biopsies and a very full history are vital; the most common is pemphigus foliaceus. Not only will large areas of the skin become crusty and infected, but also the horse will be ill. All treatments are unrewarding, although high doses of corticosteroids may appear to slow the onset of symptoms. The other main conditions in this group are bullous pemphigoid, equine sarcoidosis and generalized granulomatous disease, systemic lupus, immune-mediated vasculitis and erythema multiforme.

20.18 Photodermatitis

Photodermatitis is a complex and incompletely understood condition. It is best called 'sun-induced dermatoses'. It can then be divided into phototoxicity and photosensitization (Williams, 2018). Phototoxicity occurs in horses with white on their muzzles which will suffer from dermatitis in the summer, particularly if they are grazing in a paddock with large numbers of thistles, but this can easily be controlled with sunblock cream. It appears that the thistles physically damage the skin, as the same horse in the following year on a different pasture will not be affected. *Dermatophilus congolense* (see Section 20.11) can be isolated from the lesions, but this is a secondary invader. The white-coloured legs of the same horse will not be affected.

Photosensitization is a totally separate condition but often with a similar appearance. This is caused by either: (i) the ingestion of certain plants toxic to the liver, e.g. St John's Wort (see Section 19.37), wild carrot, buckwheat and burr trefoil; (ii) veterinary medicines affecting the liver, e.g. tetracyclines, sulfa drugs or phenothiazine; or (iii) contact with certain plants, e.g. giant hogweed or certain clovers; the clinical picture will appear the same whatever the trigger.

The affected horse must be kept out of sunlight, as all white parts will be affected; the skin, if badly affected, will remain scarred for life. Immunosuppressive doses of steroids may be helpful in severe cases, after the initial trigger has been removed. There is yet a third condition associated with sunlight, photo-aggravated vasculitis, which occurs on white parts of the legs and is often accompanied by a secondary staphylococcal infection, and therefore is painful. Clinicians should be warned that these cases do not readily resolve after bringing the horse out of sunlight, even with aggressive parenteral antibiotic therapy and local cleaning, drying and oily creams.

20.19 Pastern Dermatitis Syndrome

Often similar in appearance to photo-aggravated vasculitis (see Section 20.18), this condition is often wrongly termed mud fever. It is a multifactorial condition seen on the lower legs of all breeds of horse, and rarely has any association with mud. The underlying cause is often obscured by secondary bacterial contamination, usually *Streptococcus* spp., *Staphylococcus* spp. and *Dermatophilus* spp., and these need to be treated as well as the underlying cause, if one is known. The most likely underlying cause is *Chorioptes equi* (see Section 20.3), which can readily be seen under the low power of the microscope if brushed into a Petri dish.

Treatment of this syndrome is rather hit-and-miss, as there may be more than one underlying cause and more than one secondary infection. First, any mites present must be killed with an i/m injection of doramectin. Next, the horse is given antibiotics for a minimum of 10 days, either by injection or orally; potentiated sulfonamides are likely to be the antibiotic of choice. The scabs on the affected legs must not be picked off, but rather washed off with very dilute chlorhexidine solution; the leg is then thoroughly dried – ideally with paper towels – before covering with an oily cream. It is vitally important that the leg is dried and that no preparation is used that might harm the horse, as it will very quickly learn to resent treatment.

There are many different types of such cream, listed below alphabetically by principal active ingredient; if the first one tried does not appear to be beneficial after a few days, another should be tried:

- acriflavin;
- amoxicillin, with clavulinic acid;
- betamethasone;
- cetrimide;
- fusidic acid;
- hydrocortisone;
- lanolin; and
- silver compounds.

The condition may occur in hairy, or so-called 'feathered', horses, and in these horses treatment is likely to be more effective if the legs are clipped out, or at least the hair removed with scissors; if this is likely to upset the horse it should be sedated. If only the white limbs of the horse are affected, application of sun lotion might be considered.

20.20 Conditions of Pigmentation

Vitiligo

A common condition seen in all breeds of horse but most common in the Arab, it is also seen in the donkey. It is also termed idiopathic depigmentation, a name that defines it very well. It shows first as areas of hair that initially become depigmented – leukotrichia; this is followed by the skin becoming depigmented – leukoderma. The horse does not appear to suffer, except that some animals will become sunburnt and will need protective creams. There is no treatment, and the condition is progressive. The manner in which a horse's skin responds to trauma when it is burnt, irradiated or sutured is similar to that occurring with leukotrichia and leukoderma; it also occurs when a horse is freeze-branded.

Reticulated leukotrichia

Normally seen in the young horse, crusty lesions on the rump and back are the main signs of this condition; the crusts are then shed, leaving a hairless area, but when hair re-grows it is white. These initial crusts may be painful if a staphylococcal infection is involved; the condition will subside with or without antibiotic treatment, leaving a spotty horse. This condition is likely to be inheritable, as it is seen mainly in Arabs, Standardbreds and Quarter Horses.

Fading Arab syndrome

Seen only in the Arab breed, this is definitely an inheritable condition but, unlike vitiligo, it occurs in the newly weaned foal. All white areas turn pink as the hair is lost, these areas then becoming crusty. There is no treatment. If only a small percentage of white areas is affected the horse will be able to cope, but in the rare case with extensive damage euthanasia is the only option.

20.21 Hyperelastica Cutis

Also called cutaneous asthenia or dermatosparaxis, this probably inheritable condition is extremely rare in the horse and also rarely causes any problems. The skin on the body may be elevated in folds, causing no pain; these folds will very slowly revert to their normal position. There is no treatment.

20.22 Cutaneous Agenesis

Caused by a single autosomal recessive gene, signs are open defects of the skin on the head and legs. Euthanasia is the only option.

20.23 Congenital/Developmental Cystic Conditions of the Skin

Epidermoid inclusion cyst

Commonly known as an atheroma, this occurs in the false nostril as a spherical swelling containing thick, yellow fluid, and as it rarely causes a problem, it should be left alone. Lancing will lead to failure to heal, but sometimes aspirating the fluid is successful in reducing the size if the airway is impaired. Total removal by surgery is difficult, as there is no spare skin in the area for suturing.

Dermoid cyst

Seen as either single and multiple on the dorsal midline, this is not painful and rarely causes problems. If it bursts, however, it will be found to contain coiled hair and a sterile, cheesy exudate. A smaller, firm nodule is likely to form later at the site.

Dentigerous cyst

Also known as temporal teratoma, this occurs – as the name suggests – in the temporal area; an aberrant tooth is the source of the problem. It may well burst, discharging the dental tissue, but will remain as a small, discharging sinus. Surgical removal with no likelihood of recurrence is possible.

Linear keratosis

A focal keratinization defect that causes no problems, this is seen on the neck or rarely on the gluteal area. It should be left alone.

20.24 Atopic Dermatitis

A condition far from being understood in the horse, it is a chronic, relapsing pruritic skin disease caused by hypersensitivity to a foreign allergen; this will normally be from an outside source such as dust and forage mites but might, in rare cases, have been ingested (Table 20.3). Practitioners should eliminate all other causes before undertaking either skin tests or food elimination tests. Often cases require a multi-faceted approach to management, which may include allergen-specific immunotherapy (ASIT). The success rate of this therapy is in the order of 60%. If the allergen cannot be avoided, long-term oral prednisolone can be tried as a treatment, initially at 0.5 mg/kg every morning; the dose may have to be increased in increments up to 2 mg/kg; ideally, once the condition is under control the dose can be reduced gradually, e.g. a smaller daily dose or alternate-day medication. In some cases, antihistamine therapy is useful. See Table 20.4 for drugs which may help with equine atopic dermatitis.

20.25 Alopecia Areata

This represents a confusing condition for the practitioner, although well recognized by the pathologist. It is classified as either: (i) cicatricial, when the hair follicles are destroyed permanently and the hair will never regrow; or (ii) non-cicatricial,

Table 20.3. Some useful diagnostic techniques for selected skin conditions. Used with permission from Rendle (2017).

Presentation	Condition	Diagnostic technique of choice
Scaling	Atopy	Punch biopsy, intradermal skin testing
Scaling	Insect bite sensitivity	Punch biopsy, intradermal skin testing
Scaling	Dermatophytosis	Hair plucks, skin scrapes, fungal culture/PCR
Scaling	Dermatophilosis	Collection of crust for microscopy/culture
Scaling	Pemphigus foliaceous	Aspiration of pustules, punch biopsy with great care
Scaling	Multisystemic eosinophilic epitheliotropic disease	Punch biopsy
Scaling	Pastern dermatitis	Punch biopsy
Scaling	Leukocytoclastic vasculitis	Punch biopsy
Nodular	Bacterial folliculitis	Punch biopsy, bacterial culture of pustules of biopsies
Nodular	Sarcoid	Excisional, tru-cut or punch biopsy
Nodular	Melanoma	Excisional, tru-cut or punch biopsy
Nodular	Eosinophilic granuloma	Excisional biopsy, fine-needle aspirate may be suggestive
Nodular	Cutaneous lymphoma	Excisional, tru-cut or punch biopsy
Nodular	Mast cell tumour	Fine-needle aspiration often reveals mast cells, excisional, tru-cut or punch biopsy
Weals	Urticaria	Punch biopsy, intradermal skin testing
Ulcerative	Squamous cell carcinoma	Excisional or punch biopsy
Ulcerative	Exuberant granulation tissue	Excisional or tru-cut biopsy
Alopecia	Alopecia areata	Punch biopsy
Alopecia	Anagen/telogen effluvium	Hair plucks
Other	Oxyuris infection	Tape impressions
Other	Chorioptes and other mite/louse infestation	Tape impressions, skin scrapes, brushings

Table 20.4. Drugs that may be helpful for systemic symptomatic therapy for equine atopic dermatitis.

Glucocorticoids	Prednisolone 0.15–1.5 mg/kg PO sid induction; maintenance 0.2–0.5 mg/kg PO every other day
	Dexamethasone 0.02–0.1 mg/kg PO or injection loading; maintenance 0.01–0.02 mg/kg PO every two to three days
Antihistamines*	Hydroxyzine 1–2 mg/kg bid or tid
	Chlorophenamine 0.25–0.5 mg/kg bid
	Diphenhydramine 1–2 mg/kg bid or tid
	Alimemazine (trimeprazine) 1–2 mg/kg bid
	Cetirizine 0.2–0.4 mg/kg (or 100 mg per horse bid)
Tricyclic antidepressants*	Amitriptyline 1 mg/kg bid
	Doxepin 0.5–0.75 mg/kg bid
Phosphodiesterase inhibitors*	Pentoxifylline 10–15 mg/kg bid or tid

* = off-label use in the UK
sid = once a day; bid = twice a day; tid = three times a day; PO = per os

when the hair will grow again if the initial cause of the alopecia is corrected. Linear alopecia is an example of the former type and *Dermatophilus* infection (see Section 20.11) of the latter. Practitioners should eliminate all other causes before making a definitive diagnosis of the condition, which is untreatable.

20.26 Saddle Sores

A totally preventable condition that includes girth sores (see Fig. 20.7). It is extremely important in working horses, being caused by ill-fitting or abrasive tack. Should it occur, immediate removal of the relevant piece of tack must be carried out; the sores, which are entirely caused by the rubbing of the tack, should be treated with an oily cream. No tack should be put on that area until the sores are totally healed. The tack is then examined carefully, with all rubbing points removed or padded appropriately. Only short periods of work should be carried out initially, until the handler is totally satisfied that the sores will not recur.

20.27 Fistulous Withers

No longer a common condition, it appears to be caused by trauma followed by infection. The implicated role of *Brucella* infection is very unlikely – expected bacteriological findings are a mixed infection of *Staphylococcus* and *Streptococcus*. It is difficult to treat, not because the organisms are resistant to antibiotics but because there is very poor drainage from that area. Antibiotic treatment with penicillin, cephalosporin or potentiated sulfonamides needs to be prolonged. Obviously, the tack should be checked and kept off the horse until full healing has occurred. Mercifully, it is a rare condition these days.

20.28 Poll Evil

Very similar in appearance to fistulous withers, this condition is rare and has a different aetiology. A self-inflicted wound in the poll area is the initial sign, followed by secondary infection. Because drainage is poor healing is reputed to be delayed, but that has not been my experience, and I have found that these wounds heal quickly with good antibiotic cover.

20.29 Bird Damage

It is very hard to understand this condition, which is mainly seen in the old, debilitated donkey. Large, raw areas are formed on the back of the donkey as a result of pecking from jackdaws, crows or oxpeckers, but why the animal allows this is totally incomprehensible. If left unattended, the whole of the back will become a raw area of granulation tissue. The general condition causing the debilitation should be addressed and the raw areas covered in oily cream; pain relief with NSAIDs is indicated and, if there is any hint of infection, the animal must be given

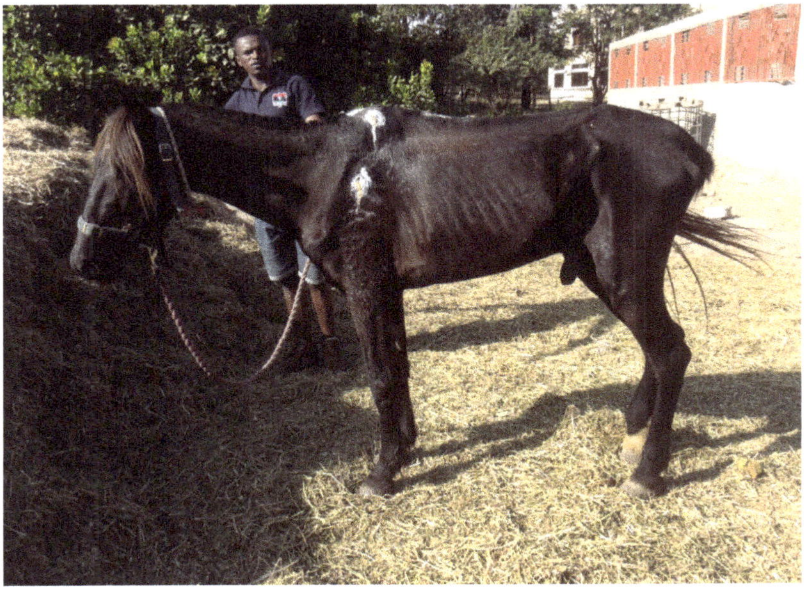

Fig. 20.7. Saddle sores.

antibiotics. Adequate stabling is required to prevent further damage.

20.30 Snake Bite

Horses are inquisitive animals, so most snake bites occur on the muzzle or face, but they will also occur on the legs if a horse treads on a snake, or on the body if it rolls on to a snake. Normally, the fang marks can be seen; depending on the type of snake and the amount of venom injected, the reaction of the horse will vary. The most dangerous sign is the massive oedema that can occur around the head and neck, which can be life-threatening if respiration is impeded; an emergency tracheostomy must be carried out in such a case, as described below.

Local anaesthetic is instilled over the trachea in the area of the 4th–5th tracheal rings. An incision about 5 cm in length is made longitudinally over the trachea – blunt dissection will easily reveal the trachea. The aim then is to remove a circular area of the ventral trachea without cutting through the whole of a tracheal ring, and this is achieved by cutting half of two adjacent rings with curved scissors. It is important that the piece of tissue to be removed is grasped with a pair of Alliss tissue forceps to prevent its inhalation into the lungs. Ideally, a purpose-made tracheostomy tube should then be fitted; however, if such a tube is not available, a piece of plastic with a flange can be inserted and sutured into position. The ideal substitute can be made by cutting the handle off a 1 l or 2 l plastic container. The tube can be removed when the oedema and respiratory restriction have lessened, and the area will heal quickly following tube removal and the insertion of two or three skin sutures.

Other reactions shown by the horse will vary with the type of snake that has bitten the horse. If the snake produces neurotoxic venom, e.g. black mamba, the horse will exhibit neurological signs; if it produces haemotoxic venom, e.g. adder or viper, the horse will show massive oedema and pain. Treatment can be specific if the appropriate antivenin is available, but this is unlikely and so the treatment should be supportive, with large doses of corticosteroids; however, the animal also should receive large doses of NSAIDs and possibly i/v fluids. Clinicians should remember that the bite itself may cause infection, so antibiotics are also given.

20.31 Specific Problems with Donkeys

Donkeys in both the developed world and the developing world are special in that they have close contact with children and therefore zoonotic diseases are particularly important. They have been domesticated for 6000 years but only arrived in the UK in AD 43 with the Roman invasion of Britain. Thus, allowances must be made as they are not fully adapted to cold and particularly wet weather (Thiemann and Sullivan, 2021). It would appear that donkeys are more prone to highly invasive equine sarcoids than horses.

20.32 Skin Diseases in Horses Where Skin Disease Occurs as Part of a Wider Systemic Disorder

- Chronic inflammatory infiltrative diseases: Sarcoidosis and multisystemic eosinophilic epitheliotropic disease.
- Autoimmune skin diseases:
  Pemphigus foliaceus, erythema multiforme, pemphigus vulgaris, bullous pemphigoid and systemic lupus.
- Immunosuppression.

References and Further Reading

Curnow, B. (2020) Diagnosis and management of the itchy horse. *In Practice* 42(1): 47–55.

Durham, A. (2019) Crusting and skin disorders in horses. *Vet Times* 49(1), 7 January: 9–11.

Knottenbelt, D.C. (2009) *Pascoe's Principles and Practice of Equine Dermatology*, 2nd edn. Elsevier Health, Philadelphia, Pennsylvania.

Kondratjeva, J., Combarros, D., Pressanti, C. and Cadiergues, M.C. (2023) What is the most effective treatment in horses with chorioptic mange? *Equine Veterinary Education* 35(3): 163–168.

Littlewood, J. (2020) Equine atopic dermatitis: Latest on diagnosis and management. *Vet Times* 6(3), 15 January: 2–4.

Mair, T. (2021) Skin lumps and bumps: Overview of sarcoids and melanomas in horses. *Vet Times* 51(15), 20 April: 6–10.

O'Brien, K. (2019) Asking the experts about skin disease. *Veterinary Practice*, 1 October, 52–57.

Pilsworth, R. and Knottenbelt, D.C. (2006) *Common Equine Skin Diseases*. Equine Veterinary Journal, Ely, UK.

Prutton, J. (2023) Summer allergies: Readying owners and yards for prevention. *Vet Times Equine Dermatology* 52(13): 6–8.

Rendle, D. (2017) Diagnosing equine skin diseases. *Vet Times* 47(15), 17 April: 8–13.

Sloet van Oldruitenbough-Oosterbaan, M.M. and Grinwis, G.C.M. (2018) Viral skin diseases in the Netherlands. *Equine Veterinary Education* 30(10): 558–563.

Sloet van Oldruitenborgh-Oosterbaan, M.M. and Knottenbelt, D.C. (2002) *The Practitioner's Guide to Equine Dermatology*. Libre Publishing, Leeuwarden, Netherlands.

Thiemann, A. and Sullivan, R. (2021) Guide to common skin disorders in donkeys. *In Practice* July/August.

Williams, P. (2018) Sun induced dermatoses in the horse. *Equine Health* 42 (July/August): 29–31.

21

Harness and Tack

Abstract

Various pieces of tack are described in this chapter, together with types of bit. Their uses are described.

21.1 Halter and Headcollar

There is considerable confusion surrounding the identification of these pieces of tack. In the UK and the Republic of Ireland, a halter is a rope that passes behind the ears and round the nose, and is also the lead rope; normally, the halter will tighten when the lead rope is pulled. A headcollar, on the other hand, is made of leather or nylon; it is like a bridle but without headband or bit. There are other more sophisticated headcollars designed to train the horse to accept commands when being led.

Foals can be trained from the first day of life by fitting a 'foal slip', which is usually made of leather and fits closely around the head. As the foal will be growing rapidly it should be constantly adjusted so that it is *never* too tight.

Halters, by their design, always have a length of rope to assist the handler but headcollars do not, and so should always have a lead rope attached whenever the horse is being handled. The horse must never be allowed to get away from the handler, but it can, if nervous, be given some headroom before being brought back under control.

21.2 Bridle

Although normally used to exert more control on the horse and sometimes very sophisticated, in reality the bridle is quite simple. It consists of a 'headpiece' that goes over the poll behind the ears, and has two parts: one runs under the throat to buckle on to the opposite side, and is called the throat latch (this stops the bridle slipping off the front of the head); the other is attached to two lower half-cheekpieces, which attach the headpiece to the bit. The bit can then be attached to a lead rope and the horse led with the added control of a bit in its mouth; an example of a bit used just for this purpose is the Chifney bit, and this is really all that is required for a bridle.

Bridles can be made more sophisticated by adding a browband, this running from the upper half-cheekpieces across the forehead, with the further addition of a noseband, which may be a simple band around the nose under the upper cheekpieces with a buckle on the ventral aspect. There is a strap over the poll – the noseband headpiece – to stop the noseband slipping down. More sophisticated nosebands are also available,

DOI: 10.1079/9781800624283.0021

e.g. the dropped noseband type, which fits below the bit. A flash may also be fitted to the standard noseband, fastened with a buckle below the bit.

The reins are fastened to the bit; some bridles will have blinkers attached, which should lie behind and to the side of the horse's eyes, to prevent the horse being distracted by the cart or other activities (see Fig. 21.1).

21.3 Bit

Five types of bit are available:

- snaffle;
- pelham;
- double bridle;
- gag; and
- bitless bridle.

These are the basic types you need to know. You can work out the mechanics of any bit, but you do not need to know the names of all the variations – there are several thousand! All five types put pressure on one or more of seven points on the horse's head:

- commissures of the lips;
- bars;
- tongue;
- chin;
- poll;
- roof of the mouth; and
- nose.

Snaffle

Applying pressure mainly to the commissures of the lips and the bars, with certain adaptations it can also put pressure on either the poll or tongue. There are many misconceptions surrounding this type of bit: a straight bar is a snaffle, and a snaffle does not have to be jointed; however, if it is, it can put pressure on the tongue through the nutcracker action. It may also have a link, e.g. French link, which is a *less* severe modification, as it does not have such a marked nutcracker action. The attachment to the bit is through the cheekpieces, which may be loose rings, e.g. the loose ring snaffle; cheekpieces may have a solid, lozenge-shaped attachment,

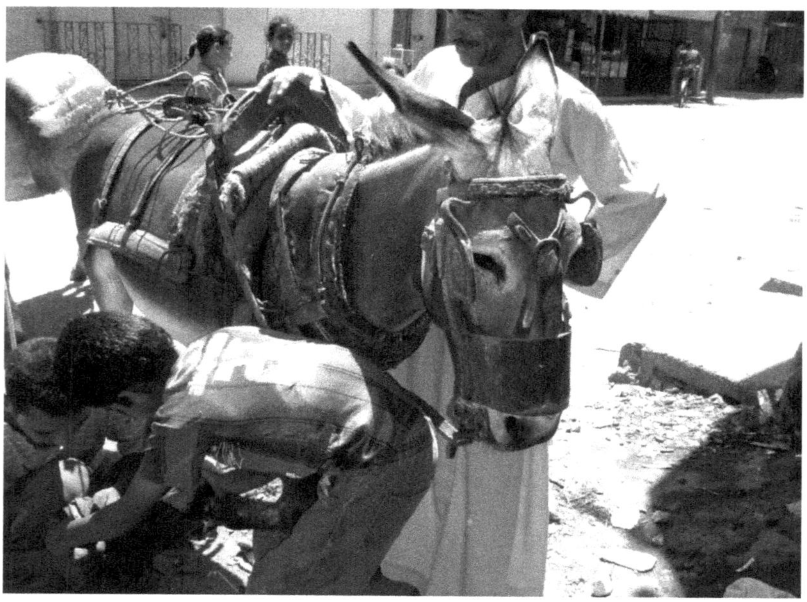

Fig. 21.1. An example of elaborate blinkers.

e.g. the eggbutt snaffle, and attachment rings can be multiple. In some instances, the rein attachment can be arranged to put pressure on the poll, e.g. the three-ringed snaffle. Further confusion is added by the fact that an alternative name for the snaffle is the bradoon.

Pelham

Although applying pressure mainly to the bars and the chin, like the snaffle this can be constructed by an arrangement of the reins to put pressure on the poll. Basically, it has a bar and chain under the chin (termed a port), the bar capable of being shaped to accommodate the tongue.

Double bridle

In reality, this is just a combination of a snaffle and a pelham; when used with double reins this can be used to put varying pressure on the lips, bars, tongue and poll.

Gag

The main pressure from this bit is on the poll, since the reins run through the attachment of the bit and up to the poll. However, depending on the configuration, there will also be pressure points elsewhere.

Bitless bridle

As the name suggests, there is no bit in the mouth, the main pressure being on the nose. The bitless bridle is often called a hackamore.

Problems with the bit

Practitioners are often asked to check a horse's mouth, as the handler is experiencing problems with control. A full oral examination should be carried out, as described in Section 10.7. Any relevant dental problems must then be corrected. A good history is taken, since that will often give the practitioner clues as to the source of the problem. Does the horse rear when asked to come into collection or to stop? This is particularly indicative if the horse is said to have 'no brakes'. Is the horse reluctant to take a rein contact on either or both turns? In my experience, a horse that bucks rarely has a problem with the bit.

Apart from dental signs, the practitioner should look for any painful sites on the head, particularly the seven points of contact as described earlier. Correct placement of the bit is next on the checklist. With the tack on, tightness of all the bridle straps should be checked; it must be remembered that a normal snaffle bit should only have 1 cm to spare on either side of the mouth. Last the type of bit is checked for severity. If there are any areas of ulceration, these will be re-examined 10 days after completion of any dentistry, to check for adequate healing. When any sores are found on the commissures of the lips, I normally advise twice-daily application of a human preparation called Orabase, which is marketed for chapped lips and oral ulceration. Another type of human medication of which there is a wide selection, used to treat haemorrhoids, can also be applied to affected areas.

Aspects of control involving tack can be found in Chapter 3.

21.4 Harness

The harness allows the horse to work by pulling various horse-drawn vehicles or implements (Fig. 21.2), e.g. a plough; horses may also pull logs and even boats. The harness must fit correctly and not rub or cause any pain. When fitting and examining harnesses of any sort, the practitioner must always have the horse's welfare uppermost in their mind.

There are two types of harness, the first being the breast strap or, as it is sometimes called, the breast collar, which is used for light work such as drawing a small cart, sleigh or carriage. This type places the weight of the load on to the sternum, near to the trachea. Heavy loads must not be drawn by this type of harness, as the sternum is not the strongest part of the skeleton, with resulting pressure on and constriction of

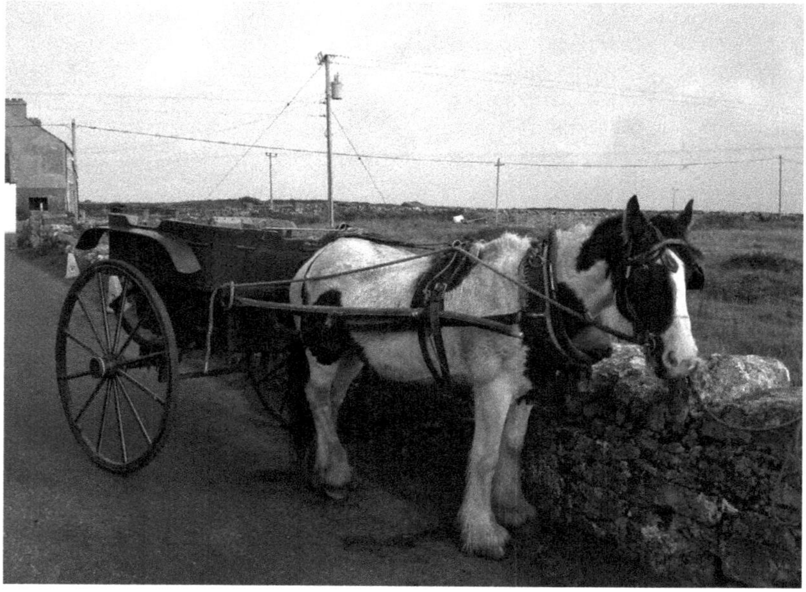

Fig. 21.2. A simple harness.

the trachea. That might reduce the horse's air supply or cause long-term damage to the trachea. The breast collar is a padded strap that passes across the breast and is attached to the traces or straps that draw the load. A swingletree can be used, so that each shoulder can pull evenly; this device, known as a singletree in North America, is a wooden or metal bar inserted to balance the drawing forces on each side.

In contrast, the second type of harness, called the collar and hames harness, places the weight of the load onto the horse's shoulders – the trachea is not involved, so the horse can use all its weight and strength. The collar is a padded loop fitting closely around the neck, having a pointed top fitting closely to the crest of the horse's neck. Because of this shape, it has to be passed over the horse's head the wrong way up before turning in the area of the cranial neck to rest close to the caudal neck. The hames fit on the outside of the collar to take the full weight of the load, while the traces or tugs attach the load to the hames.

In both types of harness there is a saddle on the horse's withers (this is nothing like a riding saddle) and a girth around the belly. The saddle has two purposes: (i) it takes the weight of the traces, which for the heavy horse may actually be chains; and (ii) it also has rings, called tenets, to prevent the reins leading from the bit from slipping down to the horse's side. The reins may be either leather or rope, and they may all be linked when several horses are harnessed together, so that the driver need hold only one set.

Unless the horse is pulling a very fine harness attached to a very light gig or cart with good brakes, it will require a breeching. This is a strap around the horse's haunches allowing it to set back and slow a vehicle; the breeching is usually hooked to either the shafts of a single cart or the pole of a double cart. If the horses are in tandem or if there are four horses, only the rear horse or horses will need a breeching; it is these horses that will be required to slow and brake the vehicle, while the front horse or horses – the leader or leaders – can only pull but not brake.

A horse pulling a vehicle with shafts will also have a belly band, which passes loosely under the belly of the horse, outside of the girth. It prevents the shafts from rising up, which is especially important on a two-wheeled vehicle, where the weight on the rear of the vehicle may tip up the front.

To complete the harness there is a back band, which is a strap passing through the harness saddle to join the belly band at either side; it takes the weight of the shafts or the pole. In a cart harness the belly band is replaced by a chain running in a groove in the harness saddle, this chain being hooked to the shafts on either side.

In a two-wheeled vehicle the shafts are fixed to the vehicle to hold it level. The back band is said to be a sliding band, i.e. when the vehicle is on a side-slope and one shaft is higher than the other, the back band is allowed to slide sideways through the harness saddle. In this way the horse can walk upright without strain on the harness. A four-wheeled vehicle normally has a fixed back band; the shafts or pole must be allowed to hinge both upward and downward, to allow the horse and vehicle to pass over hillocks or dips. Often the shafts are independently hinged, and on a side-slope these will each hinge to follow the horse, and therefore a sliding back band is not needed. However, if a sliding back band is used with independent shafts, it might allow one shaft to ride higher than the other, and so for such shafts the back band is normally fixed to the harness saddle. On other types of four-wheeled vehicle the two shafts hinge together, and a sliding back band is needed as for two-wheeled vehicles.

There are other items of harness not essential, but possibly forming part of the whole apparatus. The surcingle is sometimes used to replace the harness-saddle and girth in a light configuration. The false martingale is a strap attached to the centre of the collar, passing between the front legs, to hold the collar in position; it is called a false martingale as, unlike a riding harness, it does not attach to the reins. The crupper is a soft-padded loop passing under the tail; it is attached to either the saddle or surcingle to stop that slipping forward. Shaft tugs are loops attached to the back band to hold up the shafts of a vehicle in fine harness. In a two-wheeled vehicle these are stiff, leather loops fitting fairly loosely around the shafts to allow flexibility as the horse and the vehicle move against each other. In four-wheeled vehicles with independently hinged shafts, the tugs are buckled tightly around the shafts so they move with the horse; tugs are not needed in cart harness, since the hooks attach directly to the shafts.

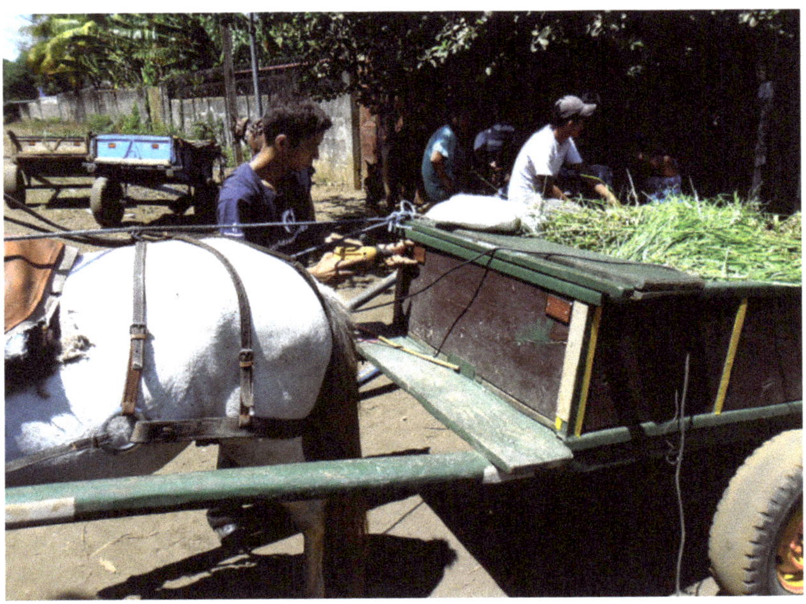

Fig. 21.3. Reflectors fitted on carts by World Horse Welfare were a game-changer in Nicaragua.

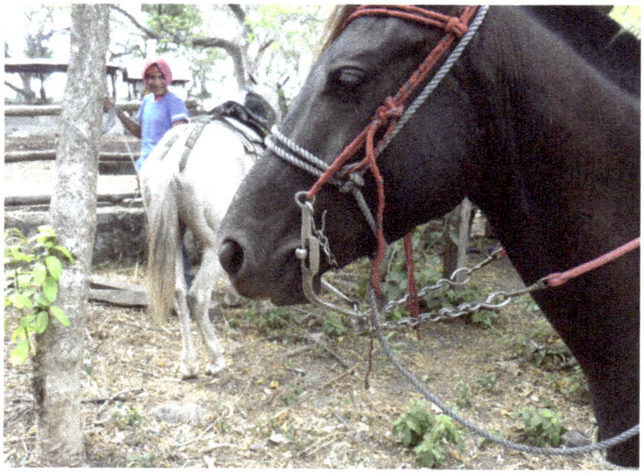

Fig. 21.4. An unnecessary overly severe leverage bit.

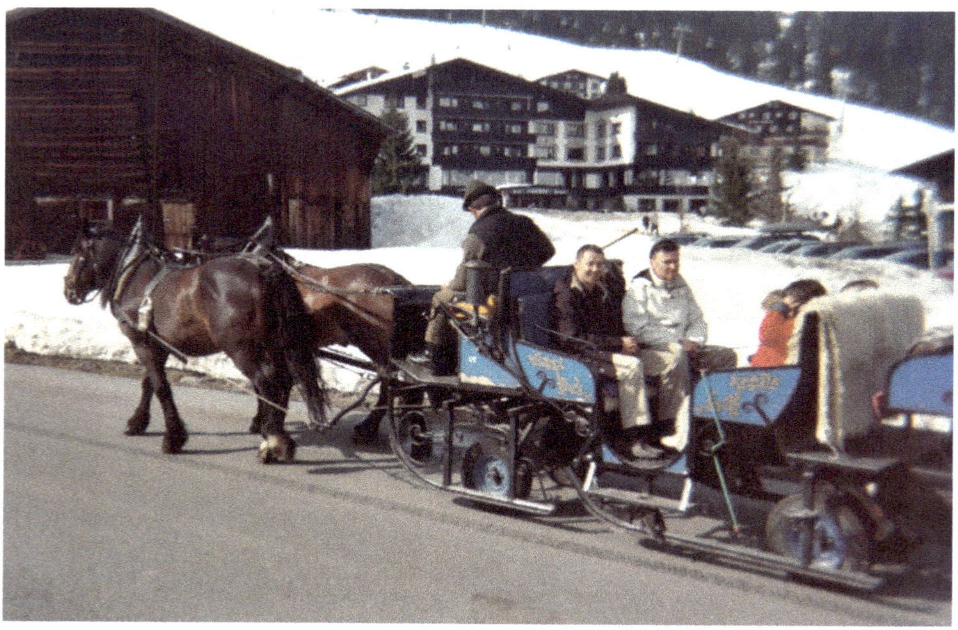

Fig. 21.5. Strong well-muscled horses are able to pull a heavy cart.

In certain situations, the faeces from the working horse are wanted by the driver as manure, or there may be laws that forbid the dropping of faeces. In these cases, the cart has a canvas bag called a 'dung catcher' attached to the shafts, just behind the horse at hock level; it is very important that this is adjusted properly so that it catches the dung but does not chafe the horse.

Further Reading

Hartley-Edwards, E. (2004) *The Complete Book of Bits and Bitting*. David and Charles, Newton Abbot, UK.
McBane, S. (2002) *The Essential Book of Horse Tack and Equipment*. David and Charles, Newton Abbot, UK.

Index

Note: The page numbers in *italics* and **bold** represent figures and tables respectively.

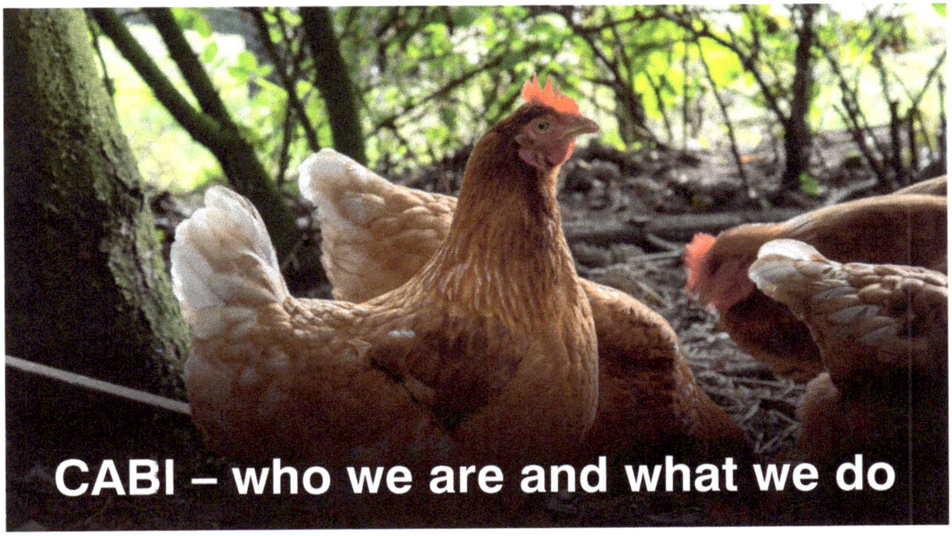

This book is published by **CABI**, an international not-for-profit organisation that improves people's lives worldwide by providing information and applying scientific expertise to solve problems in agriculture and the environment.

CABI is also a global publisher producing key scientific publications, including world renowned databases, as well as compendia, books, ebooks and full text electronic resources. We publish content in a wide range of subject areas including: agriculture and crop science / animal and veterinary sciences / ecology and conservation / environmental science / horticulture and plant sciences / human health, food science and nutrition / international development / leisure and tourism.

The profits from CABI's publishing activities enable us to work with farming communities around the world, supporting them as they battle with poor soil, invasive species and pests and diseases, to improve their livelihoods and help provide food for an ever growing population.

CABI is an international intergovernmental organisation, and we gratefully acknowledge the core financial support from our member countries (and lead agencies) including:

UKaid from the British people | Ministry of Agriculture People's Republic of China | Australian Government Australian Centre for International Agricultural Research | Agriculture and Agri-Food Canada | Ministry of Foreign Affairs of the Netherlands | Schweizerische Eidgenossenschaft Confédération suisse Confederazione Svizzera Confederaziun svizra Swiss Agency for Development and Cooperation SDC

Discover more

To read more about CABI's work, please visit: **www.cabi.org**

Browse our books at: **www.cabi.org/bookshop**,
or explore our online products at: **www.cabi.org/publishing-products**

Interested in writing for CABI? Find our author guidelines here:
www.cabi.org/publishing-products/information-for-authors/

www.ingramcontent.com/pod-product-compliance
Lightning Source LLC
LaVergne TN
LVHW071337210926
848486LV00003B/162